IMMUNIZATION

IMMUNIZATION
THE REALITY BEHIND
THE MYTH

Walene James

FOREWORD BY
Robert S. Mendelsohn, M.D.

SECOND EDITION
Revised and Updated

BERGIN & GARVEY
Westport, Connecticut • London

Library of Congress Cataloging-in-Publication Data

James, Walene.
   Immunization : the reality behind the myth / Walene James ;
foreword by Robert S. Mendelsohn. — 2nd ed., rev. and updated.
     p. cm.
   Includes bibliographical references and index.
   ISBN 0–89789–359–X (H.C. : alk. paper). — ISBN 0–89789–360–3
(P.B.)
    1. Immunization—Complications. 2. Immunization of children—
Complications. 3. Natural immunity. 4. Alternative medicine.
I. Title.
    [DNLM: 1. Immunization—adverse effects. 2. Immunization—in
infancy & childhood. 3. Immunity, Natural. 4. Holistic Health.
QW 800 J29i 1995]
RA638.J34   1995
614.4'7—dc20
DNLM/DLC
for Library of Congress   94–36206

British Library Cataloguing in Publication Data is available.

Library of Congress Catalog Card Number: 94–36206
ISBN: 0–89789–359–X (H.C.)
ISBN: 0–89789–360–3 (P.B.)

First published in 1995

Bergin & Garvey, 88 Post Road West, Westport, CT 06881
An imprint of Greenwood Publishing Group, Inc.

Printed in the United States of America

The paper used in this book complies with the
Permanent Paper Standard issued by the National
Information Standards Organization (Z39.48–1984).

10 9 8 7 6 5

To awakening people everywhere:
May your choices be conscious

The ills from which we are suffering have had
their seat in the very foundation of human thought.

—Teilhard de Chardin

Contents

Illustrations

Foreword

Immunizations?

Immunization: The Reality Behind the Myth is just that! Of course, it provides the most up-to-date, completely and authoritatively documented, comprehensive critique of vaccines. From Pasteur's smallpox scam to vaccine-linked AIDS, Walene James's book is the state-of-the-art statement on vaccine damage. And its early chapters should legitimately terrify every parent whose child faces immunizations as well as everyone who already has been so victimized.

But, true to its title, *Immunization* delivers far more than a scientific indictment of the "holy water" of modern medicine's idolatrous, deadly religion. Walene James leads us through the matrix of modern medical mistakes responsible for the blind acceptance of vaccines. She introduces readers to unknown scientists including Bechamp and Virchow who provide the antidote to the germ theory of disease.

And beyond that, James offers sensible advice to those who already have been damaged. Not content with only destroying old myths, she provides optimism and hope by her commonsense prescriptions for wise, healthful living.

Elegance of style is an additional bonus. For example, James compares modern vaccines—laden with formaldehyde, mercury, dog kidney tissue—with the "eye of newt and toe of frog" added to the brew of Macbeth's witches. She wisely comments: "Is it too impudent to suggest that man has long had a love affair with decomposing animal proteins, noxious potions that ward off the demons of ill fortune?"

Immunization: The Reality Behind the Myth will open the eyes of those who still believe in the religion of modern medicine. It will strengthen those who have left that religion. And to protect every human being right from the start—this book is the most valuable gift you can present to the mother of a newborn baby.

—Robert S. Mendelsohn, M.D.

Author, *Confessions of a Medical Heretic*

Preface to the Second Edition

When I first began writing *Immunization: The Reality Behind the Myth,* I soon realized that the vaccination issue was much larger than vaccinations per se. It was as though a hologram opened up for me, and I saw in the very small the very large, for the vaccination issue touches the very core of who we are and what we stand for as a nation. It also gives us a glimpse into the kind of world we seem bent upon creating.

"Family treasure doesn't come in through the front gate," goes the old Zen saying. Its modern counterpart might be, "It is a rule of thumb." Paul Hawken said, "the more you see a product advertised, the more of a ripoff it is."[1] Putting these two statements together, we could say that that which intrudes upon us through the media is least valuable and that which has real value is usually hidden or, at least, must be searched for. By these tokens, how would the vaccination business fare?

Hardly a month, or even a fortnight, goes by that we don't hear of the virtues and importance of vaccines. Celebrities extol them; editors, reporters, and news broadcasters refer to them as though their value were beyond question; parents of unvaccinated children are assumed to be negligent, ignorant, or poverty-stricken. Vaccination has, indeed, become part of our tribal mores, and to question its validity is "politically incorrect," if not an outright faux pas, and, in some circles, even a sacrilege.

This custom has become not only a tribal imperative that storms through the front gate but an industry that expands and proliferates into more and more areas of our lives. "Not just for kids. Immunize!" At the bottom of the bookmark was the adult immunization schedule. A poster on the wall of the library read: "Shots are not just for kids." The new childhood immunization schedule has two new vaccines, each to be given three times before the child is 6 months old. And there are vaccines ''in the works'' for every conceivable condition, from fat to contraception—even chemical carcinogens.

A friend of mine was unable to get a job for which she was very well qualified because she refused vaccinations. An unvaccinated high school senior in a personal belief exemption state was forced to stay home and miss graduation exercises because the health department declared an epidemic. A child was removed from her kindergarten classroom because her vaccination record was incomplete. And on August 19, 1981, the state, in the person of a social worker, rang our doorbell and informed us that a member of our family, a young person in excellent health, was required by law to submit to vaccinations, an invasive medical procedure not guaranteed to be either safe or effective. This coercive aspect of vaccinations became the impetus that led me to write this book.

From the political and ethical standpoint alone, vaccination is easily the most important public health issue facing us today. It is also a telling symbol of where we are in consciousness.

When I wrote the first edition of *Immunization: The Reality Behind the Myth*, I stated that my purpose was to open minds rather than fill them and that therefore I focused on principles rather than details and technical minutiae. This is still my purpose or, rather, part of it. As stated in the preface to the first edition: ''Unless data and ideas resonate against a background of larger principles, they remain small and inert, unable to pass beyond the single track of thesis-antithesis.... This field of larger principles ... must be brought into focus before the facts within it can be given life and thus become part of a living culture.'' It is my hope that bringing these unifying principles into focus will facilitate consciousness raising and that the smaller and less salutary will give way to the larger and more salutary.

This is how I, personally, came to my own nonvaccinating position, which is why a considerable portion of this book is devoted to discussing other, more ''beautiful'' approaches to health maintenance. When I didn't have my own children vaccinated, it was not because I had studied and agonized over each vaccine but because I had studied other healthcare philosophies and modalities that were more empowering and made better sense to me. But like most excursions into healthcare heterodoxy, I was driven by my own desperate search to heal a condition for which conventional medicine offered only palliatives. (My experience is briefly discussed in Chapter 4.)

But, it seems, most people are still locked into the diseasescare, diseasefight model of conventional medicine and need the ''authority'' of medically sourced facts. This newer edition, therefore, has many more of these kinds of facts as well as two new chapters—Chapters 7 and 14—along with an expanded and updated section on AIDS (Chapter 8). Chapter 7 discusses some of the more recent discoveries of several biomedical scientists whose work further refines and clarifies the paradigm-breaking discoveries of the earlier scientists discussed in Chapter 5. One of these scientists has developed a more assertive and creative model of the immune system than the merely reactive model most of us are familiar with. Another scientist points to several important physiological functions of childhood diseases as well as an important physiological function of disease in general. Chapter 14 was written in response to suggestions from friends that I outline a strategy for avoiding vaccinations, other than the legal one, which can be expensive as well as short-range because vaccination laws change. Three levels of strategies are discussed as well as more little-known facts about disease, vaccination, and politics.

The tone of this newer edition is stronger, more unequivocating than the tone in the first edition. Why? Because the political climate has become more unfriendly and intolerant of those who choose to stay off the vaccination bandwagon, and oppressive, dictatorial laws have followed. The trend is dangerous. The reader will also notice that I have substituted the word *vaccination* for the word *immunization* in as many places as seemed feasible for reasons explained in Chapter 3.

As stated earlier, our confrontation with the compulsory vaccination laws of Virginia occasioned the writing of this book. The story of that encounter and its aftermath—including three court hearings—is told in Chapters 10 and 11. Because tape recorders weren't allowed in court, I wrote down what happened immediately afterward. The story in these two chapters is taken from a diary I kept during this period and from notes I kept of important encounters during the next few years.

Because the case received considerable publicity, both local and national, I found myself besieged with requests for information on the subject of childhood vaccinations. I discovered people were starving for information: They were looking for something more than propaganda and the official line given them by their pediatricians and their health departments. Part I of this book, Chapters 1 through 4, was written in response to this need. It explores some of the mythology of vaccination—its vaunted safety, effectiveness, and responsibility for the decline in infectious diseases—and suggests other, more natural ways of creating immunity.

The more I talked with people, however, the more I realized the need for reorientation, that is, for a more salutary and liberating way of thinking about our bodies and the microorganismic life outside and within them. It isn't enough to hand people reports on the degree of harmfulness and/or ineffectiveness of specific vaccines and have them leave, hoping for better ones to come down the pike. The fear of the unknown, the "dread" disease, is still there, and the weighing of the dangers of the vaccine versus the dangers of the disease still haunts them. Hence, Part II of this book.

Part II, Chapters 5 through 9, explores the subject of vaccination on a deeper level—its theoretical premises, the germ theory of disease, disease seen from other perspectives, and the mental-emotional-aesthetic implications of a particular healthcare philosophy. Chapter 5, the most technical and a pivotal chapter in the book, tells of a little-known controversy between two scientists that took place over 100 years ago and subsequent research that supports the findings of one of these scientists, a man unknown to most of us. If his discoveries and their implications had become "establishment," the world would be a far healthier place to live, and health care would be a fraction of its present cost. And there would be no vaccinations.

Part III, Chapters 10 through 14, deals with the implications of a monolithic, coercive healthcare system for a democratic society. Chapters 10 and 11 tell what happened to us when we tried to say "No thanks" to that system. Others have told similar stories.

Because we are immersed in a sea of communications media—and are living in a "moneytheistic" technocracy—propaganda and misinformation are primary facts of life. Nowhere is this better illustrated than in the area of vaccination. Therefore, I included a chapter on propaganda and general semantics as applied to health care. If we are to mature as individuals and as a nation, we need to develop perceptiveness and discrimination. Recognizing propaganda and misinformation is part of this process. In the healthcare field, it can be a matter of health or disability—or even life or death. "If humanity is to pass safely through its present crisis on earth," Buckminster Fuller reminds us, "it will be because a majority of individuals are now doing their own thinking."[2] This chapter—and indeed this book—is a step in that direction.

Chapter 13 projects us into a multioptioned, open-ended healthcare system, bringing together much of what has been implied throughout the book. If we want change, we must have vision. We must be able to see and give energy to "the way we want it to be." Chapter 14 outlines what we need to do to actualize our vision and reclaim our heritage—freedom.

The subject of vaccination has been considered controversial. But what is *controversy*? The word itself comes from the Latin meaning "turned opposite." That which is controversial is turned opposite a dominating structure, in this case, establishment medicine. In a free and open society, there would be no such label as "controversial," only disagreement within an open forum of ideas and options. There would be no one mainstream but many streams, each meeting different needs.

Likewise with the word *alternative* as in "alternative" medicine. What if we called Spanish "alternative English"? The enthnocentrism—or is it chauvinism?—would be ovious.

A word about myself: I am a former high school English teacher with the Los Angeles City Schools, not a healthcare professional. This I consider an advantage because I don't have years of indoctrination in a particular point of view to unlearn, nor do I have a job or license that can be threatened for speaking out. The late John Holt, a leading humanistic educator, took pride in pointing out that he never took an education course. He felt he had the advantage of not having his perceptions clouded with a lot of preconceptions—and misconceptions.

About some of the challenges in writing this book: First, the biggest challenge, of course, was making difficult, technical material easy and interesting to read. To that end I have defined technical terms when I needed to use them; however, I have used as little medical terminology as possible, retaining just enough to give the reader a sense of authenticity and the flavor of "medicalese." Second, although I point out some of the fallacies of relying on statistics to support an argument, I use them. Why? Because they are a tool, and numbers still impress people. I have tried, however, to use just enough cases to make my point, though many more could be cited. Third, because of the "sensitive" position of some of the people referred to in this book, I was not given permission to use their names and have used either a fictitious name (so designated) or have simply referred to them as a "woman," a "doctor," and so on. And finally, I did not attempt to write the proverbial "balanced" exposition. The "other side" is so available, so much a part of our culture that to give it more quarter in a book of this nature would be superfluous.

But the more compelling—and real—story of vaccination takes us behind and beyond its facts and fictions and into the field of consciousness that births them. To grasp this second story we have to be able to read the mirror it holds up to us. What does the following mirror tell us about ourselves?

To show audiences the medical model of the immune process, I used to hold up a large, colored illustration from *Discover* magazine (1987). Tanks, bombers, launch pads, trucks, ambulances, and factories were all emerging from the central factory—the bone marrow. The caption on the left said to "picture the bone marrow as a massive factory that makes all the machinery a country needs to defend itself, from the tanks and bombers that battle the enemy to the trucks that carry supplies to the front and the ambulances that treat and transport the wounded."[3]

Has this battlefield mentality transformed external battlefields into internal ones? What do war models of physiological processes reveal about our consciousness? Like the bone marrow "factory" above, everything emerges from consciousness: the character of our relationships (including our relationship to the natural world), the character of our institutions, and the way we experience the world. This is the story behind the story and the real mythology of vaccination. (The word *myth* has two meanings: (1) that which isn't true and (2) that which is profoundly and universally true.)

When Einstein was asked what he thought the most important question was that human beings needed to answer, he replied, "Is the universe a friendly place or not?"[4] It is my hope that after reading this book you will be able to answer "Friendly" and that vaccinations and particularly forced vaccinations, will be seen as a vestige of an earlier, less mature consciousness—an emperor without any clothes but with the power to destroy.

NOTES

1. Paul Hawken, quoted by William Dufty in *Sugar Blues* (New York: Warner Books, 1975), p. 143.

2. Buckminster Fuller, quoted by Ronald Gross in flier advertising *The Independent Scholar's Handbook* (New York: The Scholars' Bookclub, 1986).

3. Gina Kolata, "Immune Boosters," *Discover* (September 1987).

4. Albert Einstein, quoted by A. Robert Smith, in *Venture Inward*, (January/February, 1994): 25.

Acknowledgments

I wish to express my gratitude to the following:

My daughter Tanya and my grandson Isaac, whose confrontation with the Virginia Beach courts provided the impetus for writing this book.

Clinton Miller of the National Health Federation, whose advice and moral support during the litigation process and whose encouragement during the early drafts of the manuscript were invaluable.

My daughter Ingri, whose sustained interest and insistence that this material reach people helped keep me going.

Dr. Robert S. Mendelsohn, courageous pioneer in awakening the public to the harmful but lucrative superstitions of modern medicine, for writing the foreword.

Jim Bergin, publisher, Ann Gross, editor, and the rest of the staff at Bergin & Garvey for their valuable suggestions.

To the editorial staff of Greenwood Press for their patience, professionalism, and deference to the author's wishes.

The late Dr. Gina Cerminara for her beginning and advanced courses in general semantics, and Alice Lynton of the Los Angeles City School Districts Division of Secondary Education for the section on critical reading and propaganda in Operational Aid R63, September 1963.

The many wonderful people who contributed material for this book, especially: Drs. Michael McLean, D.C., and Patricia McLean, D.C.; Dr. Kristine Severyn, Ph.D.; Barbara Mullarkey, Ingri Cassel, Kristine Rosemary, Desiree B. Craig, Heidi-Rose Dane, Paul Johnson, Clinton Miller, Joseph Nuccio, Adella Scott Wilson, Sue Eldredge, Victoria Heasley, Brenda Hardison and Robin Jackson.

And finally to my husband Paul, who edited and midwifed this book. Without his continuing guidance and encouragement, this book would never have reached completion.

Note to the Reader

Who has not dreamed of a disease-free world? The fountain of youth and eternal wellness have been one of the perennial dreams of humankind. The question this book poses is, Does our present course of action—the proliferation of disease categories, disease specialists, and disease technologies such as drugs and vaccines—bring us closer to the realization of this dream? Or is it realizable or even desirable?

Vaccination was chosen as the focus of this book partly because it epitomizes our present fragmented, adversarial approach to understanding and relating to disease processes. But for many readers the greatest value of this book will be its elucidation of ways to think about and respond to "diseasescare" and how to answer the question, Should we have our child vaccinated?

PART I   Deprogramming

Those who lack all idea that it is possible to be wrong can learn nothing except know-how.

—Gregory Bateson,
Mind and Nature

1   The Tyranny of What Everyone Knows*

Any action that is dictated by fear or by coercion of any kind ceases to be moral.

—Mahatma Gandhi,
Ethical Religion

UBIQUITY AND ADDICTION

Our age has been called the information age. It could also be called the misinformation age. With the advent of electronic technology, it is now possible to inform/misinform more people than at any time in history. Embedded in the bits and pieces of information/misinformation with which we are bombarded are parts of the larger continent of "what everyone knows," the conventional wisdom of the culture that philosophers call "premises" or "basic assumptions." Because this conventional wisdom shapes and even determines our perceptions and interpretations of the world, we might say that "what everyone knows" sits in the control room of our collective psyche. Its power derives largely from our unconsciousness of it; therefore, reexamining what everyone knows is part of the process of becoming conscious and empowered human beings.

In our culture, *healing* and *health* have become practically synonymous with the practice of medicine and its administration of drugs, surgery, radiation, and vaccination. This last ritual is the focus of this book. It was chosen because (1) of a personal confrontation with the compulsory immunization laws of the state

*Title of an article in *Network Review*, September 1984.

of Virginia; (2) of all the practices of modern medicine, this "sacrament" is the most blindly and aggressively pursued; and (3) the assumptions upon which this practice is based are the same assumptions behind much of the destructiveness and wastefulness of modern medicine. This destructiveness and wastefulness extend far beyond the parameters of medicine itself.

So ubiquitous has medical enterprise and rubric become that it is difficult to open a newspaper or magazine without encountering some article eulogizing some aspect of technological medicine—for example, medical advice; medical "breakthroughs"; melodramas of disease and disability in which modern technological medicine comes to the rescue; organ transplants; and futuristic projections involving exotic technology such as cloning, cryonics, and so on. Even the problems of medically oriented health care, such as skyrocketing costs, are discussed as though the real problems were peripheral, for example, gouging billing practices, fee splitting, unnecessary operations, or incompetent surgeons. Does it ever occur to us that the real problem might be within the medical system itself, its basic premises concerning the nature of man and, specifically, his relation to the conditions of health and disease? Because of the monopolistic position of the medical profession in our present healthcare system, these premises are firmly embedded in our culture.

When we think of a doctor, particularly a family doctor, the image of a medical doctor automatically comes to mind. Is this because only the medical philosophy of health and disease is taught in public institutions and carried in the media? Is it because only medical doctors are permitted to be public health officers, and with few exceptions, only a medical doctor's professional opinion is recognized in a court of law? Or is it because only drug-oriented research is supported by taxpayers' money, and drugs, the right hand of modern medicine, are seen as the panacea for most of our ills? From cancer to rape, the drug answer is heralded and sought. Like the great flood, the medicodrug consciousness inundates most of the civilized world, and the immunization ritual is, for most of us, our initiation into lifelong addiction to the medicodrug establishment.

This drug consciousness fuels our current crises in health care, drug abuse, and violence. From a recent news broadcast: 35 to 45 percent of our drug problem is related to pharmaceutical drugs.[1] Add to this the vaccination bandwagon, which continues to expand into new territories, and, as we shall see, we have a major contributor to our crises in health, drugs, and violence. The question then becomes, Can we possibly emerge from these crises without first emerging from the tunnel of the pharmaceutical fix?

"Remaining unimmunized for childhood diseases is a risk no child should face," reads a folder from our health department. The same folder also tells us that "health experts warn that unless more young children are immunized, widespread epidemics could take place once again."[2] "Epidemics are certain to occur if the immunity level of the population is not maintained by immunizing children" reads another folder from our health department.[3] Still another folder features grotesque cartoons personifying "Dangerous Childhood Diseases." We

see "Mean-ole Measles," "Dippie Diphtheria," and "Locky Lockjaw" grim-
acing at us when we open the folder. The caption next to "Rolly Polio," who
is sitting in a wheelchair holding up one of his crutches, tells us: "See that you
and everyone around you has taken the oral polio vaccine." "Whoopy Whooping Cough," "Dippie Diphtheria," and "Locky Lockjaw" remind us to get
booster shots, to return periodically for that all-important "protection." "Everyone, 1 year to 101 years needs a booster every 10 years," Dippy Diphtheria
reminds us.[4] Other folders from the health department describe the seriousness
and high fatalities of various childhood diseases. The number of children permanently damaged by immunizations is minuscule, they assure us, and a small
price to pay for that "protection" that has all but "wiped out" these terrible
scourges.

"Thanks to vaccination, smallpox has been virtually banished from the
globe—a triumph of a historic public-health crusade," reads an editorial in our
local newspaper. This same editorial urged the state legislature to "immunize
immunizations" from legal loopholes that would allow a child to "escape"
immunizations because of parental objection. It pointed out how "measles and
measles encephalitis are now on the defensive in the United States—a situation
directly attributable to mass immunization of the young." Again we are reminded that "whenever an epidemic of a childhood disease occurs, the outbreak
is nearly always traceable to a falloff in inoculations."[5]

Again, the power of vaccines to rescue us from the scourge of "dread"
disease is eulogized: "Elena Jenkins, 10, owes her life to a new vaccine," reads
a picture caption in a recent article titled "How Vaccines May End Infections
Forever."[6] "Expanded immunization—using newly improved vaccines" will
"prevent the six main immunizable diseases from killing an estimated 5 million
children a year and disabling 5 million more," James Grant, executive director
of the United Nations International Children's Emergency Fund (UNICEF), tells
us.[7]

New vaccines and vaccine technology are further heralded: "Pioneering Doctor Predicts 1 Vaccine for Several Diseases."[8] "Unborn Children Can be Immunized Via the Mother."[9] And from the front page of our local newspaper:
"Scientists Hail New Chickenpox Vaccine."[10]

And so the wisdom of the culture broadcasts that disease is an unmitigated
evil, a dangerous enemy that must be attacked and destroyed. Vaccines, it tells
us, are miracle weapons that rout the invaders and save us from being conquered
by them. They are one of the heroes in man's eternal struggle against the ter-
rifying threat of disease, disability, and death.

UBIQUITY AND COERCION

"The children, kicking and screaming, were taken away from the parents and
given smallpox vaccinations."[11]

"Our three school age children were suspended from a local public school district in Arkansas . . . for breaking the state immunization law. . . . The judge, without deliberation, pronounced Stephen [the father] guilty of truancy and fined him $750 plus court costs and appeal fees."[12]

A hundred years ago penalties were more severe: " . . . a mandatory [vaccination] law . . . with the threat of prison as well as the seizure of the goods of persons refusing to comply."[13]

Here in Virginia the front page of our local newspaper reminds us: "No shots, no school. Students who can't prove they have been immunized against contagious childhood diseases shouldn't expect to start school Monday."[14]

It's tough to argue with ubiquity, especially when it is armed with the police powers of the state. If a parent objects to his child being vaccinated, officialdom assures him that the benefits outweigh the risks. If he persists in his refusal, he is told he is putting his child in jeopardy. Finally, if pressure doesn't work, coercion often will. If "right" is obvious and unequivocal, then forcing the right on others is doing them and society a service.

Parents who choose not to vaccinate their children have been denied access to medical care—even emergency medical care, Medicaid, schools, and head start programs (see Chapter 11). Maryland "encourages" parents to vaccinate their children by docking welfare checks $25 a month for each child not receiving "proper health care," which includes scheduled vaccinations.[15]

Has the medical-pharmaceutical industry become the state-sanctioned church? A number of writers have noted the similarity of the medical profession to a priesthood and have observed that medicine and government are as interlocked today as were the church and state during the Middle Ages. For example, Drs. Robert Mendelsohn and Thomas Szasz refer to the "Church of Modern Medicine" and the "therapeutic state," respectively.[16,17] Dr. Szasz notes the similarity of the therapeutic state to the theocratic state of the Middle Ages. Is history doomed to repeat itself? Do the evils we think we have abolished in one age return in a different guise in another?

When ubiquity reigns, a culture becomes stuck in a stance, and interpretations of reality that are at variance with the dominant stance are locked out. For instance, in the 1983 congressional hearings on vaccinations—S. 2117—Congress refused to let scientists opposed to vaccinations testify before the committee.[18] Ten years later the show was repeated (see Chapter 11).

Maybe we need to open the door and start asking questions—pointed, "unthinkable" questions:

Is a coercive, "closed-shop" healthcare system, such as described here, a contradiction in terms? Is it possible that vaccinations are not a good idea? Is it possible that the premises upon which they are based are faulty? Is it possible that the decline of infectious diseases might have little or nothing to do with the near-universal practice of vaccination? Is it possible that the increase in chronic and degenerative disease is related to the parallel increase in the practice of mass vaccination?

To answer yes to any of these questions is to invite vigorous opposition and defensiveness from the medical community. Because of its enormous investment—ego as well as monetary—in this practice, this community will resist answers that threaten its image and position. But the door to discovery is opened by knowing how to ask questions and not being afraid to look at the answers.

NOTES

1. *Morning Edition*, WHRV-FM, April 8, 1993.

2. "Protect Them from Harm" (folder published by the Virginia State Department of Health, Richmond, VA). I picked up the literature from the health department on Independence Boulevard in Virginia Beach, summer 1982.

3. "Questions and Answers on Polio" (folder published by the Virginia State Department of Health, Richmond, VA). From the health department in Virginia Beach, summer 1982.

4. "PARENTS—State Law Requires . . . Immunization Against Dangerous Childhood Diseases" (folder published by the Southland Corporation in Cooperation with the Virginia State Department of Health).

5. "Immunize Immunizations," *Virginian-Pilot*, November 27, 1981, p. A14.

6. Earl Ubell, "How Vaccines May End Infections Forever," *Parade*, February 12, 1984.

7. James Grant, "Simple, Available and Effective Interventions," *A Shift in the Wind* 18 (May 1984): 7.

8. "Pioneering Doctor Predicts 1 Vaccine for Several Diseases," *Virginian-Pilot*, November 9, 1983.

9. "Unborn Children Can Be Immunized Via the Mother," *Washington Post*, September 14, 1983.

10. "Scientists Hail New Chickenpox Vaccine," *Virginian-Pilot*, May 31, 1984.

11. Donna Kudabeck and Stephen Kudabeck, "Opposing Compulsory Immunizations," *Health Freedom News*, April 1984, p. 21.

12. Ibid.

13. Harold Buttram et al., *The Dangers of Immunization*, The Humanitarian Society, Quakertown, PA, 1979, p. 41. Statement refers to a law passed in England in 1867.

14. Lisa Hogberg, "No Shots, No School," *Virginia Beach Beacon*, August 28, 1983.

15. Diane Tenant, "A Healthy Risk," *Virginian-Pilot/Ledger-Star*, August 14, 1993.

16. Robert Mendelsohn, *Confessions of a Medical Heretic* (Chicago: Contemporary Books, 1979).

17. Sarah E. Foster, "Up Against The Birth Monopoly," *Reason*, September 1982, p. 26.

18. Interview with Clinton Miller, "Vaccination Concerns," *Spotlight*, June 4, 1984.

2 Are Immunizations Harmless?

> Civilization means, above all, an unwillingness to inflict unnecessary
> pain. Within the ambit of that definition, those of us who heedlessly
> accept the commands of authority cannot yet claim to be civilized men.
> —Harold J. Laski,
> as quoted by Stanley Milgram
> in *Obedience to Authority*

THE FOUR CORNERSTONES

"The judge said that I must present evidence before the next hearing that vaccinations are harmful, or he would have to order shots for Isaac," my daughter Tanya told me. He told her to turn in the evidence to the prosecuting attorney at least two weeks before the date of the next hearing. We turned in almost 90 pages of scientific evidence and opinion attesting to the harmfulness of vaccinations. Much of the material in this chapter is taken from that body of evidence and opinion. Since Tanya was taken to court in 1981 for refusing to have her son vaccinated, much new material has surfaced. I have included as much of this material as possible.

Briefly, the four cornerstones upon which the practice of vaccination rests are: (1) Vaccinations are relatively harmless; (2) vaccinations are effective; (3) vaccinations were primarily responsible for the decline in infectious diseases; and (4) vaccinations are the only practical and dependable way to prevent both epidemics and potentially dangerous diseases.

Let's examine each of these premises (in this and the next two chapters).

Later, we will examine their implications as well as the mind-set that makes each of these assumptions not only possible but an almost inevitable way of perceiving and interpreting certain data.

VACCINES IN GENERAL

The theory of vaccination states that by giving a person a mild form of a disease via the use of immunizing agents, specific antibodies are produced that will protect the organism when the real thing comes along. "This sounds simple and plausible enough except that it doesn't quite work that way," Dr. Alec Burton reminds us.[1] For instance, vaccines, of themselves, as we shall discover, produce a variety of illnesses, some of which may be considerably more serious than the disease for which they were given. These vaccine-induced diseases may involve "deeper structures, more vital organs, and [have] less of a tendency to resolve spontaneously. Even more worrisome is the fact that they are almost always more difficult to recognize," Dr. Richard Moskowitz points out.[2]

Besides introducing foreign proteins, and even live viruses into the bloodstream, each vaccine has its own preservative, neutralizer, and carrying agent, none of which are indigenous to the body. For instance, triple antigen DPT (diphtheria, pertussis, and tetanus) contains formaldehyde, mercury (thimerosal), and aluminum phosphate (*Physicians' Desk Reference*, 1980), all of which are toxic to the human body. The packet insert accompanying the vaccine (Lederle) lists aluminum potassium sulfate, thimerosal (a mercury derivative), and sodium phosphate—all toxic to the human body. The packet insert for the polio vaccine (Lederle) lists monkey kidney cell culture, lactalbumin hydrolysate, antibiotics, and calf serum. The packet insert (Merck Sharp & Dohme) for the MMR (measles, mumps, and rubella) vaccine lists chick embryo and neomycin, which is a mixture of antibiotics. Chick embryo, monkey kidney cells, and calf serum are foreign proteins, biological substances composed of animal cells, that, because they enter directly into the bloodstream, can become part of our genetic material. (Normal animal cells—as well as plant cells—shed DNA [deoxyribonucleic acid], which is then taken up by other cells in the body.)[3] These foreign proteins as well as the other carriers and reaction products of a vaccine are potential allergens and can produce anaphylactic shock. "Any person who dies within 15 minutes to a day after taking the vaccine could be suffering from a personal sensitivity, an allergy to the vaccine which is unrelated to the 'dead' viruses therein, most researchers concede."[4] This statement was made in reference to the swine flu vaccine; however, the principle applies to all vaccines.

Another problem with vaccines is that they go directly into the bloodstream without "censoring by the liver," Dr. William Albrecht tells us.

If you take water into your system as drink, it goes into your bloodstream directly from the stomach. But if you take fats, they move into your lymphatic system. When you take other substances like carbohydrates and proteins, they go into the intestines, and from there are passed through the liver, as the body's chemical censor, before they go into the blood and the circulation throughout the body. Most of your vaccination serums are proteins, and are not censored by the liver. Consequently vaccinations can be a terrific shock to the system.[5]

Injections of foreign substances—viruses, toxins, and foreign proteins—into the bloodstream, that is, vaccinations, have been associated with diseases and disorders of the blood, brain, nervous system, and skin. Rare diseases such as atypical measles and monkey fever as well as such well-known disorders as premature aging and allergies have been associated with vaccinations. Also linked to immunizations are diseases such as cancer, leukemia, paralysis, multiple sclerosis, arthritis, SIDS (sudden infant death syndrome),[6] and most recently, AIDS (acquired immunodeficiency syndrome) (see Chapter 8). Let's look at the packet inserts of some of the more common vaccines.

MMR AND POLIO VACCINES

From the packet inserts (Lederle; Merck, Sharp & Dohme) accompanying the polio and MMR (measles, mumps, and rubella) vaccines, we learn that paralytic diseases have been on rare occasions associated with polio vaccine and that "significant central nervous system reactions such as encephalitis and encephalopathy" can occur after injection with measles, mumps, and rubella vaccine. Reports of ocular palsies, Guillain-Barré syndrome, and subacute sclerosing panencephalitis have occurred after measles vaccination. These are admittedly rare reactions, but some of the more common reactions, which can be "expected to follow administration of monovalent vaccines given separately," are "malaise, sore throat, headache, fever, and rash; mild local reactions such as erythema, induration, tenderness and regional lymphadenopathy; parotitis, orchitis, thrombocytopenia and purpura; allergic reactions such as wheal and flare at the injection site or urticaria; and arthritis, arthralgia and polyneuritis." From Dr. Robert Mendelsohn we learn that measles vaccine can cause "neurologic and sometimes fatal conditions such as ataxia (discoordination), retardation, hyperactivity, aseptic meningitis, seizures, and hemiparesis (paralysis of one side of the body)."[7] According to an article in *Science*, in early 1970 the HEW (Department of Health, Education and Welfare) reported that "as much as 26 percent of children receiving rubella vaccination in national testing programs developed arthralgia and arthritis." Many had to seek medical attention, and some were hospitalized to test for rheumatic fever and rheumatoid arthritis."[8] "The British journal *Medical Hypothesis* reported in 1988 in a study of 200 patients with chronic Epstein-Barr virus syndrome [debilitating fatigue] that the disease was attributable to the live rubella virus found in the vaccine."[9]

The Centers for Disease Control (CDC) reports the following side effects of mumps vaccination: parotitis (inflammation of the parotid glands); allergic reactions, including rash, pruritus, and purpura; and central nervous system (CNS) involvement such as fever, seizures, unilateral nerve deafness, and encephalitis within 30 days of mumps vaccination.[10]

In short and in plain language, the MMR and polio vaccines can produce the following pathologies: brain damage; paralysis; nerve inflammation; disease of the lymph glands; inflammation of the testicles and glands near the ear; partial deafness; skin disorders—rashes, tenderness, hardness, itchiness, and discoloration; blood disorders; allergies; arthritis; and chronic fatigue syndrome.

DPT VACCINE

From the packet insert (Lederle) for the DPT (diphtheria, pertussis, and tetanus) vaccine we learn that "symptomology related to neurological disorders" and "excessive screaming syndrome" can follow administration of pertussis antigen. From the *Physicians' Desk Reference* (1980, p. 1866) we learn that DPT can cause "fever over 103°, convulsions . . . alterations of consciousness; focal neurologic signs, screaming episodes; . . . shock; collapse; thrombocytopenic purpura." Under "Side Effects and Adverse Reactions" are listed: "1. Severe temperature elevations—105° or higher. 2. Collapse with rapid recovery. 3. Collapse followed by prolonged prostration and shock-like state. 4. Screaming episodes. . . . 5. Isolated convulsions with or without fever. 6. Frank encephalopathy [brain damage] with changes in the level of consciousness, focal neurological signs, and convulsions with or without permanent neurological and/or mental deficit. 7. Thrombocytopenic purpura [blood and skin disorder]. The occurrence of sudden infant death syndrome [SIDS] has been reported following administration of DPT."

"The whooping cough vaccine (a component of the triple antigen DPT) has such a high percentage of neurologic complications, including death. (*sic*) Several physicians I know (myself included) do not give it at all," Dr. Mendelsohn tells us.[11] "Dr. Edward B. Shaw, a distinguished University of California physician, has stated (*JAMA* March 1975): 'I doubt that the decrease in pertussis (whooping cough) is due to the vaccine which is a very poor antigen and an extremely dangerous one, with many very serious complications.' "[12]

Some researchers from Australia have pointed to other serious problems with pertussis vaccine. Drs. Glen Dettman, Archie Kalokerinos, and Munro Ford have pointed to evidence linking pertussis vaccine with the later appearance of asthma and hayfever.[13] Dr. John Fox, of the University School of Medicine, has warned that the risk of paralytic complications may occur with vaccines against measles, polio, whooping cough, and tetanus.[14]

"Many children have suffered horrible and permanent side effects from this vaccine," investigative reporter Lea Thompson said on the *Today* show (April 20, 1982). She was referring to the DPT shots given to children but particularly to the pertussis (whooping cough) component. This 20-minute segment on the *Today* show featuring Thompson was excerpted from the hour-long documentary *DPT: Vaccine Roulette* that I later saw (1982). This documentary featured children who had been permanently brain damaged as a result of DPT shots. The pictures were pathetic: twisted, uncontrollable bodies, anguished parents, and medical bureaucrats—with three exceptions—repeating the official lines: "The benefits of the vaccine, in my view, far outweigh the risks" and "Much more is to be gained by immunizing the children with the current vaccines with its limitations, than by allowing our children to be exposed to contracting Pertussis."[15]

Some interesting statistics emerged; however, these figures are very conservative because doctors seldom report reactions, and what does get reported is the result of some special study commissioned by the government. A recent study at the University of California at Los Angeles (UCLA) estimates that as many as 1 in every 13 children had persistent high-pitched crying after the DPT shot. "This may be indicative of brain damage in the recipient child," Dr. Bobbie Young said. Later on he said, "You know, we start off with healthy infants, and we pop 'em not once, but three or four times with a vaccine . . . the probability of causing damage is the same each time. My greatest fear is that very few of them escape some kind of neurological damage out of this."

One child in 700 has convulsions or goes into shock. "These reactions sometimes cause learning disabilities or brain damage," Thompson said. These figures represent only the reported effects occurring within 48 hours after the administration of the vaccine. Since no follow-up studies were done on children after this period, and many doctors are reluctant to admit that there is a causal relationship between the administration of the vaccine and later neurological disorders—probably because of malpractice suits, as well as not wanting to "be wrong"—the side effects of this vaccine are very underreported.

An even more recent figure on the reaction to the DPT vaccine indicates that 1 in 100 children react with convulsions or collapse or high-pitched screaming. One out of 3 of these—that is, 1 in 300—will remain permanently damaged. According to the testimony of the assistant secretary of health, Dr. Edward Brandt, Jr., before the U.S. Senate Committee on May 3, 1985, every year 35,000 children suffer neurological reactions because of this vaccine.[16] A still more damaging figure is that more than 1 out of 175 children who receive the full DPT series suffered severe reactions. Dr. Keith Block arrived at this figure after decoding the "double talk" in an article in *Pediatrics* (November 1981) entitled "Nature and Rates of Adverse Reactions Associated with DPT and DT Immunizations in Infants and Children."[17]

Perhaps the most disturbing statement that most seriously damages the case for compulsory immunization comes from the DPT documentary mentioned above. In an interview with Food and Drug Administration (FDA) official Dr. John Robbins, he states: "I think if you as a parent brought your child to a doctor for a DPT shot and the doctor said to you initially, 'Well, I have to tell you that some children who get this vaccine get brain damaged,' there's no question as to what your reaction would be. As a responsible parent you would say, 'I wish not to take this vaccine.' "

What about the D and T components of the DPT vaccine? Many people, including most doctors, consider only the P component "problematical." The 1993 *Physicians' Desk Reference* (pp. 1230–1231) gives the same warnings, contraindications, and possible reactions to the DT as to the DPT. Some of the possible reactions to either the diphtheria or tetanus vaccine include skin rashes, hardness, tenderness, abscess formation, pallor, coldness, drowsiness, vomiting, anorexia, arthralgia (pain in joints), persistent crying, hyporesponsiveness, and more serious complications involving the central nervous system—encephalopathy (brain damage), Guillain-Barré syndrome (paralysis), convulsions, and anaphylactic shock. In Poland, researchers reported that 13 of 17 children who were given DT vaccinations showed significant changes in their electroencephalograms and the appearance of seizure activity for the first time or intensification of previously present seizure activity.[18]

Because many people think that tetanus booster shots are important, we might mention some of the reactions to this vaccine that have been reported in various medical journals. One study showed that tetanus booster vaccinations caused T lymphocyte blood count ratios to temporarily drop below normal, the greatest decrease occurring up to two weeks later. These altered ratios are similar to those found in people with AIDS.[19] Other reactions reported are (1) demyelinating neuropathy (degenerating condition of the nervous system), (2) hemolytic (blood-destroying) anemia, (3) recurrent abscess formation, (4) paralysis, (5) anaphylaxis (shock), (6) numbness, (7) tingling, and (8) emotional instability.[20]

In terms of precise numbers and percentages, it's difficult to assess the number of vaccine-related injuries in the United States because doctors seldom report them. For instance, a study of rubella vaccine injuries revealed that fewer than 10 percent of doctors report injuries. Even with this underreporting, it was found that 45 percent of women develop complications—usually arthritic—following rubella vaccination.[21]

Medline, the National Library of Medicine database, has 1,778 citations on the adverse effects of vaccinations and immunizations,[22] but, again, we can't be sure just how extensive—in terms of numbers and percentages—these adverse effects are. In the next section—and elsewhere in this book—we will discover that these injuries are probably far more extensive than the data presented so far suggest.

LONG-TERM EFFECTS

What about the subtle, long-term effects of vaccination? Because these are hard to quantify and prove, most doctors dismiss them, but there is not only highly suggestive inferential evidence for these effects but some rather "hard" scientific evidence as well. Bear in mind that vaccinations were introduced on a mass scale during the last century before the development of molecular biology and the discovery that the immune system includes the brain-mind. This latter means that states of mind—attitudes, emotions, and beliefs—directly affect immunocompetence. In fact, the brain has been called the major immune organ. This has profound implications for any kind of coercive medical treatment such as compulsory vaccinations.

Although many doctors, even during the last century, denounced vaccinations as inherently damaging, only rather recently has specific evidence surfaced suggesting that vaccinations damage (1) the immune system, (2) the central nervous system, (3) the autonomic nervous system, and (4) the spirit-mind-body connection. Let's begin by looking at evidence suggesting damage to the immune system.

The Immune System

Weakens Total Immune Response. By focusing exclusively on increased antibody production—which is only one aspect and by no means the most important aspect—of the immune process, vaccinations isolate this function and allow it to substitute for the entire immune response, Dr. Moskowitz points out. Because vaccines "trick" the body so that it will no longer initiate a generalized inflammatory response, they accomplish what the entire immune system seems to have evolved to prevent. They place the virus directly into the blood and give it access to the major immune organs and tissues without any obvious way of getting rid of it. These attenuated viruses and virus elements persist in the blood for a long time, perhaps permanently. This in turn implies a systematic weakening of the ability to mount an effective response not only to childhood diseases but to other acute infections as well.[23] According to Dr. Moskowitz and others, childhood diseases are decisive experiences in the physiologic maturation of the immune system that prepare the child to respond promptly and effectively to any infections he or she may acquire in the future. The ability to mount a vigorous, acute response to infectious organisms is a fundamental requirement of health and well-being.[24]

Viral Persistence. The long-term persistence of viruses and other foreign proteins within the cells of the immune system has been implicated in a number of chronic and degenerative diseases. For instance, a major article appearing in the *British Medical Journal* titled "Multiple Sclerosis and Vaccination," pointed out what German authors have described as the apparent provocation of multiple sclerosis (MS) by vaccinations against smallpox, typhoid, tetanus, polio, tuberculosis and diphtheria. Also mentioned was another researcher, Zintchenko, who in 1965 reported 12 patients in whom multiple sclerosis first became evident after a series of anti-rabies vaccinations.[25]

The mechanism of this provocation of degenerative disease by vaccines is suggested by the article "Measles Virus Infection Without Rash in Childhood Is Related to Disease in Adult Life" (*Lancet*, January 5, 1985). When researchers in Denmark examined the histories of people who claimed not to have had measles in childhood and yet had blood antibody evidence of such an infection, they found that some had been injected in childhood with measles vaccine after exposure to the infection. This may have suppressed the disease which was at the time developing in their bodies. A high proportion of these individuals were found in adult life to have developed immunoreactive diseases such as sebacious skin disease, tumors, and degenerative disease of bone and cartilage. These include cancer, MS, lupus erythematosus (skin disease), and chondromalacia (softening of the cartilage).

The researchers theorize that the body neutralizes the invading virus by burning up the cells that contain these viruses. This incineration takes place at the site of the spots or rash that characterizes measles. The measles vaccine prevents this rash from forming, and the virus survives in the body, causing havoc later.[26]

A number of researchers are pointing to latent viruses in the body that when activated cause damage to the myelin sheath surrounding the nerves. (Myelin is the tough, protective, fatty, waterproof substance that coats the nerves like insulation on an electric wire.) This can lead to multiple sclerosis and other diseases of the nervous system. For instance, Dr. H. Weaver reported in *Medical News* that "circulating antibodies are responsible for some destruction of the myelin sheath in MS. Moreover, cell culture tests reveal that an unidentified blood protein destroys the myelin, but when the protein factor is removed, the myelin is rapidly repaired." Dr. Weaver goes on to say that a delayed autoimmune reaction in the central nervous system may be involved, probably from prior infection such as measles and mumps.[27] (We learned earlier that vaccines introduce foreign proteins directly into the bloodstream, thereby bypassing the digestive and immune organs.)

"When polio shots became popular, I thought I had seen the last of that disease," an orthopedic specialist told Dr. Marshall Mandell. "Instead, I see dozens more children with one leg slightly shorter, some groups of muscles mildly damaged, a back twisted, or some other abnormality due, I believe, to the infection caused by the live polio virus."[28]

Genetic Transfer. In March 1976 at a Science Writer's Seminar sponsored by the American Cancer Society, Robert W. Simpson, professor of virology at Rutger's University, presented a paper that pointed out that

immunization programs against flu, measles, mumps, polio and so forth, may actually be seeding humans with RNA [ribonucleic acid] to form latent proviruses in cells throughout the body. These latent proviruses could be molecules in search of diseases, including rheumatoid arthritis, multiple sclerosis, systemic lupus erythematosus, Parkinson's disease, and perhaps cancer.[29]

Dr. Wendell D. Winters, a UCLA virologist, communicated similar findings at the same seminar.[30] "Immunization may cause changes in the slow viruses, changes in the DNA mechanism, as being studied by Dr. Robert Hutchinson at the University of Tennessee in Nashville."[31]

Live viruses, the primary antigenic material of vaccines, are capable of surviving or remaining latent within the host cells for years, without provoking acute disease. They do this by attaching their own genetic material as an extra particle or "episome" to the genome (half set of chromosomes and their genes) of the host cell and replicating along with it. This allows the host cell to continue its own normal functions for the most part but imposes on it additional instructions for the synthesis of viral proteins.[32] "The persistence of live viruses or other foreign antigens within the cells of the host therefore cannot fail to provoke auto-immune phenomena, because destroying the infected cells is now the only possible way that this constant antigenic challenge can be removed from the body."[33] Some of the diseases that have been implicated in this provocation of autoimmune phenomena are herpes, shingles, warts, tumors (both benign and malignant) and diseases of the central nervous system such as various forms of paralysis and inflammation of the brain.[34]

If the components of the immune system were designed to help the organism discriminate "self" from "nonself," as a number of researchers believe, then latent viruses, autoimmune phenomena, and cancer would seem, according to Dr. Moskowitz, to represent different aspects of chronic immune failure, wherein the immune system cannot recognize its own cells as unambiguously its own or eliminate parasites as unequivocally foreign.[35] By the same token, we might say that the inability of the immune system to distinguish between harmful and harmless substances in the environment, as in the case of allergies, constitutes another aspect of chronic immune failure.

Cells infected with viral particles, specifically viral RNA integrating with cell DNA, are known as *proviruses* or *molecular intermediates*. These proviruses can lie dormant in cells throughout the body and be activated at a later stage, triggering the degenerative diseases cited earlier. Live viruses in vaccines are not the only problem, however. We now know that genetic transfer of information occurs between (1) bacteria of different species, (2) bacteria and higher plants and animals, and (3) cells of higher organisms. This process of shedding genetic material (DNA and RNA) by the cells of one species and its subsequent absorption by another species is known as *transcession*. One of the questions that has been raised is, Does transcession from bacteria to our own cells explain the heart damage that can occur after rheumatic fever and similar bacterial infections? That is, is the immune system reacting to its own cells, producing an alien RNA?[36]

Transcession explains why the body's immune system cannot distinguish between foreign invaders and its own tissues and begins to destroy itself. This autoimmune phenomenon, which characterizes degenerative diseases such as cancer, leukemia, MS, and rheumatoid arthritis, prompted Dr. Mendelsohn to ask, "Have we traded mumps and measles for cancer and leukemia?"[37] In fact, Dr. Mendelsohn referred to vaccinations as medical time bombs.

Some researchers have suggested that "the harm from viral vaccines may not be so much the viruses themselves as from the fact that, having been cultured in animal tissues, they become carriers of animal genetic material or patterns" and that these "live attenuated viruses used for vaccines would implant foreign, alien material derived from animal culture tissues into the human genetic system.''[38]

Even omitting possible viral contamination and transcession from animal cells used to culture vaccines, a number of researchers have suggested that

by means of vaccination into the blood stream, of a variety of virus and bacterial materials, mankind has indeed managed to engage in a massive experiment in genetic engineering. The repercussions of this will be felt for generations as the latent provirus cells, and other cells whose DNA has been altered, begin to produce the inevitable consequences of their presence.[39]

Thymus Damage and Immune Exhaustion. Recent research points to the relationship of vaccinations to thymus gland damage and immunological inertia. This could be part of the explanation for the increase in degenerative diseases.

The immune system produces two functionally distinct kinds of lymphocytes (white blood cells): (1) the B cells, which mature largely in the bone marrow and produce antibodies for the control of bacterial infections, and (2) the T cells, which originate in the bone marrow but mature in the thymus gland. The T cells protect us from intracellular disorders such as

cancer, virus infections, foreign grafts or transplants, tuberculosis, and various intracellular infections. According to sophisticated research . . . at the Arthur Research Corporation, Tucson, Arizona and other centers . . . the effects of childhood vaccine programs on the T-lymphocytes . . . indicate that the immune system becomes ''Substantially committed'' after the routine series of vaccines. In other words, a substantial portion of immune bodies (T-lymphocytes) becomes committed to the specific antigens involved in the vaccines. Having become committed, these lymphocytes become immunologically inert, incapable of reacting or defending against other antigens, infections, or diseases. These findings would tend to indicate that the immunological reserve is substantially reduced in many children subjected to standard vaccine programs.[40]

Other researchers have stated that routine childhood vaccinations are likely to use 30 to 70 percent of the total immunological reserve or capacity, whereas the immunity conferred by the experience of having the disease uses only 3 to 7 percent of the total immune capacity.[41] This is not surprising when we remember that before our present vaccines came into use, the usual childhood diseases were nearly always scattered at random throughout childhood, leaving little impact on the healthy child. With vaccines, however, ''the system is challenged with massive amounts of concentrated antigen injected directly into the body, or, as in the case of the oral Sabin polio vaccine, with rapid penetration from the intestines into the blood stream. Such challenges, according to an increasing body of scientific evidence, cannot help but have an unwanted effect on the immune system and its reserves.''[42]

The thymic hormone *thymosin*, produced by the medullary epithelial cells within the thymus gland, is necessary for the maturation, differentiation, and function of T lymphocytes throughout the body. Abnormalities in the secretory role of the thymus in production of thymosin are associated with a wide variety of immunodeficiency, autoimmune, and neoplastic diseases. For example, patients with various types of cancers, leukemias, lupus erythematosis, and rheumatoid arthritis usually show impairment of their thymus-dependent immune systems.[43]

Recent investigation in which postmortem examinations were carried out on thymus glands from adult natives in India and Peru showed that the thymus gland did not atrophy in the adult natives, at least not to the extent usually found and reported in the United States. It has long been considered a normal or natural process for the thymus gland to go into rapid atrophy following puberty. The suggestion has been made that the atrophy of the thymus gland found in most adults in the United States is the result of massive vaccination programs.[44]

When the thymus gland is removed from experimental animals, there is an increased incidence of tumor formation following exposure of animals to chemical carcinogens and tumor viruses as well as a shortened latency period of tumor development. "Spontaneous cancer development in old age may also be related to declining thymus function and immune responses in old age, at least in those instances in which the cancer cells contain foreign antigens."[45]

Well-known author, lecturer, and health activist Betty Lee Morales writes that her parents, who were naturopathic doctors, predicted 50 years ago that cancer would be epidemic in her lifetime as a delayed result of mass vaccinations.[46] Dr. Robert Mendelsohn extends this idea when he says, "I think that most of the degenerative diseases are going to be shown to be due to x-rays, drugs, and polluted food, additives, preservatives and immunizations."[47]

"With all our discoveries about the effects on the human body of ingesting substances not found in nature, one thing we ought to know by now is that many of these toxins—and vaccinations are toxins by definition—kill slowly or kill only after the lapse of significant periods of time," Nicholas von Hoffman said in his *Washington Post* column.[48]

Central Nervous System

Have you ever wondered why the DPT or DT vaccine is not given to anyone over age 7? (The 1993 *Physicians' Desk Reference* warns against it.) Why? Because of the high rate of neurological damage and other reactions associated with it, Dr. George Wootan tells us. "It may be that the vaccine is no less dangerous for younger children but that we fail to recognize much of the damage it does. For example, some of the learning disabilities we see in children of school age may actually be signs of neurological damage suffered during a vaccine reaction."[49]

Dr. Wootan isn't the first doctor to suggest that our current epidemic of learning disabilities might be connected to childhood vaccination programs. Reports of a possible connection between vaccinations and neurological damage resulting in varying degrees of learning disabilities have appeared for many years. For instance, in 1973 Drs. Phillip Landrigan and John Witte linked hyperactivity and brain damage to the live measles vaccine,[50] and in 1985, Harris Coulter and Barbara Loe Fisher presented compelling evidence in their book *DPT: A Shot in the Dark* linking the pertussis vaccine to various kinds of neurological damage, including death.[51] But it wasn't until 1990 with the publication of Harris Coulter's thoroughly documented book *Vaccination, Social Violence and Criminality: The Medical Assault on the American Brain* that the case was arrestingly made for the link between vaccination and the later appearance of such neurological disorders as autism, hyperactivity, learning disabilities, and mental retardation. Autism, minimal brain damage, and the sociopathic personality "represent a continuum of neurologic damage due to encephalitis which in the overwhelming majority of cases is from vaccination."[52] The sociopathic criminal, for instance, who treats his victims as objects rather than human beings, is a milder form of the radical alienation of the autistic.

These disorders, now called "developmental disabilities," affect about 20 percent of American children—one youngster in five. "This is a stupifying figure," Coulter tells us. "If some foreign enemy had inflicted such damage on our children, we would declare war. But . . . we have inflicted it on ourselves. And we persist in it to this day."[53] These are serious charges, to be sure, but Coulter supports them with some very persuasive data. The rise in illiteracy, semiliteracy, mental retardation, and criminality correlates with the increase in childhood vaccination programs. This increase includes not only the number of children vaccinated but the number of vaccines they receive. Paralleling this increase in neurological damage is the increase in "activity-limiting chronic conditions" such as childhood respiratory diseases and ear and eye diseases.

A case in point: When Congress passed the Immunization Assistance Act in 1965, more and more states, during the next few years, extended their vaccination programs and made them mandatory. Four or five years later physicians encountered "a whole new group of neurologically defective 4- and 5-year-olds. A 1986 National Health Interview Survey found that between 1969 and 1981 "activity-limiting chronic conditions" in persons younger than 17 increased by an inexplicable 44 percent, . . . almost all the increase occurred between 1969 and 1975!" Most of these conditions can readily be associated with postencephalitic syndrome. Childhood respiratory diseases increased 47 percent, childhood asthma increased 65 percent, deaths from asthma in children aged 5 and older also increased; "mental and nervous system disorders" increased 80 percent; nonpsychotic personality and mental disorders such as behavioral disorders, hyperactivity, and drug abuse went up 300 percent; and diseases of eyes and ears went up 120 percent.[54]

Poverty was not a major cause because the increase was virtually identical in both high- and low-income families, nor were conditions not associated with vaccine damage such as injuries, genitourinary disorders, infectious or parasititic diseases, deformities, and diseases of the circulatory system. These remained stationary during this time or actually declined.[55]

Numbers and percentages of disabled children—many with multiple learning disabilities—have more than doubled from 1960 to 1980 (from 1 million to 2 million).[56]

Physiologic Mechanisms of Developmental Disabilities. The one common denominator of developmental disabilities is nearly always related to demyelination of the cranial nerve fibers. Either impairment of the process of myelination or destruction of myelin results in cranial nerve palsies. Because the function of the cranial nerves is to carry information to the brain and to help the brain control sensory organs and muscles, the cranial nerves affect how we process information. When myelin is missing, nerve impulses are short-circuited. This impairment of cranial nerve function results in various kinds of thinking, perceiving, learning, and behavioral disorders.

Brain and Spinal Cord Involvement. Autopsies after postvaccinal encephalitis show lesions in the white matter of the brain and spinal cord with complete or partial destruction of the myelin sheaths within the lesions.[57]

At the time of birth, myelination has just begun and in some nerves it doesn't begin until 8 months of age or later. Myelination proceeds at different rates in different neurologic areas for the next 15 years; in some nerves, however, myelination continues to age 45! In the brain, myelination begins with the phylogenetically older parts (those areas which humans share with lower animals) and then moves to the phylogenetically more recent parts (which distinguish humans from animals). Since the cerebral hemispheres and the cerebral cortex (the locus of memory and higher activities of the mind) are the more recent developments of the brain, they are the last to be completely myelinated—in the fifth year of life or later.[58]

Anything that interferes with myelination hinders the child's neurologic development and maturation. Vaccination-associated encephalitis during the first year of life could easily interrupt the myelination process and thus cause neurological damage. And what about demyelination, that is, the removal of myelin after it has been deposited? Charles M. Poser of the Harvard Medical School Department of Neurology said that almost any "vaccination can lead to a noninfectious inflammatory reaction involving the nervous system . . . often associated with demyelination."[59] Actually, it has been known since the 1920s that encephalitis, including that caused by vaccination, can cause demyelination.[60]

An allergic reaction to vaccinations can cause demyelination; conversely, an allergic state predisposes to the development of encephalitis after vaccination. Autistic, hyperactive, and minimally brain-damaged children manifest a high degree of allergic reactions. In fact, "⅘ of autistic children and adults have 'severe allergies.' "[61]

What about the neurologic defectives who make a disproportionate contribution to the rising tide of crime and violence in America? Postencephalitic symptoms predisposing to violence include (1) a low threshold of frustration and the "uncontrollable impulse"; (2) emotional blunting—the inability to feel and empathize with others; and (3) naked aggression and a fascination with violence and cruelty. Because these emotional disabilities express themselves on a spectrum from near normal to pathological, for each institutionalized postencephalitic, hundreds of others remain at large. Let's look at a few statistics suggestive of how these disabilities can be expressed in a social context.

The murder rate doubled between 1960 and 1980. Between 1970 and 1980, arson rose 325 percent. Officially reported rapes have risen five times in 25 years. Between 1969 and 1979, female adolescent crime increased from 12 percent to 48 percent, approximately equal to the rate in male adolescents. Women are participating in violent crime in an unprecedented way. From 1976 to 1986, reported cases of child abuse increased 200 percent. Between 1977 and 1988, the U.S. prison population doubled; in California, it tripled.[62]

We now have the highest violent crime rate in the industrial world.[63] We also have "the most immunized child in history."[64] By age 2, nearly every American child has been vaccinated against seven or eight diseases and usually three or four times for some of them. We might note that "most of the world, even those countries with compulsory vaccination laws . . . allow parents to choose whether to vaccinate their children. . . . With few exceptions, those denying this right are former Communist East Bloc countries,"[65] as well as a number of states in the United States.

Explanations for this rising tide of social violence and "developmental disabilities" have been almost entirely psychological and sociological. This has been misleading, Coulter suggests, primarily because it excludes other factors such as the contribution postvaccinal encephalitis makes to the very sociological and psychological factors being studied. Examples: Poverty—hyperactive adolescents cannot keep jobs; illiteracy—dyslexic children cannot study; social violence—uneducated youth without jobs have nothing else to do; alcoholism and drug addiction—people with neurological disorders must find escape somewhere.[66]

If poverty, which has been almost universally cited as the culprit, is the cause, why is violence three times higher today than it was in 1933 during the depths of the depression? And why is it six times higher than it was during the 1940s?[67] If lack of maternal warmth is the primary culprit, as some psychotherapists claimed, why did autism first appear among the most "educated" parents? These parents are the ones most likely to take their child to the pediatrician for the latest in "medical advances," which would include the latest in shots. Coulter notes that "autism emerged in the United States at a time when vaccination against whooping cough was becoming increasingly popular and widespread." He also notes that autism became more evenly distributed throughout the population after federally funded vaccination programs in the 1960s made vaccines more available.[68] Today, over 4,500 new cases of autism occur every year in the United States.[69]

"The same correlations between autism and childhood vaccination programs may be found in other countries as well,'' investigative journalist Neil Miller points out. ''In Japan, the first autistic child was diagnosed in 1945.'' After the war, when the United States occupied Japan, a mandatory vaccination program was established. ''Today, hundreds of new cases of autism are diagnosed in Japanese children every year.''[70]

The same pattern appears in Europe and England: In the 1950s, Europe received the pertussis vaccine; in the same decade, the first cases of autism appeared. In England the pertussis vaccine wasn't promoted on a large scale until the late 1950s. In 1962, the National Society for Autistic Children in Britain was established.[71]

We are now into the second generation of a vaccine-damaged population. Could the steep rise in child abuse—reported cases increased 120 percent from 1981 to 1991[72]—be related to the ''short fuse'' and low threshold of tolerance of a vaccine-damaged parent interacting with the hyperactivity and low threshold of frustration of the vaccine-damaged child?

Autonomic Nervous System

Respiratory Disorders. Medical folk wisdom used to hold that ''no child ever dies of asthma,'' but ''since the 1960s there has been an 'epidemic' of asthma deaths among young persons in the United Kingdom, New Zealand, Australia, and the United States.'' Breathing difficulties such as SIDS and asthma are due to impairment of the cranial nerves governing respiration.[73] As we learned earlier, cranial nerve palsies are the physiologic substrate of postencephalitic syndrome.

Heart Damage. For many years, reports of deaths from vaccinations of military recruits have surfaced. Did you know that the most common cause of deaths in Air Force recruits is myocarditis (inflammation of the heart muscle) and that this has, in many cases, been linked to vaccinations? In a Finnish study, postvaccination EKG (electrocardiogram) changes of myocarditis were seen in 3 percent of asymptomatic recruits.[74]

Glandular Damage. In a sense, we are our glands. Because our glands work together to control mind-body functions, we can't really speak about the functioning of one gland without recognizing the contributions of all other glands. Earlier we spoke of the possible links between vaccinations and thymus gland damage as well as the link between vaccinations and allergies, this latter now affecting fully 50 percent of the population.[75] Did you know that this increasing allergic sensitization of the American population not only is linked to childhood vaccinations but is a predisposing factor for the development of encephalitis from both the vaccines and the childhood diseases for which they were given? ''Prior to 1900, encephalitis from childhood diseases was almost a negligible danger. After 1920, it was encountered more and more frequently.''[76]

Allergies have been called stress diseases and as such involve the adrenal glands. (Vaccinations, themselves, are stressful to the body.) Natural therapies that include nutritional support for the adrenal glands have usually been successful. I speak from personal experience and the experience of many people I have known.

In some postencephalitic cases, appetite disturbances leading to bulimia, anorexia, and obesity have been observed. Great increases in weight indicate derangement of the pituitary, hypothalamus, and thyroid. In one case of rapid weight gain after vaccine damage, the thyroid was almost completely destroyed.[77]

Sexual disorders such as hypersexuality (compulsive and excessive sexual activity), hyposexuality (mechanical, unfeeling sex), and confused sexuality (bisexuality and homosexuality) are sometimes part of the postencephalitic syndrome.[78] Could these disorders be related to glandular disturbances, or could they—particularly hypersexuality—be one of the many ways the postencephalitic compensates for the many disadvantages he or she experiences in his or her encounters with the world?

Spirit-Mind-Body Connection

What if I were to suggest that childhood diseases can be interpreted as healing crises, opportunities to cleanse and heal the body? What if I add that circumventing childhood diseases via vaccinations can lead to problems later on such as sclerotic (hardening) degenerative diseases (cancer, rheumatoid arthritis, multiple sclerosis, etc.)? This understanding of inflammatory diseases is similar to many schools of natural healing such as classical naturopathy and homeopathy. But now, what if I add that childhood diseases are opportunities to "exercise" the immune system, "maturing struggles" whereby "the higher self [soul] remodels the body in accordance with spiritual ideals"?[79] Disease can then be seen as a positive, transformative experience. The role of the physician is to support the body with homeopathic medicines and to engage the patient's mind toward awareness of what needs to be done in consciousness, that is, learning the lesson the illness is trying to teach. What if I then add that if the soul is not present at the immunological boundary (where the self meets the notself), then biological chaos breaks loose and disease develops?[80] These are some of the ideas of anthroposophical medicine, founded in the early 1920s by Austrian scientist and psychic Rudolf Steiner.

Anthroposophical medicine is not an alternative to the prevailing Western medical model but an expansion of it to include soul and spirit. Without this inclusion, medicine will remain a "soulless technology that removes only symptoms."[81]

Could anything be more soulless than trying to coerce immunity and healing? Could anything be more alien to the spirit of healing than the coerced assembly line? And what about the tunnel vision engendered by a monolithic "healthcare" system with near-exclusive command of information resources to promote its particular point of view? Because tunnel vision seriously limits our thinking and perception of possibilities—and therefore, options—it is mentally and spiritually handicapping. And yet this is the system we have bought into.

What about the high-pitched screaming—or sometimes extreme apathy—of a vaccine-damaged baby that occurs within 48 hours after vaccination? Besides indicating neurological damage taking place, could it also be—at least in part— the soul's recognition that the physical vehicle into which it has projected has now been damaged to such a degree that it will allow for only a limited range of experience in this dimension? And what about the violent outbursts and unpredictable attacks, including attacks against self, of many postencephalitics? Could their rage be an expression of the ego's—or possibly the soul's—frustration at finding itself imprisoned in a physical vehicle that precludes its full expression?

One violent and hostile 16-year-old, who started biting himself at 14 months, said, "I hate the way I am. How long am I going to have to be this way? Is it forever?"[82] Another postencephalitic said, "All my life I have been frustrated with my disability—like I am imprisoned in a body that won't do what I want it to do."[83] Another case I know personally is a child adopted at birth and subject to near-uncontrollable rudeness and temper tantrums, who asked her mother, "Mommy, what's wrong with me? How did I get this way?" She was not referring to her tantrums but to her learning impairment, of which she was becoming acutely aware since starting first grade. After the mother tried to explain that they're working on getting the two sides of her brain to talk to each other a little better (she was undergoing repatterning and movement therapy), the daughter was silent. After a while she told her mother that her birth mother had drunk "something smelly, stinky when I was inside her body, and it hurt my body when it was trying to grow." The mother was stunned, because further questioning revealed that it was like that "stinky stuff Uncle Fred drinks." The mother knew that the birth mother had smoked and taken heavy amounts of antibiotics when she was pregnant, and she had reason to suspect that she consumed alcohol as well. She, a single parent, had never spoken a word about this to her daughter. Since the child had never been vaccinated and had none of the childhood diseases except for a mild case of chickenpox when she was 7, the problem was clearly prenatal. In fact, six medical and educational specialists had identified it as such. The case is particularly poignant because the daughter is very intelligent, intuitive, and attractive but has difficulty processing and retaining information as well as coordinating the fine muscle movements that make reading and writing possible.

These stories illustrate, it seems to me, that there is a very conscious being— a soul—in these neurologically damaged bodies. In fact, in this last case, when I told the mother that the child's rages were probably the result of the child's frustration with her essential self's or soul's inability to make the necessary connections with the physical vehicle to allow for its full expression, she replied, "That's it exactly!"

Is the positivistic, reductionist model of medical orthodoxy a model whose time has passed?

MORE CASUALTIES

Two Australian doctors, Glen Dettman and Archie Kalokerinos, felt so strongly about the destructive effects of vaccines that in 1976 they began a worldwide campaign to warn people against all vaccines: "Vaccines are killing children. There's no doubt about it. We've got figures to show it. It's damaging them, and in the United Kingdom there is now a society for parents of vaccine-damaged children," they said in an interview with Jay Patrick.[84]

The *British Medical Journal* (February 1976) published the following letter from Rosemary Fox, secretary of the Association of Parents of Vaccine-Damaged Children:

Two years ago, we started to collect details from parents of serious reactions suffered by their children to immunizations of all kinds. In 65 percent of the cases referred to us, reactions followed "triple" vaccinations. The children in this group total 182 to date; all are severely brain damaged, some are also paralyzed, and 5 have died during the past 18 months. Approximately 60 percent of reactions (major convulsions, intense screaming, collapse, etc.) occurred within 3 days and all within 12 days.[85]

One of the leading bacteriologists of our time and professor of bacteriology at the London School of Hygiene and Tropical Medicine, Sir Graham S. Wilson wrote in his book *The Hazards of Immunization*:

The risk attendant on the use of vaccines and sera are not as well recognized as they should be. . . . The late Dr. J. R. Hutchinson, of the Ministry of Health, collected records of fatal immunological accidents during the war years, and was kind enough to show them to me. I was frankly surprised when I saw them to learn of the large number of persons in the civil and military population that had died apparently as the result of attempted immunization against some disease or other. Yet, only a very few of these were referred to in medical journals. . . . And further, when one considers that such accidents have probably been going on for the last 60 or 70 years, one realizes what a very small proportion have been described in the medical literature of the world.[86]

From West Germany we read of more vaccination casualties. A reader writing to *Organic Consumer Report* (June 13, 1968) mentions an article that appeared in *Medical World* which stated that about 3,000 children each year suffer varying degrees of brain damage as the result of smallpox vaccination. This same writer mentions another medical journal in which Dr. G. Kittel reported that in the previous year smallpox vaccination damaged the hearing of 3,296 children in West Germany, and 71 became totally deaf. Hearing loss was reported by Dr. William Albrecht, who said in the article quoted earlier in this chapter that a typhoid shot he received made him stone deaf in one ear as well as deathly ill at the time of the shot.

Thus far our discussion has revolved around numbers and nomenclature, making it too easy to forget that these abstractions represent people, real human tragedies. So to flesh out our discussion, let us look briefly at a few case histories compiled by Lily Loat, for many years secretary of the National Anti-Vaccination League of Great Britain.

Dennis Hillier, a healthy English boy who excelled in running, swimming, football, and other games, died in October 1942 of a rare form of encephalitis, some two months after his second inoculation. He had reacted to an initial inoculation with slightly confused speech, but no one had connected this reaction with the inoculation. In describing the case, Dr. W. Russell Brain said at a meeting of the Section of Neurology of the Royal Society of Medicine in February 1943, "The patient, a boy of eleven, developed symptoms after anti-diphtheria inoculation." After mentioning several other cases of nervous disorders and poliomyelitis occurring within a few days after inoculation against diphtheria, he added, "the relation of the infection to the inoculation was at present unsettled."

Christine Timms, a 13-month-old English child who had not been ill since birth, died in February 1949, five days after she had been inoculated against diphtheria. The pathologist said the death was due to septicemia due to septic tonsilitis.

A 5-year-old child, Sylvia Harrison Laplage, died in July 1949, a few days after inoculation against diphtheria. The death certificate gave the cause of death as "Toxaemia of unknown origin."[87]

It goes on, case after case. Rarely is the cause of death ever listed as vaccinia. Asthma, acute lymphatic leukemia, streptococcal cellulitis, tubercular meningitis, and infantile paralysis are some of the causes of death listed on the death certificates.

More graphic descriptions of children dying—frequently after terrible suffering—from the effects of vaccination can be found in Eleanor McBean's book *The Poisoned Needle.* Many of the cases have accompanying photographs of the children showing gaping wounds, festering sores, sightless eyes, and withered limbs as the result of vaccination. By the side of a picture of a beautiful baby girl we read:

Margaret Ann, the only daughter of Mr. and Mrs. Donald W. Gooding, of Wolsey, Essex, England, was pronounced a perfect baby by the doctor when she was born. This beautiful and healthy infant was vaccinated at the age of 4 months. The first two injections didn't take so a third was given, after which inflammation of the brain developed within 5 days. She was taken to the hospital where she remained for many weeks. At the age of 13 months she was blind and could not learn to walk. She also developed digestive disturbances and convulsions.[88]

Interviews with over 100 parents of vaccine-damaged children and stories of the subsequent medical cover-ups are reported in *DPT: A Shot in the Dark* by Harris L. Coulter and Barbara Loe Fisher. A few of the interviews are published in detail; all are heartbreaking—beautiful, healthy babies killed or damaged for life. One mother, for example, whose son died 33 hours after his first DPT shot, confronted her pediatrician and was met with denials, even though she pointed out to him that her first son had the same reaction after his shot. The coroner also tried to deny any connection, writing on the death certificate "death due to irreversible shock" even after the mother explained in detail what had happened. "He said he couldn't write down on the death certificate that Richie had died from a DPT reaction because 'the state's standing on immunizations would be in an uproar.' "[89]

Almost 40 years ago I remember reading of scores of vaccinated children who were stricken with polio and many who died during the Salk vaccination campaigns of 1955. Leonard Scheele, surgeon general at the time, told an American Medical Association (AMA) convention in 1955, "No batch of vaccine can be proved safe before it is given to children."[90]

More recently, I read a case of a girl turned into a "vegetable" (postvaccinal encephalitis) from a smallpox vaccination.[91] I remembered Jack Ashley, a member of the British Parliament, saying that vaccination has turned some children into "cabbages." "Over a 25-year period, 300 children in Britain had been deafened, blinded, or suffered permanent brain damage after immunization against whooping cough, diphtheria and tetanus. Happy healthy children have been turned into cabbages within a few days."[92] "Dozens of children die each year, and thousands are severely harmed and crippled for life, as a direct result of vaccinations," Dr. Paavo Airola tells us.[93] Is it any wonder that some doctors have called vaccinations "legalized child abuse"?[94]

At this point, one might ask, How does such a destructive practice manage to survive for so long? The answer is simple: The equation "Disease prevention equals vaccination" and its corollary "Mass immunization programs equal prevention of epidemics" are writ large in the public mind. I won't go into the complexities of who is responsible for this public image except to suggest that those who make money from this practice—namely, the medical/pharmaceutical industry—are clearly implicated. But, as we shall soon discover, more than money is involved.

NOTES

1. Alec Burton, "The Fallacy of the Germ Theory of Disease" (presentation given at the convention of the National Hygiene Society, Milwaukee, WI, 1978).

2. Richard Moskowitz, "The Case Against Immunizations," p. 10; reprinted from the *Journal of the American Institute of Homeopathy* 76 (March 1983).

3. *World Medicine*, September 22, 1971, pp. 69–72; *New Medical Journals Limited* (London, England: Clareville House), pp. 26–27; reprinted in part in Harold Buttram et

al. *The Dangers of Immunization* (Quakertown, PA: Humanitarian Publishing Company, 1979), pp. 20–25.

4. Jay Patrick, "The Great American Deception," *Let's Live*, December 1976, p. 58.

5. *Organic Consumer Report*, December 4, 1962.

6. *Physicians' Desk Reference*, 1980, p. 1866; *Organic Consumer Report*, April 19, 1977; *Organic Consumer Report*, April 29, 1969. Also see the works of Drs. Robert Mendelsohn, Richard Moskowitz, Paavo Airola, Glen Dettman, Archie Kalokerinos, and others, many of whose works are referred to in this and other chapters.

7. Robert Mendelsohn, *Confessions of a Medical Heretic* (Chicago: Contemporary Books, 1979), pp. 142–145.

8. *Science,* March 26, 1977, p. 9; reported by Donna Benson, "Vaccine Aftermath," *Health Freedom News*, July–August 1984, p. 29.

9. *Medical Hypothesis*, 1988; reported by Richard Leviton, "Who Calls the Shots?" *East West Journal*, November 1988, p. 52.

10. Mendelsohn, *Confessions*, p. 4.

11. Robert Mendelsohn, "Vaccinations Pose Hazards, Too," *Idaho Statesman*, December 19, 1977.

12. *Journal of the American Medical Association*, March 10, 1975, p. 1026.

13. Archie Kalokerinos and Glen Dettman, "A Supportive Submission," *The Dangers of Immunization* (Australian edition of *The Dangers of Immunization* by Harold Buttram et al., ibid.) (Warburton, Victoria, Australia, 1979), p. 74.

14. Archie Kalokerinos and Glen Dettman, " 'Mumps' the Word But You Have Yet Another Vaccine Deficiency," *Australasian Nurses Journal*, June 1981, p. 17.

15. *DPT: Vaccine Roulette*, documentary, 1982. Drs. Edward Mortimer (American Academy of Pediatrics) and John Robbins (FDA, Bureau of Biologics) are quoted respectively.

16. Betty Kamen, "A Shot in the Dark," *Health Freedom News*, May 1985, p. 38.

17. Marian Tompson, "Another View," in . . . *The Risks of Immunizations and How to Avoid Them*, by Robert S. Mendelsohn (Evanston, IL: The People's Doctor Newsletter, 1988), p. 31.

18. R. Mendelsohn, *The Risks of Immunizations*, p. 71.

19. *New England Journal of Medicine*, November 26, 1981, pp. 1307–1313; cited by Neil Z. Miller; *Vaccines: Are They Really Safe and Effective?* (Santa Fe, NM: New Atlantean Press, 1993), p. 32.

20. Mendelsohn, *Immunizations*, pp. 41, 42, 71.

21. TV, *20/20*, aired third or fourth Sunday in January 1990.

22. Christopher Kent and Patrick Gentempo, Jr., "Immunizations: Fact, Myth, Speculations," *ICA International Review of Chiropractic*, November-December 1990.

23. Moskowitz, *Case Against Immunizations*, p. 15.

24. Ibid., p. 14. Also, anthroposophical medicine explicates similar ideas. See latter part of this chapter as well as Leviton's interview with Philip Incao, "Who Calls the Shots?" p. 53. The idea that diseases need to be expressed rather than suppressed (with drugs and vaccines) is not foreign to homeopathy and naturopathy also. (See Part II of this book.)

25. *British Medical Journal*, April 11, 1967, cited by Leon Chaitow, *Vaccination and Immunization: Dangers, Delusions and Alternatives* (Essex, England: C. W. Daniel, 1987), pp. 105–106.

26. *The Lancet*, January 5, 1985; ibid., pp. 107–109.

27. *Medical News*, May 22, 1967; Chaitow, *Vaccination and Immunization*, p. 107.

28. Adelle Davis, *Let's Have Healthy Children* (New York: Signet, 1981), p. 273; rev. Marshall Mandell, M.D.

29. Moskowitz, *Case Against Immunization*, p. 23.

30. Betty Lee Morales, "What's Your Problem?" *Let's Live*, December 1976.

31. Robert Mendelsohn, "More Confessions," interview, *Herbalist New Health*, July 1981, p. 60.

32. Moskowitz, *Case Against Immunizations*, p. 15.

33. Ibid.

34. Ibid.

35. Ibid., p. 16.

36. Harold Buttram and The Humanitarian Society with supportive submissions by Archie Kalokerinos and Glen Dettman, *The Dangers of Immunization* (Warburton, Victoria, Australia: Biological Research Institute, 1979), p. 27. The entire chapter entitled "Vaccinations: Sowing the Seeds of Genetic Change," pp. 26–31, discusses this transfer phenomenon. Also, Dr. Mendelsohn has a discussion of proviruses in *The Risks of Immunizations*, p. 28.

37. Robert Mendelsohn, "The Medical Time Bomb of Immunization Against Disease," *East West Journal*, November 1984, p. 48.

38. Buttram et al., *The Dangers of Immunization*, p. 65.

39. Chaitow, *Vaccination*, p. 104.

40 Buttram et al., *The Dangers of Immunization*, p. 49.

41. *Immunizations, Special Edition* (Santa Fe, NM: Mothering Publications, 1984), cited by Cynthia Cournoyer, *What About Immunizations? Exposing the Vaccine Philosophy* (Santa Cruz, CA: Nelson's Books, 1991), p. 28.

42. Buttram et al., *The Dangers of Immunization*, (Quakertown, PA: The Humanitarian Society, 1979), p. 59.

43. Ibid., p. 45.

44. Ibid., pp. 45–46.

45. Ibid., p. 47.

46. Morales, "What's your Problem?"

47. Mendelsohn, interview by Ron Kotulak in *Public Scrutiny*, March 1981, p. 22.

48. Nicholas von Hoffman, "Free Immunity Shots: Pros and Cons," *Washington Post*, November 28, 1977.

49. George Wootan and Sarah Verney, *Take Charge of Your Child's Health* (Oak Park, IL: Crown Books, 1992); cited in Barbara Mullarkey's column "Viewpoints," *Wednesday Journal*, January 27, 1993.

50. Phillip Landrigan and John Witte, "Neurologic Disorders Following Live Measles Virus Vaccination," *Journal of the American Medical Association* 223 (March 26, 1973): 1459.

51. Harris L. Coulter and Barbara Loe Fisher, *DPT: A Shot in the Dark* (New York: Harcourt Brace Jovanovich, 1985).

52. Harris L. Coulter, *Vaccination, Social Violence and Criminality: The Medical Assault on the American Brain* (Berkeley, CA: North Atlantic Books, 1990), p. 250.

53. Ibid., pp. xiii–xiv.

54. Ibid., pp. 257–258.

55. Ibid., p. 258.

56. Ibid.

57. Ibid., p. 158.

58. Ibid., pp. 155–156.

59. Ibid., p. 156.

60. Ibid., p. 157.

61. Ibid., pp. 152–153.

62. Ibid., pp. 172–175.

63. Ross Perot, National Press Club, WHRV-FM, March 18, 1993.

64. Coulter, *Vaccination*, p. xi.

65. Kristine M. Severyn, "Vaccines May Do More Harm Than Good," *Dayton Daily News*, May 19, 1992, p. 7A. Countries considered "free" that have compulsory vaccination laws have an "escape" clause, that is, a personal belief exemption.

66. Coulter, *Vaccination*, p. 260.

67. Ibid., p. 173.

68. Ibid., pp. 51–53.

69. Ibid., pp. 49–50.

70. *Nagoya Medical Journal* 46 (1984): 35; reported by Miller, *Vaccines: Are They Really Safe and Effective?* (Santa Fe, NM: New Atlantean Press, 1993), p. 53.

71. Coulter, *Vaccination*, p. 50.

72. American Humane Association and the National Committee for Prevention of Child Abuse; reported by Vicki Kemper, "A Tough Cop on the Trail of Hope," *Utne Reader*, March-April 1993, p. 76.

73. Coulter, *Vaccination*, pp. 69–70. Also, on the Gary Null Show (WNIS-AM, July 3, 1994), cardiologist Cass Igram said that there is now a higher death rate from asthma for young people and adults than at any time in human history.

74. Mendelsohn, *The Risks of Immunizations*, p. 83.

75. Coulter, *Vaccination*, p. 151.

76. Ibid., p. 160.

77. Ibid., p. 109.

78. Ibid., pp. 89–92.

79. Leviton, "Who Calls the Shots?" p. 56.

80. Richard Leviton, "What Does Illness Mean?" *Yoga Journal*, November-December 1991, p. 101.

81. Otto Wolff, M.D., quoted by Richard Leviton, "The Promise of Anthroposophical Medicine," *East West Journal*, July 1988, p. 56.

82. Coulter, *Vaccination*, p. 45.

83. Ibid., p. 129.

84. Patrick, "Great American Deception," p. 57.

85. Cited by Paavo Airola, *Everywoman's Book* (Phoenix, AZ: Health Plus Publishers, 1979), p. 281.

86. Ibid., p. 284.

87. Lily Loat, *The Truth About Vaccination and Immunization* (London: Health for All, 1951), pp. 53–55.

88. Eleanor McBean, *The Poisoned Needle* (Mokelumne Hill, CA: Health Research, 1956), p. 78.

89. Coulter and Fisher, *DPT: A Shot in the Dark*, p. 10. A later version of this book— *A Shot in the Dark* (Garden City, NY: Avery, 1991)—reveals the coroner did finally sign a death certificate for Richie stating that he died from "irreversible shock" due to a "probable reaction to DPT."

90. "Vaccination—Compulsory or Choice?" *Organic Consumer Report*, October 3, 1978. p. 1.

91. "Rachel's Tragedy," *The Washington Post*, September 9, 1981, p. A–195.

92. *Organic Consumer Report*, "Organic Seeds for Thought," Cabbage Heads—London, England, (from a reader's letter), April 19, 1977, p. 2.

93. Paavo Airola, "Nutrition Forum," *Let's Live*, December 1976.

94. Glen Dettman and Archie Kalokerinos, "Immunizations—What Are Your Rights?" *Toorak Times* (Victoria, Australia), October 11, 1981.

3 Are Immunizations Effective? (The Statistical Mill)

Ignorance is not not knowing but knowing what isn't so.

—Mark Twain

If you find yourself thinking like everyone else, you better reform.

—Will Rogers,
American humorist

THE DECLINE OF INFECTIOUS DISEASES

Do vaccines protect us from the disease for which they are given? This question might seem absurd on the face of it, given the near disappearance of many infectious diseases for which vaccines are given credit. A closer look, however, at the effectiveness of vaccines, as well as a look at some of the methods of gathering and interpreting statistical data, reveals some interesting discrepancies.

Are vaccinations primarily responsible for the decline of infectious diseases? Actual statistics and records from around the world show that infectious diseases—for example, smallpox, diphtheria, whooping cough, and scarlet fever—began to disappear long before immunizations ever came on the scene.[1] According to the *World Health Statistics Annual*, 1973–1976, Vol. 2, there has been a steady decline of infectious diseases "in most 'developing' countries regardless of the percentage of immunizations administered in these countries. It appears that generally improved conditions of sanitation are largely responsible for preventing 'infectious' diseases."[2]

What about the decline in tuberculosis, chickenpox, scarlet fever, typhus, typhoid, and the plague for which there are no routine immunizations? A number of researchers, including distinguished biologist Rene Dubos, have pointed out that infectious diseases disappeared as the result of sanitation and public water supplies. Other researchers have included improved personal hygiene and better distribution and increased consumption of fresh fruits and vegetables.[3] When Dr. Jonathan Miller was interviewed on the *Dick Cavett Show* (February 4, 1981), he pointed to improved ventilation and drainage, along with nutrition, as being the primary determinants responsible for the decline in the death rate. (He also said that in the past 50 years modern medicine has made such an insignificant contribution to human health and longevity that the enormous expense incurred for developing and administering treatments was hardly worth it.)

An article with the droll title " 'Mumps' the Word But You Have Yet Another Vaccine Deficiency" appeared in the *Australasian Nurses Journal* in June 1981 in which Dr. Glen Dettman and Dr. Archie Kalokerinos discuss not only the new mumps vaccine being promoted but the efficacy of all vaccines. Besides pointing out that 90 percent of the so-called killer diseases had all but disappeared when immunizations were introduced on a large scale (see Figure 1), they say that

since the introduction of routine immunisations we now have an ever alarming increase of degenerative diseases and maladies, but worse still, the diseases we are supposed to be protected from still occur, probably in larger numbers than we might have expected them to, had we simply allowed the declining disease rate as exemplified by the graph to continue.

The doctors also point to an editorial that appeared in *Lancet* (January 12, 1980) which states that the BCG (bacille Calmette-Guérin) vaccine (tuberculosis vaccine) was a failure and that there was a greater incidence of tuberculosis in the vaccinated. In another article, these same doctors mention that in their own country of Australia where tuberculosis vaccinations were given, some of the strain of bacteria mutated, killing around 600 children.[4]

The recitation of statistics that provaccinationists love to use to "prove" the effectiveness of mass immunization programs are classic examples of post hoc reasoning, the fallacy of "after therefore because of" (post hoc ergo propter hoc). "Permitting statistical treatment and the hypnotic presence of numbers and decimal points to befog causal relationships is little better than superstition," Darrell Huff tells us in his delightful little book *How to Lie with Statistics*. After pointing out some humorous examples of positive correlations of unrelated events made to appear as though they were causally related, he says that "scantier evidence than this—treated in the statistical mill until common sense could no longer penetrate it—has made many a medical fortune and many a medical article in magazines, including professional ones."[5]

Figure 1
The Immunization Myth?

Figure 1 below was presented at the Presidential address of the British Association for the Advancement of Sciences (Porter, 1971), and Figure 2 appeared in an article published in Scientific American, written by Professor John Dingle (1973). These two countries are widely separated, but the conclusions are similar.

England & Wales: Deaths of children under 15 years attributed to scarlet fever, diphtheria, whooping cough and measles (Porter, 1971).

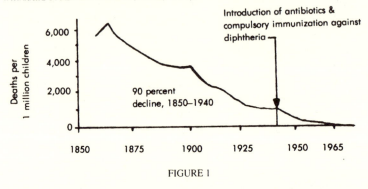

FIGURE 1

Declining death rates attributable to infectious diseases of infancy and childhood, such as tuberculosis (upper curve) and typhoid fever (lower curve). No immunization against TB has been adopted in the U.S. The effectiveness of typhoid vaccine is questionable (Dingle, 1973).

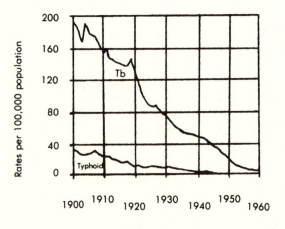

FIGURE 2

Source: Harold Buttram et al., The Humanitarian Society, *The Dangers of Immunisation*, Biological Research Institute, (Warburton, Victoria, Australia: 1979).

Before a causal relationship can be established between any two events, the following criteria must be satisfied:

1. *Controls.* Was there a control group? What were the controls used?
2. *Variables.* What were the variables? Were they controlled?
3. *Size and duration.* Were the number of participants and the duration of the experiment adequate?

In other words, when a causal relationship is implied, we must ask ourselves, What other factors are involved, and what are the controls?

Polio

Let's look at the statistical mill itself. The case of poliomyelitis is particularly instructive since its apparent decline cannot be explained by such developments as sanitation, public water supplies, and ventilation. In fact, it is a disease that occurs only among the most civilized peoples with the highest standards of sanitation, and the like, being unknown among preliterate cultures that have been relatively untouched by civilization.

Jonas Salk, the discoverer of the Salk polio vaccine, has been called the "twentieth-century miraclemaker" and the savior of countless lives.[6] We read glowing reports of the dramatic decrease in poliomyelitis in the United States as a result of the Salk vaccine. For instance, the Virginia State Department of Health distributes a folder that tells us that polio vaccines have reduced the incidence of polio in the United States from 18,000 cases of paralytic polio in 1954 to fewer that 20 in 1973–1978. A recent article in *Modern Maturity* states that in 1953 there were 15,600 cases of paralytic polio in the United States; by 1957, due to the Salk vaccine, the number had dropped to 2,499.[7]

During the 1962 congressional hearings on H.R. 10541, Dr. Bernard Greenberg, head of the Department of Biostatistics of the University of North Carolina School of Public Health, testified that not only did polio increase substantially (50 percent from 1957 to 1958 and 80 percent from 1958 to 1959) *after* the introduction of mass and frequently compulsory immunization programs, but statistics were manipulated and statements made by the Public Health Service to give the opposite impression.[8]

For instance, in 1957 a spokesman for the North Carolina Health Department made glowing claims for the efficacy of the Salk vaccine, showing how polio steadily decreased from 1953 to 1957. His figures were challenged by Dr. Fred Klenner, who pointed out that it wasn't until 1955 that a single person in the state received a polio vaccine injection. Even then, injections were administered on a very limited basis because of the number of polio cases resulting from the vaccine. It wasn't until 1956 "that polio vaccinations assumed 'inspiring' proportions." The 61 percent drop in polio cases in 1954 was credited to the Salk vaccine when it wasn't even in the state! By 1957, polio was on the increase.[9]

Other ways polio statistics were manipulated to give the impression of the effectiveness of the Salk vaccine were:

1. *Redefinition of an epidemic.* More cases were required to refer to polio as epidemic after the introduction of the Salk vaccine (from 20 per 100,000 to 35 per 100,000 per year).

2. *Redefinition of the disease.* In order to qualify for classification as paralytic polio-myelitis, the patient had to exhibit paralytic symptoms for at least 60 days after the onset of the disease. Prior to 1954 the patient had to exhibit paralytic symptoms for only 24 hours! Laboratory confirmation and the presence of residual paralysis were not required. After 1954, residual paralysis was determined 10 to 20 days and again 50 to 70 days after the onset of the disease. Dr. Greenberg said that "this change in definition meant that in 1955 we started reporting a new disease, namely, paralytic poliomyelitis with a longer lasting paralysis."

3. *Mislabeling.* After the introduction of the Salk vaccine, "Cocksackie virus and aseptic meningitis have been distinguished from paralytic poliomyelitis," explained Dr. Greenberg. "Prior to 1954 large numbers of these cases undoubtedly were mislabeled as paralytic polio."[10]

Another way of reducing the incidence of disease by way of semantics—or statistical artifact, as Dr. Greenberg calls it—is simply to reclassify the disease. From the *Los Angeles County Health Index: Morbidity and Mortality, Reportable Diseases*, we read the following:

Date	Viral or Aseptic Meningitis	*Polio
July 1955	50	273
July 1961	161	65
July 1963	151	31
September 1966	256	5

The reason for this remarkable change is stated in this same publication: "Most cases reported prior to July 1, 1958, as non-paralytic poliomyelitis are now reported as viral or aseptic meningitis."[11] In *Organic Consumer Report* (March 11, 1975), we read, "In a California Report of Communicable Diseases, polio showed a zero count, while an accompanying asterisk explained, " 'All such cases now reported as meningitis.' "

There have been at least three major polio epidemics in the United States, according to Dr. Christopher Kent. "One occurred in the teens, another in the late thirties, and the most recent in the fifties." The first two epidemics simply went away like the old epidemics of plague. Around 1948, the incidence of polio began to soar. (Interestingly, this is when pertussis—whooping cough—vaccine appeared, Dr. Kent points out.) It reached a high in 1949, with 43,000 cases, but by 1951 had dropped to below 28,000. In 1952, when a government-subsidized study of polio vaccine began, the rate soared to an all-time high of well over 55,000 cases. After the study, the number of cases dropped again and continued to decline as they had in the previous epidemics. "This time, however, the vaccine took the credit instead of nature."[12]

The cyclical nature of polio is again illustrated by the remarks of Dr. Alec Burton at the 1978 meeting of the Natural Hygiene Society in Milwaukee, Wisconsin. Some years ago at the University of New South Wales in Australia, statistics were compiled that showed that the polio vaccine in use at the time had no influence whatsoever on the polio epidemic. Polio comes in cycles anyway, Dr. Burton said, and when it has been "conquered" by vaccines, and a disease with identical symptoms continues to appear, doctors look for a new virus because they know the old one has been "wiped out." "And the game goes on," he added.[13]

When Dr. Robert Mendelsohn was asked about the possibility of childhood diseases—particularly polio—returning if the vaccinations were stopped, he replied: "Doctors admit that forty percent of our population is not immunized against polio. So where is polio? Diseases are like fashions; they come and go, like the flu epidemic of 1918."[14]

On a 1983 *Donahue* show ("Dangers of Childhood Immunizations," January 12), Dr. Mendelsohn pointed out that polio disappeared in Europe during the 1940s and 1950s without mass vaccination and that polio does not occur in the Third World, where only 10 percent of the people have been vaccinated against polio or anything else.

Returning to the congressional hearings referred to earlier (H.R. 10541), we read that in 1958 Israel had a major "type I" polio epidemic *after* mass vaccinations. There was no difference in protection between the vaccinated and the unvaccinated. In 1961, Massachusetts had a "type III" polio outbreak and "there were more paralytic cases in the triple vaccinates than in the unvaccinated."[15]

In a letter published in the *Journal of the American Medical Association (JAMA)*, January 21, 1956, which was inserted into these same hearings, Dr. Herbert Ratner pointed out that because poliomyelitis is such a low-incidence disease, this complicates the evaluation of a vaccine for it. He also said that there is "a high degree of acquired immunity and many natural factors preventing the occurrence of the disease . . . in the Nation at large."[16]

Dr. Richard Moskowitz adds that the virulence of the poliovirus was low to begin with.

Given the fact that the poliovirus was ubiquitous before the vaccine was introduced, and could be found routinely in samples of city sewage whenever it was looked for, it is evident that effective, natural immunity to poliovirus was already as close to being universal as it can ever be, and *a fortiori* no artificial substitute could ever equal or even approximate that result.[17]

MMR and DPT

What about the rest of the standard repertoire of vaccines for children in the United States—measles, mumps, rubella, diphtheria, whooping cough, and tetanus? Since we have concerned ourselves so far with large numbers and population studies, let's look briefly at a few small-scale studies.

"The World Health Organization did a study and found that while in an unimmunized, measles-susceptible group of children the normal rate of contraction of disease was 2.4 percent; in the control group that had been immunized, the rate of contraction rose to 33.5 percent."[18] On a 1983 *Donahue* show ("Dangers of Childhood Immunizations," January 12), Dr. J. Anthony Morris pointed out that in a recent measles epidemic in Dade County, Florida, most of the cases occurred in vaccinated children.

"In a 1978 survey of 30 states, more than half of the children who contracted measles had been adequately vaccinated. Moreover, according to the World Health Organization, the chances are about fifteen times greater that measles will be contracted by those vaccinated for them than by those who are not."[19]

Let's look again at the statistical mill with regard to measles. From 1958 to 1966, the number of measles cases reported each year dropped from 800,000 to 200,000. The drug industry claims this drop was due to vaccinations; however, there are some interesting discrepancies: First, the incidence of measles has been declining steadily for the past 100 years. Second, it wasn't until 1967 that the live vaccine that is presently used was introduced because the killed virus vaccine that came out in 1963 was found to be ineffective and potentially harmful. Third, a survey of pediatricians in New York City revealed that only 3.2 percent of them were actually reporting measles cases to the health department. And fourth, in 1974, the Centers for Disease Control (which has promoted the current measles vaccine) determined that there were 36 cases of measles in Georgia, but the Georgia state surveillance system reported 660 cases that same year.[20]

The statistical mill is worth looking at with respect to whooping cough "epidemics." Because physicians have a stake in vaccination programs, "there is a natural tendency to underreport whooping cough when it occurs in a vaccinated population, and to overreport it when it appears to be occurring in an unvaccinated population," Harris Coulter and Barbara Loe Fisher report. When vaccination rates decline, physicians tend to diagnose pertussis "every time a baby clears his throat," Dr. Mendelsohn tells us. Within a few months after *DPT: Vaccine Roulette* was aired (April 1982), the states of Maryland and Wisconsin reported whooping cough "epidemics." The Maryland state health officials implied that this rise in cases was the result of parents seeing the documentary and not having their children vaccinated. The cases in both the Maryland and Wisconsin "epidemics" were analyzed by J. Anthony Morris, an expert on bacterial and viral diseases. In Maryland, he found laboratory confirmation in only 5 out of the 41 cases, and all of them had been vaccinated! In Wisconsin, he found laboratory confirmation in only 16 out of 43 cases, and all but 2 had been vaccinated.[21] The formula seems to be: If you want to sell vaccines—and visits to the doctor—create epidemics.

The effectiveness of whooping cough vaccine has been reported to be about 50 percent. Of 8,092 cases of whooping cough reported in the *British Medical Journal*, 36 percent were immunized and 30 percent unimmunized.[22] Hardly 50 percent protection.

What about rubella? Dr. Stanley Plotkin, professor of pediatrics at the University of Pennsylvania School of Medicine, states, "It is clear that vaccination of children (for rubella), which has only been done for several years, is not very successful as a policy." Thirty-six percent of adolescent females who had been vaccinated against rubella lacked evidence of immunity by blood test, he points out. In another study reported by the University of Minnesota, a high serological (pertaining to serums) failure rate was shown in children given rubella, measles, and mumps vaccine.[23]

A large proportion of children are found to be seronegative (no evidence of immunity in blood tests) four to five years after rubella vaccination.[24] In another study, 80 percent of army recruits who had been immunized against rubella came down with the disease. The same results were shown in a consecutive study that took place at an institution for the mentally retarded.[25]

Cook County, Ill., hospital decided to immunize one-half of the nursing staff and not the other half. Diphtheria broke out soon afterward among the immunized cases, not the others. It invaded both halves, both the immunized and the unimmunized, and the total of cases was much higher among the supposedly immunized cases than among those not immunized.[26]

During a 1969 outbreak of diphtheria in Chicago, four of the sixteen victims had been "fully immunized against the disease," according to the Chicago Board of Health. Five others had received one or more doses of the vaccine, and two of these people had tested at full immunity. In another report of diphtheria cases, three of which were fatal, one person who died and fourteen out of twenty-three carriers had been fully immunized.[27]

Sometimes diphtheria has increased to epidemic proportions *after* the introduction of mass compulsory vaccination. For instance, diphtheria increased by 30 percent in France, 55 percent in Hungary, and tripled in Geneva, Switzerland, *after* the introduction of mass compulsory vaccination. "In Germany, where compulsory mass immunization was introduced in 1940, the number of cases increased from 40,000 per year to 250,000 by 1945, virtually all among immunized children. . . . On the other hand, in Sweden, diphtheria virtually disappeared without any immunizations."[28] "In major U.S. epidemics during the past decade, the diphtheria immunization had failed to demonstrate effectiveness in terms of cases or deaths."[29]

Could the real reason vaccination promise and performance seem so contradictory is that the vaccination premise itself is faulty? As stated earlier, the theory of vaccination postulates that the use of immunizing agents produces a mild form of a disease for which specific antibodies are formed that will protect the body when the real thing comes along. As we saw, it doesn't quite work that way. Dr. Alec Burton points out, for instance, that there are children with agammaglobulinemia, which means that they are incapable of producing antibodies, yet these children develop and recover from measles and other zymotic (infectious or contagious) diseases almost as spontaneously as other children.

He describes an interesting study in England that was carried out in 1949–1950 and published by the British Medical Council in May 1950 in their report #272. The study investigated the relation of the incidence of diphtheria to the presence of antibodies. Since diphtheria was epidemic at or just prior to the time of the study, the researchers had a large number of cases to investigate. The purpose of the research was to determine the existence or nonexistence of antibodies in people who developed diphtheria and those who did not but were in close proximity to those who did, such as physicians, nurses working in hospitals, family, and friends. The conclusion was that there was no relation whatsoever between the antibody count and the incidence of disease. The researchers found people who were highly resistant with extremely low antibody counts, and people who developed the disease who had high antibody counts. The study was finally abandoned because of the extremely conflicting data.[30]

The mystery begins to unravel when we look at the work of Drs. Glen Dettman and Archie Kalokerinos. In one of their articles they quote Dr. Wendel Belfield of San Jose, California, who says, "Antibodies are not needed when the primary immunological defense (leukocytes, interferon, etc.) is functioning at maximum capacity. . . . Antibody production appears to occur only when the ascorbate level, in the primary defense components are at low levels thereby permitting some viruses to survive the primary defense."[31]

Smallpox

No discussion of immunization would be complete without including smallpox since the World Health Organization (WHO) is now claiming that their global smallpox immunization campaign has rid the world of smallpox. One dissenter, Arie Zuckerman, who is a member of the WHO's advisory panel on viruses, warned against the smallpox vaccine, saying, "Immunization against smallpox is more hazardous than the disease itself." We now have "monkeypox," which, according to the weekly epidemiological record of WHO (54 [1979]:12–13), is clinically indistinguishable from smallpox.[32]

The chicanery sometimes used in compiling vaccination statistics is discussed in much of the literature distributed by the National Anti-Vaccination League in Britain. For instance, "the Ministry of Health itself has admitted that the vaccinal condition is a guiding factor in diagnosis."[33] This means that if a person who is vaccinated comes down with the disease he is "protected" against, the disease is simply recorded under another name; for example, "in the thirty years ending in 1934, 3,112 people are stated to have died of chicken-pox, and only

579 of smallpox in England and Wales. Yet all authorities are agreed that chicken-pox is a non fatal disease.''[34] In other words, people who have been vaccinated for smallpox and later come down with the disease are classified in the health records as having chickenpox. ''This has been admitted by English medical officers of health, and the Ministry of Health has twice stated in answer to questions in Parliament that vaccination is one factor in the diagnosis of these cases.''[35]

George Bernard Shaw said, ''During the last considerable epidemic at the turn of the century, I was a member of the Health Committee of London Borough Council, and I learned how the credit of vaccination is kept up statistically by diagnosing all the revaccinated cases (of smallpox) as pustular eczema, varioloid or what not—except smallpox.''[36]

The cycles of mandatory vaccinations for smallpox and the terrible smallpox epidemics that followed would take many pages to chronicle, so let's just look at a few samples: ''For more than fifty years the populations of Australia and New Zealand (with the exception of the armed forces in time of war) have been practically unvaccinated, and they have been more free from smallpox than any other community.'' ''The most thoroughly vaccinated countries are Italy, the Philippine Islands, Mexico and what was formerly called British India. And all of these have been scourged with smallpox epidemics.''[37]

''Our U.S. Government staged a compulsory vaccination campaign in the Philippines which brought on the largest smallpox epidemic in the history of that country with 162,503 cases and 71,453 deaths, all vaccinated. That was between 1917 and 1919.''[38]

In England the ''ghastly epidemic of 1871–1872 broke out after 13 years of voluntary inoculations, followed by 18 years of a mandatory program, backed up by four years of Draconian [very severe] punishments'' for those refusing vaccinations, writes Fernand Delarue in his book *L'intoxication vaccinale*. At the time of the epidemic's outbreak, 90 percent of the population was believed to have been vaccinated.[39]

''Japan started compulsory vaccination against smallpox in 1872 and continued it for about 100 years with disastrous results. Smallpox increased every year. By 1892 their records showed 165,774 cases with 29,979 deaths, all vaccinated. In Australia where they had no compulsory vaccination they had only 3 deaths from smallpox in 15 years.''[40]

But the answer to the riddle of smallpox—and polio—is found in the next chapter.

FROM ACUTE TO CHRONIC DISEASE

As we have seen, statistical argument can be deceptive, so let's suppose that disease can be prevented by artificial immunization. (This is the practice of injecting toxic substances into the body as opposed to natural immunization that occurs as the result of natural infection and/or certain living habits that we shall discuss later.) There is, however, a very disturbing question we should ask our-selves: Could artificial immunization suppress disease symptoms arising from imbalances—for example, biochemical deficiencies and toxicity—and drive the disease deeper into the body where it might later manifest in more dangerous and disabling ways? I am reminded of what Dr. William Howard Hay said in this connection:

And if you have been dealing as I have with the derelicts from all over the world for 30 years, you would find an almost fatal relationship between this history of vaccination and some failing that follows this for many years that has kept a person from being as well as he should have been.[41]

Dr. Richard Moskowitz states the case more specifically:

It is dangerously misleading, and, indeed, the exact opposite of the truth to claim that a vaccine makes us ''immune'' or *protects* us against an acute disease, if in fact it only drives the disease deeper into the interior and causes us to harbor it *chronically*, with the result that our responses to it become progressively weaker, and show less and less tendency to heal or resolve themselves spontaneously.[42]

In a later article, Dr. Moskowitz suggests that because vaccinations do not produce genuine immunity, the terms *vaccinated* and *unvaccinated* be substi-tuted for the terms *immunized* and *unimmunized*. How do vaccinations work? Immunosuppressively, as Dr. Moskowitz and other researchers have suggested.[43]

Vaccines have been called potential allergens because they introduce foreign proteins directly into the blood without digestion or ''censoring by the liver.'' When we remember that one of the chief causes of allergies is the presence of undigested proteins in the blood, the connection between vaccinations and al-lergies becomes apparent. In Chapter 9 we shall discuss in more detail how vaccinations, along with other drugs, reroute acute illnesses into their chronic form.

Vaccines have also been called drugs because, like drugs, they are inherently toxic and work on the principle of *suppression* rather than *expression*, as do natural therapies. This suppression of symptoms prevents the body-mind from discharging what needs to come out and only compounds the problem, as we will learn in Chapters 8 and 9. Also, the expression of symptoms is part of the full immunological response which is necessary for the development of true immunity (see Chapter 7).

Perhaps the only real difference between vaccines and drugs is that drugs work to suppress present symptoms and vaccines work to suppress *possible* future symptoms. Orthodoxy regards this latter as immunity, but evidence sug-gests it is immune suppression.

Perhaps a fairly straightforward illustration of how vaccines can work to sup-press rather that prevent disease can be found in the example of measles. Although outbreaks of measles continue to occur among supposedly immune schoolchildren, the peak incidence of measles now occurs in adolescents and young adults where the risk of pneumonia and demonstrable liver abnormalities has increased substantially to well over 3 percent and 2 percent, respectively.[44]

The syndrome of "atypical measles"—pneumonia, petechiae (skin blotching), edema, and severe pain—not only is difficult to diagnose but is often overlooked entirely. Likewise, symptoms of atypical mumps—anorexia, vomiting, and erythematous (red) rashes, without any parotid (near the ear) involvement—require extensive serological testing to rule out other concurrent diseases.[45]

As with measles, outbreaks of mumps and rubella among supposedly immune schoolchildren continue to be reported. Again, however, both these diseases, which are essentially benign, self-limited diseases of childhood, are being transformed by a vaccine into considerably less benign diseases of adolescents and young adults. In the case of mumps, the chief complication is epididymoorchitis (acute inflammation of the testicles), which occurs in 30 to 40 percent of males affected after the age of puberty. This usually results in atrophy of the affected testicle. Mumps can also "attack" the ovary and pancreas.[46]

When rubella occurs in older children and adults, it can produce not only arthritis (as can the vaccine), purpura (skin discoloration), and other severe systemic disorders but also "congenital rubella syndrome" (damage to the developing embryo during the first trimester of pregnancy), the very disease the vaccine was designed to prevent.[47]

ARTIFICIAL VERSUS NATURAL IMMUNITY

When immunity to a disease is acquired naturally, the possibility of reinfection is only 3.2 percent, journalist Marian Tompson tells us. If the immunity comes from a vaccination, the chance of reinfection is 80 percent.[48] In one study of military recruits, the rubella reinfection rate was 80 percent compared with 4 percent in naturally immune individuals.[49]

Dr. William Howard Hay has pointed out that in any epidemic of communicable disease only a small percentage of the population contracts the disease. Most people are naturally immune; so if a man who has been vaccinated does not contract the disease, that really proves nothing. If he had not been vaccinated, the chances are he would not have contracted the disease anyway. We have no way of knowing. In a sense, we have destroyed our evidence.[50]

"Just because you give somebody a vaccine, and maybe get an antibody reaction, doesn't mean a thing. The only true antibodies, of course, are those you get naturally," Dr. Dettman said in an interview with Jay Patrick. "What we're doing is interfering with a very delicate mechanism that does its own thing. If nutrition is correct, it does it in the right way. Now if you insult a person in this way and try to trigger off something that nature looks after, you're asking for all sorts of trouble, and we don't believe it works."[51] (For more on developing natural immunity and why vaccinations don't produce true immunity, see Chapter 7.)

"Natural diseases are a lot safer than acute artificial complications," Dr. Mendelsohn reminds us.[52]

Perhaps the strongest statement against the effectiveness of artificial immunization comes from Dr. Hay.

It is nonsense to think that you can inject pus [from smallpox vaccine] . . . into a little child and in any way improve its health. . . . There is no such thing as immunization, but we sell it under the name—immunization. . . . If we could by any means build up a natural resistance to disease through these artificial means, I would applaud it to the echo, but we can't do it. The body has its own methods of defense. These depend on the vitality of the body at the time. If it is vital enough, it will resist all infections; if it isn't vital enough it won't and you can't change the vitality of the body for the better by introducing poison of any kind into it.[53]

Before leaving the question of vaccine effectiveness, let's look at the monorail—or is it a disease scary-go-round?—that we seem to be on, as well as the pivotal argument for mandating vaccinations.

VACCINATIONS FOR VACCINATIONS?

Do we now have vaccinations for diseases caused by vaccinations?

Did you know that poliomyelitis has long been associated with vaccinations, particularly the diphtheria and whooping cough vaccinations? From studies in England and Australia, reported in the *Los Angeles Mirror*, May 30, 1951, doctors found more children under 5 years old developed polio within a month after vaccinations for whooping cough and diphtheria than nonvaccinated youngsters.[54] An article in *Time* magazine, June 25, 1951, titled "Polio Precaution," stated: "Researchers on three continents have reported that when a child after recent inoculation contracts the paralyzing form of polio, the paralysis seems most likely to strike the injected arm or leg. For that reason New York City's Department of Health suspended diphtheria and whooping cough inoculations at its 76 child health stations until October 1."[55]

Dr. William Frederick Koch stated the case more strongly: "The injection of any serum, vaccine or even penicillin has shown a very marked increase in the incidence of polio—at least 400 percent. Statistics on this are so conclusive, no one can deny it."[56]

Now we have polio vaccines—Salk and Sabin—both of which have been known to cause polio. In fact, a virologist with the CDC, Dr. Larry Schonberger, has said that polio caused by the vaccine has become more common than the natural virus.[57] As we said earlier, most of these cases are filed under viral or aseptic meningitis, another disease that can be caused by vaccinations. One researcher found clear connections between DPT injections and the increase of meningitis diseases.[58] Now we have the meningitis vaccine (Hib) to prevent meningitis. A Minnesota study showed that the vaccine increases the risk of meningitis fivefold![59]

What about cancer? This, too, has long been associated with vaccinations, as has its variant, leukemia. An article in *Medical News* (March 26, 1956) asks the question, "Is lymphatic leukemia a 'man-made' disease?" It goes on to point out that a group of medical researchers at the University of Utah Medical School believe that in some instances it is. "These scientists believe that immunizing agents used to prevent certain childhood diseases, or drugs to treat others, might actually enhance the development of lymphatic leukemia."[60]

In 1974, Dr. Frederick Klenner wrote to Kalokerinos and Dettman in Australia: "Many here voice a silent view that the Salk and Sabin vaccine, being made of monkey kidney tissue, has been directly responsible for the major increase of leukemia in this country."[61] In his book *You Can Master Disease*, published in 1952, Dr. Bernard Jensen quotes British, Canadian, and American doctors, including cancer specialists, who point to a definite link between vaccinations and cancer.[62] The more recent discoveries of researchers linking cancer to vaccinations—discussed in Chapter 2—are not new, only more precisely and scientifically articulated.

Scientists are now trying to find vaccines not only for cancer but for allergies, MS, and arthritis, diseases again associated with vaccines. AIDS (another variant of cancer) is perhaps the most obvious example of the disease scary-go-round. Vaccines and drugs have been clearly implicated as primary causes of AIDS, but they are also part of the official solution (see Chapter 8).

Worth mentioning is the new "China syndrome," reported in *Science* (July 5, 1991), which has been appearing in significant numbers in China and Latin America—7,000 cases reported in Latin America between 1987 and 1990. These new paralytic syndromes are like polio in that they "attack the motor neurons of the spinal cord and prevent it from generating nerve impulses." But it *can't* be polio because "the children who get it have already been vaccinated against poliovirus." Researchers have speculated that it might be Guillain-Barré syndrome (GBS), a disease, as we said earlier, known to be caused by vaccination. But what later researchers from Johns Hopkins University found was not GBS but a brand-new disease—medical "virgin territory."[63] Are we now going to work on developing a vaccine for this "new" kind of motor paralysis?

There is talk of finding vaccines for every conceivable kind of human inconvenience—colds, dental caries, slimming, contraception, even environmental toxins, venoms, and chemical carcinogens.[64] What will be the long-term effects of these new vaccines and what new diseases will we encounter next?

Did you know that the United Nations has committed $150 million to develop a "supervaccine" to provide immunity against 30 childhood diseases with a single shot?[65]

Perhaps Emil Chartier said it best: "Nothing is more dangerous than an idea when it is the only one we have."[66]

COMMUNITIES OF IMMUNITIES?

It's called "herd" immunity, and it means that if enough members of a population are vaccinated, everyone will be "protected." Even though epidemiological studies have proven this theory to be false, this argument is trotted out again and again by political medicine to justify mandatory vaccination programs. No one seems to think, if vaccinations are really immunizations—that is, they produce immunity to the diseases for which they are given—it wouldn't make any difference whether anyone else was vaccinated or not. We've already seen how herd immunity theories don't work with respect to smallpox and diphtheria epidemics, so let's look for a moment at a few of the other childhood diseases.

In a 1986 outbreak of measles in Corpus Christi, Texas, 99 percent of the children had been vaccinated, and more than 95 percent were purportedly immune.[67]

"In 1984, 27 cases of measles were reported at a high school in Waltham, Massachusetts, where over 98 percent of the students had documentary proof of vaccination. In 1989, an Illinois high school with vaccination records on 99.7 percent of its students reported 69 cases over a three-week period. These reports fail to mention the surprisingly low number of measles cases in unvaccinated students."[68]

In 1987, the CDC reported 2,440 cases of measles among vaccinated children.[69]

Study after study points unerringly to clusters of vaccinated children who have contracted measles.[70] But one of the more stark instances of vaccine failure occurred in 1989 in Ohio where 72.5 percent of the 2,720 reported cases of measles occurred in vaccinated persons. That's 1,972 cases! Eighty percent of these cases occurred in persons 15 years of age and older (when the disease tends to be more serious). This reflects the experience of other states.[71] The other vaccinations have high failure rates as well.

According to the *Journal of Pediatrics* (1989), one study showed a 55 percent failure rate for pertussis vaccine.[72]

In 1986, in Kansas, 1,300 cases of pertussis were reported. Of the patients whose vaccination status was known, 90 percent were "adequately" vaccinated.[73]

"According to the Ohio Department of Health, half of the reported Ohio whooping cough cases [from 1987 to 1991] were in vaccinated persons—in cases where vaccinations status was known."[74]

In 1971, in Casper, Wyoming, a rubella epidemic occurred one year after 84 percent of the city's schoolchildren had been vaccinated against rubella (91 of the 125 cases occurred in vaccinated children).[75]

When it was first evident that vaccinations failed to produce immunity, booster shots were "invented." For instance, several states have recently mandated documentary proof of MMR revaccination before a child can enter seventh grade. Why? The original dose didn't work, so another one will.

When revaccinations don't work, it's because everyone isn't vaccinated. We need "herd" immunity. This means that there are enough people in the community (herd?) who are immune by virtue of either having had the disease or having had a vaccination that "took." This latter means that there is a sufficiently high antibody count to render the person immune. Never mind that there are studies which suggest that antibody count has little to do with producing immunity and, in fact, may indicate immune weakness.[76] Never mind that a vaccinated person, according to this reasoning, whose vaccination didn't "take" (who didn't "respond properly") could be part of the "reservoir of disease" just like the unvaccinated. Nevertheless, everyone must be vaccinated to "protect" everyone else. Even though admittedly vaccines are not 100 percent effective and some children are damaged, they must be "sacrificed" for the good of the community.

Never mind that this thinking contradicts the premises of vaccination. The benefits *must* outweigh the risks. Vaccines *must* be effective. Reports of adverse reactions and ineffectiveness *must* be dismissed or attacked. Why? Because the American medical establishment long ago committed its reputation and credibility to mass vaccination programs. With its "deep pockets" and ready—and near-exclusive—media access to promote its vaccination programs and counter criticism of them, it has created an almost irresistible momentum to support the vaccinal fix.

So pervasive is this momentum that biomedical researchers are looking for a vaccine for AIDS. Never mind the contradiction that the purpose of a vaccine is to produce disease-specific antibodies but AIDS (HIV [human immunodeficiency virus]) antibodies are supposed to be a sign of infection.

I'm reminded of something Weller Embler said, "it is easy to believe what one wants to believe. Facts are not so stubborn and brutal as we have been led to think, and one can get information which will support his wishful thinking without much trouble.... Deep inner desires will cause outward facts to suffer rare changes; wanting things desperately enough will change the face of reality altogether." Embler goes on to point out that along with the gathering of information "the making of judgements is often conditioned by prejudice toward those judgements which it will benefit us personally to make.... If our interests are at stake ... we can prefer the monstrous to the beautiful and good."[77]

NOTES

1. Robert Mendelsohn (speech given at the National Health Federation Conference in Orlando, FL, February 1980). Other researchers who have pointed out the same thing include: Paavo Airola, *Everywoman's Book* (Phoenix, AZ: Health Plus, 1979), p. 274,

Rene Dubos, *Mirage of Health* (Garden City, NY: Anchor Books, 1961), pp. 30, 31, 70, 129, 130; Harold Buttram et al., *The Dangers of Immunization*. (Quakertown, PA: The Humanitarian Society, 1979), pp. 48–56; Archie Kalokerinos and Glen Dettman, " 'Mumps' the Word But You Have Yet Another Vaccine Deficiency," *Australasian Nurses Journal*, June 1981; also Dettman and Kalokerinos interviewed by Jay Patrick, "The Great American Deception," *Let's Live*, December 1976, p. 57.

2. Leonard Jacobs, "Menage," *East West Journal*, September 1977, p. 15. The *World Health Statistics Annual* is published by the World Health Organization, Geneva, Switzerland.

3. See authors cited in note 1. Also, an interesting study by W. J. McCormick, "The Changing Incidence and Mortality of Infectious Disease in Relation to Changed Trends in Nutrition," *Medical Record*, September 1947, credits the increased consumption of vitamin C–rich foods, particularly citrus and tomatoes, as well as improved nutrition and hygiene with the decline of infectious diseases.

4. Dettman and Kalokerinos interviewed by Patrick, "The Great American Deception," p. 57.

5. Darrell Huff, *How to Lie with Statistics* (New York: W. W. Norton, 1954), chap. 8, pp. 98–99.

6. Joan S. Wixen, "Twentieth-Century Miraclemaker," *Modern Maturity*, December 1984–January 1985, p. 92.

7. Ibid.

8. House Committee on Interstate and Foreign Commerce, *Hearings on H.R. 10541*, 87th Cong. 2nd sess., May 1962, p. 94.

9. "The Disturbing Question of the Salk Vaccine," *Prevention*, September 1959, p. 52.

10. *Hearings on H.R. 10541*, pp. 94, 96, 112.

11. Christopher Kent, "Drugs, Bugs, and Shots in the Dark," *Health Freedom News*, January 1983, p. 26.

12. Ibid.

13. Alec Burton, "The Fallacy of the Germ Theory of Disease" (presentation given at the convention of the National Hygiene Society, Milwaukee, WI, 1978). This isn't as far-fetched as it might appear. In 1960, New Orleans had an outbreak of a disease much like mild, noncrippling polio—muscle pains, headache, slurred speech, weakness, fatigue—which often persists for years. They named it Iceland disease because it was first discovered by two Reykjavik doctors. See J. D. Ratcliff, "Sleep: How Much Do You Need," *Readers Digest* (August 1965), p. 90. Could Iceland disease be another case of atypical polio caused by the vaccine? (See discussion of vaccine-caused atypical diseases later in this chapter.)

14. Robert Mendelsohn, interview with Alice Karas, *Herbalist New Health*, July 1981, p. 61.

15. *Hearings on H.R. 10541*, p. 113.

16. Ibid., p. 89.

17. Richard Moskowitz, *The Case Against Immunizations* (reprinted from the *Journal of the American Institute of Homeopathy* 76 [March 1983]: 21).

18. Airola, *Everywoman's Book*, p. 279.

19. Robert Mendelsohn, "The Medical Time Bomb of Immunization Against Disease," *East West Journal*, November 1984, p. 49.

20. Marian Tompson, "Another View," *The Risks of Immunizations and How to*

Avoid Them (Evanston, IL: The People's Doctor Newsletter by Robert S. Mendelsohn, 1988), p. 8.

21. Harris L. Coulter and Barbara Loe Fisher, *DPT: A Shot in Dark* (New York: Harcourt Brace Jovanovich, 1985), pp. 164–168.

22. Airola, *Everywoman's Book*, p. 272.

23. Robert S. Mendelsohn, *The Risks of Immunizations and How to Avoid Them* (Evanston, IL: The People's Doctor Newsletter, 1988), p. 10.

24. Ibid.

25. Airola, *Everywoman's Book*, p. 276.

26. William Howard Hay, M.D., address before the Medical Freedom Society, Pocono, PA, June 25, 1937, and read into the minutes of the U.S. House of Representatives by the Honorable Usher L. Burdick of North Dakota.

27. Robert Mendelsohn, *Confessions of a Medical Heretic* (Chicago: Contemporary Books, 1979), p. 143.

28. Airola, *Everywoman's Book*, p. 277.

29. Mendelsohn, *The Risks of Immunizations and How to Avoid Them*, p. 12.

30. Burton, "The Fallacy of the Germ Theory." For a more detailed, technical discussion of this study, see Leon Chaitow, *Vaccination and Immunization: Dangers, Delusions and Alternatives* (Essex, England: C. W. Daniel, 1987), pp. 41–43.

31. Archie Kalokerinos and Glen Dettman, "A Supportive Submission," *The Dangers of Immunisation* (Australian edition of Harold Buttram et al., *The Dangers of Immunisation* [Quakertown, PA: The Humanitarian Society, 1979]). Australian edition published by the Biological Research Institute, Warburton, Victoria, Australia, pp. 79–80.

32. Ibid., p. 75.

33. M. Beddow Bayly, *The Case Against Vaccination* (London: Wm. H. Taylor & Sons, June 1936), p. 4.

34. Ibid., p. 5.

35. Lily Loat (address given before the English Annual Session of the American Medical Liberty League); reprinted in "Philosophy of Health," *Truth Teller*, January 1927.

36. Eleanora McBean, *The Poisoned Needle* (Mokelumne Hill, CA: Health Research, 1956), p. 64.

37. Lily Loat, *The Truth About Vaccination and Immunization* (London: Health for All, 1951), p. 28.

38. Buttram et al., *The Dangers of Immunization*, p. 42.

39. Ibid., p. 41.

40. Ibid., pp. 41–42.

41. Hay, *Congressional Record*.

42. Moskowitz, *Case Against Immunizations*, p. 13.

43. Richard Moskowitz, "Unvaccinated Children," *Mothering*, Winter 1987.

44. Moskowitz, *Case Against Immunizations*, p. 9.

45. Ibid., p. 10.

46. Ibid., pp. 9, 10, 18, 19.

47. Ibid., p. 19.

48. Tompson, "Another View."

49. Mendelsohn, *The Risks of Immunizations and How to Avoid Them*, p. 3.

50. Hay, *Congressional Record*. The actual percentage of persons (prior to 1937)

affected by the epidemics for which we now have vaccinations are (1) not more than 10 percent of the general population and (2) not more than 15 percent of the childhood population in the case of diphtheria.

51. Patrick, "The Great American Deception," p. 3.

52. Alice Karas, interview with Robert Mendelsohn, "More Confessions," *Herbalist New Health*, July 1981, p. 60.

53. Hay, *Congressional Record*.

54. Reported by Bernard Jensen, *You Can Master Disease* (Solana Beach, CA: Bernard Jensen Publishing Division, 1952), p. 92.

55. Ibid.

56. *Organic Consumer Report*, October 3, 1978.

57. Mendelsohn, *The Risks of Immunizations and How to Avoid Them*, p. 27.

58. Viera Scheibner, *Vaccination: The Medical Assault on the Immune System* (Maryborough, Victoria, Australia: Australian Print Group, 1993), pp. 130–131.

59. Mendelsohn, *The Risks of Immunizations and How to Avoid Them*, p. 87.

60. Reported in the *National Health Federation Bulletin*, January 1960.

61. Kalokerinos and Dettman, " 'Mumps,' " p. 17.

62. Jensen, *You Can Master Disease*, p. 92.

63. "New 'China Syndrome' Puzzle," *Science*, July 5, 1991.

64. Mendelsohn, *The Risks of Immunizations and How to Avoid Them*, p. 95; Chaitow, *Vaccination*, p. 114.

65. Julia Helgason, "The Government Is . . . in Some Cases, Lying to Us," *Dayton Daily News*, September 12, 1993. Taken from research by Kristine M. Severyn, "Parents Should Have Freedom of Choice in Child Vaccinations," Your Opinion, *Xenia, Ohio Daily Gazette*, February 18, 1993.

66. Quoted by Theodore Roszak, *The Cult of Information* (New York: Pantheon Books, 1986), p. 95.

67. Lynne McTaggart, "The MMR Vaccine," *Mothering*, Spring 1992, p. 58.

68. Richard Moskowitz, "Vaccination: A Sacrament of Modern Medicine," *Mothering*, Spring 1992, p. 52.

69. McTaggart, "The MMR Vaccine," p. 58.

70. Ibid.

71. Severyn, "Parents."

72. *Journal of Pediatrics* 115 (1989): 686–693; reported in ibid.

73. *Vaccine Bulletin*, February 1987, p. 11; reported by Neil Z. Miller, *Vaccines: Are They Safe and Effective?* (Santa Fe, NM: New Atlantean Press, 1992), p. 33.

74. Barbara Mullarkey, "Government Support of Vaccinations Continues to Prick Parents," *Wednesday Journal*, June 9, 1993. information from Kristine Severyn, "Parents 'Shut Out' of Congressional Vaccine Hearings"

75. Tompson, "Another View," p. 31.

76. See earlier part of this chapter. Also, Cynthia Cournoyer points to several other studies showing that antibody count was not indicative of protection from the disease and, in fact, may indicate just the opposite. When the "first line of defense" (mucous membranes of the nose, mouth, and digestive tract) are fully functioning, antigens (viruses, bacteria, foreign substances) never gain access to the bloodstream, thereby never stimulating the production of antibodies. The production of antibodies, she points out,

indicates failure of the immune system. See Cynthia Cournoyer, *What About Immunizations? Exposing the Vaccine Philosophy* (Santa Cruz, CA: Nelson's Books, 1991), pp. 18–19.

77. Weller Embler, "Language and Truth," in *Our Language and Our World*, Selections from ETC.: A Review of General Semantics, 1953–58, ed. S. I. Hayakawa (New York: Harper & Brothers, 1959), pp. 378–379, 380.

4   Creating Natural Immunity

Follow principle and the knot unties itself.

—Thomas Jefferson

FIRST PRINCIPLES

If we can't prevent disease by injecting toxins into our bodies, how can we prevent it? First of all, we must begin by thinking health, rather than disease; of building or creating something desirable, rather than avoiding or destroying something undesirable. Freedom from illness is a by-product of thinking and building health, not of fighting disease. Essentially, we build health by positive thinking and balanced living. This latter includes biochemical balance that is supported by eating fresh, whole, natural foods, that is, foods that have not been refined, chemicalized, and overcooked. Both herbs and megadoses of vitamin C have been used successfully either to prevent infectious diseases or to shorten their duration and lessen their discomfort.[1]

Currently, the focus is on megadoses of vitamin C to "protect people from bacterial assaults." Other researchers prefer to think of vitamin C as helping to correct body chemistry. It is this latter interpretation that we will follow, partly because it is more constructive to think of disease as something we build from within rather than something that attacks us from without. Also, research that we will later explore supports this more endogenous—and, I think, more holistic—point of view.

THREE BOOKS

In 1939, 1949, and 1951, three books were published that not only support this more endogenous theory of disease but also made a major contribution to our understanding of how both infectious and degenerative disease are indeed built from within by our habits of living and thinking. Few people have heard of these books because they are "dangerous." Dangerous because if the ideas they contain were widely disseminated, they would topple much of the present medical-pharmaceutical establishment. The first and most dangerous book, *The Chemistry of Natural Immunity*, was written by a man who was not only a doctor of medicine but a doctor of biochemistry as well. The author, Dr. William Frederick Koch, discusses his research and presents case histories from his own medical practice. He discovered that homeopathic doses of oxidation catalysts injected at cyclical intervals along with a regimen of "fresh pure air, pure water, plenty of rest, and reasonable exercise" and a diet of whole, natural foods— "vegetable, fruit and whole grain cereal diet, avoiding coffee, tea, chocolate, alcohol, spices, tobacco"—and "the use of bowel lavage with salt water when necessary" would support the oxidation mechanism of the body and facilitate natural immunity to disease. (We can think of the oxidation process as cell respiration. When this process is blocked, disease results.)

The case histories in the book are impressive: Cancer, poliomyelitis, psoriasis, epilepsy, arthritis, allergies, toxic goiter, and the like, respond to this therapy, most with complete recoveries.[2]

The Koch treatment, as it is called, is of particular significance to me because of a personal experience I had with it. About 30 years ago (in California where I was living), I had a severe attack of asthma as a result of an unusually stressful experience.[3] I went to a medical doctor who specialized in using nutritional and other "natural" therapies, and he gave me an injection of what he said was an early form of the Koch oxidation catalysts (developed by Dr. Koch in the early years of his practice). Within a few hours after receiving the injection, I experienced a distinct feeling of euphoria and well-being. I found myself breathing deeply and having several loose bowel movements a day as though my body were discharging toxins. My asthma disappeared and has never returned. The immediacy and apparent permanence of my response were no doubt due, at least in part, to the fact that I was already living on a program very much like the one Dr. Koch recommended. Because the Koch treatment is illegal in this country, the doctor who treated me had to send to Switzerland for the Koch catalyst. The Koch catalysts are not toxic or dangerous physiologically, only dangerous politically and economically.

Our second book, *Diet Prevents Polio* by Dr. Benjamin Sandler, tells how a polio epidemic in Asheville, North Carolina, was averted when he got on the radio and warned parents not to feed their children sugar and foods containing sugar—that is, soft drinks, ice cream, candy, and the like—and to reduce consumption of fruits and fruit juices. Dr. Sandler recommended a high-protein diet with low-starch vegetables as being the best protection against low blood sugar, a condition he found made people susceptible to polio. Polio epidemics occur during the summer, he said, because this is the time people consume high-sugar foods as well as fruits and fruit juices. (Later researchers have vindicated fresh fruit and fruit juices provided they are unsweetened with refined sugar. They say, in effect, that because the sugar in these natural foods is in a different form and is accompanied by other food factors, it is metabolized in a different way than are refined sugars.) The typical polio "profile," Dr. Sandler found, is vigorous physical exertion, for example, running, hiking, swimming, coupled with high consumption of refined carbohydrates—refined flour and sugar products, particularly sugar. (Refined sugar is eight times as concentrated as flour.)[4]

That the Sandler diet does prevent polio is illustrated not only by research with rabbits and monkeys that Dr. Sandler studied and experimented with himself but by case studies of human beings and the subsequent and remarkable reduction of polio in North Carolina after his diet was publicized on the radio and in the newspapers. The incidence of polio in North Carolina dropped from 2,402 cases in 1948 to 214 cases in 1949 when the country as a whole—39 states—showed an increase in the number of cases from 1948 to 1949![5]

Another researcher, Dr. J. W. McCormick of Toronto, Canada, has pointed out that the first case of poliomyelitis was reported in Vienna one year after roller-mill white flour was first sold in that city (Vienna was the first city to install such a mill). Dr. McCormick calls polio the form of beriberi that follows the use of degerminated flour.[6]

Other researchers have linked polio to DDT (dichlorodipheny/trichloroethane) poisoning, pointing out, for instance, that American servicemen in the Philippines and elsewhere in the Far East who used "vast quantities of DDT as insecticides, had a high incidence of polio, whereas it was extremely low in the surrounding native population." Other researchers have indicted other poisons that affect the nervous system.[7] Still others have indicted the high intake of white sugar and sugar products—again, ice cream, candy bars, soft drinks—as being a primary cause of polio among U.S. servicemen stationed overseas, particularly when the native population with whom the soldiers mingled freely were free of the disease.[8]

Our third book, *Bacteria, Inc.*, tells the story of the discovery of the cause, prevention, and cure of smallpox. Author Cash Asher describes the research of distinguished medical doctor Charles A. R. Campbell who, around the turn of the century, had been recommended for the Nobel Prize. Dr. Campbell made notable contributions in researching typhoid and malaria as well as smallpox, and like malaria, he discovered that smallpox was carried by a blood-sucking insect, that the disease was neither infectious nor contagious, and that vaccinations do not prevent it. Although Drs. Campbell, J. A. Watts, and others disclosed their findings at the turn of the century, their reports were ignored.

Through a series of carefully controlled experiments, Dr. Campbell discovered that smallpox was caused by the bite of *Cimex lectularius*, the Latin name for bedbug. (Around the turn of the century, bedbugs were a common household pest. Straw-filled mattresses and straw-padded rag carpets, the natural breeding place of the bedbug, were standard household furnishings.) Dr. Campbell also discovered that the degree of severity of the disease was directly proportional to the cachexia (general ill health and malnutrition) of the patient. He spoke of "scorbutic cachexia," relating it to scurvy, "the disease caused by lack of green food," and said that "the removal of this perversion of nutrition will so mitigate the virulence of this malady as positively to prevent the pitting or pocking of smallpox."[9] In other words, eating lots of fresh greens will prevent the scarring of smallpox. My guess is that eating a balanced diet of whole, fresh foods, which would naturally include fresh greens, not only would prevent the scarification of smallpox but would lessen the discomfort and duration of this disease as it does in other diseases.

If this sounds a bit simplistic, given the enormous mystique surrounding smallpox and its prominent place in history, one need only to turn back the pages of time to eighteenth-century England to discover that the consumption of fresh fruits and vegetables was a rarity, particularly among the poorer classes who ate mostly cereal foods. An English country gentleman's dinner in 1768 would include: "A roasted Shoulder of Mutton and a plum Pudding—Veal Cutlets, Frill'd Potatoes, cold Tongue, Ham and cold roast Beef, and eggs in their shells. Punch, Wine, Beer and Cyder for drinking."[10]

Smallpox, typhus (carried by body lice), plague (carried by lice on rats), typhoid, and cholera (caused by contaminated water) have been called "filth" diseases. When we read about the great epidemics of smallpox, plague, and the like, that swept through Europe and England hundreds of years ago, killing up to three fourths of the population, as did the black plague in the fourteenth century, it is hard for us to imagine the living conditions that spawned them:

No sewers, no water closets, but instead, festering privies; excessive over-crowding, both of houses per acre and people per house; small, ill-ventilated and ill-built houses crammed into narrow courts and tortuous alleys, without adequate water supply and devoid of sanitary conveniences; lack of cleanliness owing to scarcity of water; absence of baths and laundry facilities; unpaved and ill-paved streets, which were made the receptacle for all kinds of slops and other filth. . . .

. . . in addition to constantly breathing in the horrible effluvia from the stinking heaps of rotting refuse and filth from vaults containing sewage heaps and from their own unwashed clothes and bedclothes, the poor suffered badly in periods of scarcity and want.

. . . in the seventeenth and eighteenth centuries bad harvests were almost always followed by a large increase in the number of deaths from smallpox and fevers.[11]

"History shows that famine and pestilence commonly ride together," Rene Dubos tells us. "Susceptibility to infection . . . appears to be linked in a reversible manner to the metabolic state."[12] Again, the importance of diet in building health and reducing susceptibility to disease.

Changing patterns of living produce changing patterns of disease: As straw-filled mattresses and straw-padded rag carpets were discarded along with fly-infested privies, mosquito-infested rain barrels, and food cooled in cellars rather than in refrigerators, smallpox, along with other "dirt" diseases, disappeared. Likewise, tetanus, which can be caused by a spore found in horse manure and fecal matter in general, has practically disappeared with the advent of the "horseless carriage" and the flush toilet. And now in our sanitized world we have degenerative diseases—heart trouble, cancer, arthritis, multiple sclerosis, polio, hyperkinesis, and others—due at least in part to our consumption of refined carbohydrates, devitalized and chemicalized food, exposure to agricultural and industrial poisons, and yes, vaccinations.

COVER-UP

What happened to the information contained in the three books we discussed? Why isn't this information general knowledge? In the words of Cash Asher: "Why, then, does the vaccination fetish persist? We must find the answer in economics—in the billion dollar serum industry and its correlative industry, medical practice."[13] In the television documentary *Pesticides and Pills*, which aired on Public Television in the latter part of 1981, Dr. Milton Silverman, University of California pharmacologist, said in reference to the pharmaceutical industry that it "is now grossing sales in the tens of billions of dollars a year." In two broadcasts—August 15, 1993, and May 8, 1994—Gary Null stated that the pharmaceutical industry is a $100 billion a year industry (WNIS-AM). Need I say that any business that controls such large sums of money becomes an irresistible political and economic force that puts its stamp on legislation and subsequently education. When the bedbug was exposed as the carrier of smallpox, the manufacturing of serums had grown into a profitable industry. Many states and cities had enacted laws and regulations making vaccination compulsory, and the vaccination of every child before entering school had become an established practice. Doctors were finding vaccinations a lucrative part of their practice. Is it any wonder that Dr. Campbell's attempts to communicate his discoveries were ignored?

In the case of polio and Dr. Sandler, I heard in a public lecture many years ago that hundreds of thousands of dollars worth of soft drinks, ice cream, and candy went unsold, precipitating heavy losses for the businesses involved. Referring to Asheville, North Carolina, Dr. Sandler said, "Store sales of sugar, candy, ice cream, cakes, soft drinks, and the like dropped sharply and remained at low level for the rest of the summer. One southern producer of ice cream shipped one million fewer gallons of ice cream than usual, during the first week following the release of the diet story."[14] Like Dr. Campbell, Dr. Sandler's work was ignored by public health officials and the medical community in general. I suspect pressure from big business—which includes the medical-pharmaceutical "big business"—kept the story under wraps.

The discoveries of Dr. Koch met with much more drastic action. His therapy was too revolutionary and too threatening to the medical-pharmaceutical business to be merely ignored or hushed up. He was actively persecuted and prosecuted, much as doctors are today who use laetrile or other metabolic therapies. Many years ago, I read about arrests, trials, defamation, heartache, and eventual "escape" to Brazil, where Dr. Koch spent his later years helping the Brazilian government eliminate diseases of cattle and other livestock.

THE BEST "VACCINE"

A question frequently asked is, If natural immunity is so effective, how is it that native peoples such as the North, South, and Central American Indians as well as the Polynesians frequently experienced such devastating epidemics when they first came into contact with white men? These people obviously ate "natural food," and yet when white man brought his Western civilization to them, they died in large numbers—at least according to some accounts. The key here is "brought his Western civilization to them." This civilization included not only canned, preserved, and refined foods that native people frequently accepted as gifts from the newcomers but a great deal of negativity as well, as stories of exploitation and cruelty attest. Also, their native diets, even before the advent of white man, were not always balanced, being subject to the vagaries of the weather and tribal customs. However, it does appear that as long as they lived on their native foods, they were relatively free from disease. Only when they adopted white man's foods did disease ravage their numbers.

In his book *Nutrition and Physical Degeneration*, Dr. Weston A. Price documents the results of his trip around the world to many remote areas where native peoples lived relatively untouched by modern civilization. In every case, he found that people who lived on their native diets not only were free from disease but were free from the skeletal deformities that characterized native people who had adopted white man's foods.[15]

Frequently we hear that native people succumbed to white man's diseases because they had no natural immunity, the implication being that either artificial immunization or longer and more gradual exposure would have given them that immunity. It seems, rather, that their departure from their traditional food patterns destroyed their immunity and that had they remained on a diet of their traditional foods, they would have retained their immunity.

"Even the World Health Organization has conceded that the best vaccine against common infectious diseases is an adequate diet. Despite this, they made it perfectly clear to us that they still intended to promote mass immunization campaigns," Drs. Archie Kalokerinos and Glen Dettman tell us. "Do we take this as an admission that we cannot or do not wish to provide an adequate diet? More likely it would seem, there is no profit in the constituents of an adequate diet for the pharmaceutical companies."[16]

CHILDREN "IN JEOPARDY"?

In jeopardy is a term frequently used by pediatricians to refer to an unvaccinated child. Suppose your child does contract a "dread" disease like whooping cough, diphtheria, or polio. What can you do about it that is simple, harmless, and effective? As I pointed out earlier, megadoses of vitamin C have been known both to shorten the duration of many infectious diseases as well as to lessen their discomfort. Used along with herbs, particularly alfalfa, and a non-mucous-forming diet (consisting primarily of fresh fruits and vegetables, whole grains and legumes, some fish and fowl, and no dairy or flour products), the vitamin C is rendered more effective. Let's look at a few cases where vitamin C alone was used.

According to a 1950 *Journal of the American Medical Association* article, 90 children with whooping cough were treated daily with 500 milligrams of vitamin C, intravenously and orally, for one week. After that the dose was reduced by 100 milligrams every 2 days until it was 100 milligrams a day, this last dose being continued until each child was completely recovered. Children receiving vitamin C intravenously were usually well in 15 days; those receiving vitamin C orally were well in 20 days. The disease lasted 34 days in children treated with vaccine. In three quarters of the cases when vitamin C therapy was started in the catarrhal stage, the spasmodic stage was wholly prevented.[17]

Adelle Davis used much higher potencies and administered them orally. She describes how her own children weathered most of the childhood diseases with only one day of sickness—no nausea, no vomiting, no irritability, and no missed meals. For her 5-year-old son's "one-day mumps," she began at 7 A.M. to give him 1,000 milligrams of vitamin C every hour during the day. By evening, all swelling was gone, and there was no further sign of illness. To administer this high a potency orally to a small child, it is necessary to dissolve fifty 500-milligram tablets of vitamin C in a cup of boiling water and mix it with one-fourth cup of fruit juice such as pineapple, apricot, or orange. Each teaspoonful of the solution would then contain 500 milligrams of vitamin C. Later, Adelle Davis would discover that lesser amounts of vitamin C are needed when calcium and pantothenic acid (vitamin B_5) are included in the dosage. (I, personally, have found using the entire C complex—bioflavinoids and hesperidin—more effective than just the ascorbic acid fraction.)[18]

"It is almost unbelievable how mild these childhood diseases can be when no malnutrition exists," Dr. Marshall Mandell points out, adding that both his children had all of them for approximately a half a day. When unmistakable symptoms were discovered (usually in the morning), Dr. Mandell gave them "fortified milk" (Brewer's yeast, skim milk powder, fresh or frozen fruit, and whole milk liquified in a blender) with 10,000 units of vitamin A, 250 units of vitamim E, 1 gram of vitamin C, and 50 to 100 milligrams of pantothenic acid (vitamin B₅) every hour. "By noon all signs of fever were gone, and the children were impossible to keep in bed. No meals were missed; no real sickness occurred," he tells us.[19]

If the illness seems more serious, larger doses of vitamin C can be taken. Adelle Davis describes again how her sleeping 3-year-old daughter had the classic symptoms of illness—elevated temperature, flushed and burning skin, labored breathing. She gave her 2,000 milligrams of the dissolved vitamin C in juice, and in 15 minutes, her temperature was normal. She slept soundly the rest of the night and awoke the next day "full of her usual vivacity."[20] In this case, the remarkable degree of effectiveness of this treatment is due—in large part, I think—to the fact that Adelle Davis fed her children an exceptionally healthy diet.

Amounts of vitamin C needed vary greatly according to the usual diet and tissue saturation with the vitamin as well as with the severity of the disease. Dr. Fred Klenner, for instance, describes an 18-month-old girl whose body was blue, stiff, and cold to the touch; he could neither hear her heart nor feel her pulse. The mother was convinced the child was already dead. "Dr. Klenner injected 6,000 mg of vitamin C into her blood; four hours later the child was cheerful and alert, holding a bottle with her right hand, though her left side was paralyzed. A second injection was given; soon the child was laughing and holding her bottle with both hands, all signs of paralysis gone."[21]

But even without these megadoses of vitamin C, the child who is well nourished can handle these "dread" diseases without much discomfort. My own children, who were never vaccinated, came down with whooping cough, the younger child being only 2 weeks old. Because I was nursing her, our doctor—a naturopath, chiropractor, and iridologist—said just to keep nursing her and she would be all right. I've forgotten the advice he gave for my older daughter, but I will say the disease was certainly not horrendous in the least. Annoying, inconvenient, and at times, uncomfortable—but certainly not "dread." Had I known about giving children megadoses of vitamin C, the duration of the disease could have been shortened and the discomfort of the spasmodic stage eliminated. As it was, the disease lasted six weeks, including two weeks of the spasmodic stage. Yet I heard on a TV program a couple of years ago that in England whooping cough could last three and sometimes four months! I'm sure a child fed a balanced diet of "natural" foods would not experience the disease that severely. I, along with Dr. Mendelsohn, would rather have the disease than the vaccination.

When we talk about natural foods for a small child, and particularly an infant, we are talking about breast milk, not formula milk. We are also talking about fresh fruits and vegetables (can be pureed in a blender), not canned, and whole (preferably germinated) grains, not packaged cereals.

A caveat: Because we are into the second generation of a vaccine-damaged population, mother's milk may not contain the specific antibodies to the diseases the infant is likely to contact. When natural immunity is not allowed to develop (because of vaccinations), the mother cannot pass on these protective factors to her baby. Evidence: In 1993, more than 25 percent of all measles cases were occurring in babies under a year old. "CDC officials admit this situation is likely to get worse and attribute it to the growing numbers of mothers who were vaccinated during the 1960's, '70's, and '80's."[22]

But before leaving the subject of vitamin C, let's look again at the work of Dr. Klenner, who has used massive doses of vitamin C in successfully treating patients of all ages suffering from such serious illnesses as encephalitis, meningitis, poliomyelitis, virus pneumonia, tetanus (lockjaw), and many other infections. "To extremely ill patients he would give the vitamin by injection in amounts ranging from 2 to 4 grams (2,000 to 4,000 milligrams) approximately every two to four hours around the clock, the amount and number of injections depending on the progress of each individual."[23]

This brings us to the subject of tetanus, one of the diseases most feared by parents. Because tetanus is not considered contagious, as are the other diseases discussed earlier, it was mentioned only briefly in Chapter 2.

Tetanus

Tetanus is a disorder of the nervous system caused by anaerobic (lives without air) bacteria that infect improperly cleaned wounds. The bacteria (spores, in this case) become trapped beneath the skin, where they feed on dead tissue. "Any wound containing foreign material or devitalized tissue must be considered tetanus prone, as well as crushing injuries, deep second and third degree burns, and any infected wound. . . . Many tetanus prone wounds, however, can be converted to non-prone wounds by proper cleansing and debridgement."[24] (*Debridgement* means the removal of foreign matter and excison of surrounding tissue.)

And, as we just learned, megadoses of vitamin C have been successful in treating tetanus, should it occur. (Clinton Miller, former legislative advocate with the National Health Federation, gave me the figure of 30 grams—that's 30,000 milligrams—a day.)[25]

But what are your chances of contracting tetanus? And is the vaccine effective? The answer is similar to what we discovered about the other vaccines. For instance, tetanus was steadily disappearing from developing countries long before the vaccine was introduced. Increased attention to wound hygiene was the critical factor, according to some researchers.[26] Reports of tetanus cases continue to include numbers of fully vaccinated people.[27]

Tetanus is actually a rare disease. Most of the people who get it are not children but adults over 50 years old.[28] As the comparison below shows, your child's chances of dying in an automobile accident or of tuberculosis are many times that of dying of tetanus.

U.S. Cases and Incidents, 1990[29]

	Cases	*Deaths*
Tuberculosis	25,700	18,000 (January–November)
Automobile accidents		47,900
Tetanus	64	
In 1988	53	About 10[30]

Polio

Because this is a disease that still frightens many parents, let's look at some other ways of both preventing and treating it. Most involve changing the body chemistry through diet and certain supplements. One, namely, chiropractic, involves releasing pressure on the nerves leading to the affected organs by way of chiropractic adjustments. A chiropractic organization, the Polio Foundation of California (founded in 1950), recommended a diet very similar to the Sandler diet as a preventive of polio except that along with a high-protein diet it also emphasizes fresh fruits, vegetables, and whole grains. Natural sweeteners such as honey and 100 percent maple syrup are permitted.

During the 1940s and 1950s, a number of chiropractors researched polio and discovered that if chiropractic treatment was begun during the acute phase, that is, at the onset of fever and paralysis, it could be cured in a matter of days. For instance, Dr. Edward R. Dunn, director of his own Polio Clinic in Oklahoma City, treated polio successfully for over 30 years. From hundreds of case histories, he eventually claimed a Five Day Cure for Polio. Even bulbar cases yield as readily if treatment was begun the first few hours and not later than 72 hours after the first symptoms. Even after longer periods of delay, most cases fully recovered.[31]

Food supplements have been used successfully to treat polio. For instance, Canadian physician W. J. McCormick has for many years cured polio with vitamin B therapy. Investigating the dietary history of his patients, he found that without exception the B complex was practically nonexistent in their diets. They all ate white bread, muscle meats, and potatoes to the exclusion of other vegetables.[32]

Iodine has been used successfully to both prevent and treat various paralytic diseases including polio. Dr. J. F. Edward, writing in the *Manitoba Medical Review* for June–July 1954, told of his success in treating and preventing polio with potassium iodide. He also listed 25 different references that reported the work of other doctors and veterinarians who had successfully treated and prevented various paralytic diseases, including herpes zoster and encephalitis, with potassium iodide.[33] Later, *Prevention* magazine distributed a flier describing an article Dr. Edward wrote in the *Canadian Medical Journal* (September 1, 1955) in which he not only showed that iodide could be used for treating polio but suggested that lack of iodine in the diet might be a contributing cause of this disease. *Prevention*'s editors speculate that one reason why polio might be more prevalent in hot weather is that iodine is lost in the perspiration along with other minerals.[34]

Another doctor, DeForest Clinton Jarvis, found that polio is accompanied by a disturbance in the calcium-potassium and calcium-phosphorous ratio of the blood. He successfully treated polio in both humans and animals by using, for the most part, simple, natural treatments designed to raise the blood calcium and lower the blood phosphorous. Some of these are (1) drinking a glass of water with each meal to which has been added two teaspoonfuls of honey and two teaspoonfuls of apple cider vinegar; (2) applying hot, moist applications to the affected parts; (3) drinking certain herb teas; (4) using a sedative diet—one that eliminates all wheat products, citrus fruits, and muscle meats such as beef, lamb, and pork; (5) giving injections of insulin as needed; and for adults, (6) using 10 drops of a saturated solution of potassium iodine in a glass of water after each meal. Using only kelp, a natural source of iodine, Dr. Jarvis cured a paralyzed chinchilla.[35]

Magnesium has also been used successfully to arrest polio. Dr. A. Neveu of France reported complete reversal of this disease within two days to one week, even after early arm and leg paralysis. Dr. Neveu uses magnesium chloride and claims rapid results are realized when correctly used. His formula: 20 grams (.7 ounce) of desiccated magnesium chloride added to one liter (about one quart) of water. The dose varies from 80 cc (cubic centimeters) every three hours to 125 cc every six hours. Magnesium should be used under the care of a qualified physician, Dr. Neveu advises.[36]

With all this talk about paralytic polio, we need to be reminded that actual paralysis is very rare. Ninety percent of the people who are exposed to the natural polio virus show no symptoms at all.[37]

Like Dr. Edward, famous medical clairvoyant Edgar Cayce recommended iodine as a polio preventive. He recommended using Atomidine, a solution carrying iodine in atomic form, and he gave instructions for using it both internally and externally as a wash and as a throat and nasal spray.

Also, like a number of doctors mentioned earlier, Edgar Cayce thought more in terms of preventing disease by changing body chemistry rather than by "fighting germs." He said that if the body were maintained in an alkaline condition, this would "immunize" a person against infectious diseases. When a young woman asked him, "Can immunizations against them [infectious diseases] be set up in any other manner than by inoculations?" he replied, "As indicated, if an alkalinity is maintained in the system—especially with lettuce, carrots and celery, these in the blood supply will maintain such a condition as to immunize a person." He specified that alkaline vegetables—lettuce, carrots, and celery— must be eaten every day.[38] Keeping the body alkaline, by using predominantly alkaline-forming foods[39] in the diet as a means of preventing disease, has long been taught by doctors such as Bernard Jensen who use natural therapies. And where does vitamin C fit into this picture? Vitamin C creates an alkaline ash within the body.

Vitamiln C is not necessarily the sine qua non of natural or drugless healing.

Other natural substances such as herbs have been used successfully in treating—and preventing—"infectious" diseases.[40] Just plain alfalfa—tablets or capsules—have been used successfully to prevent whooping cough as well as to build stronger bodies in children.[41] And of course, garlic is an old folk remedy for preventing infectious diseases.

Certain food supplements have also been helpful in preventing serious injury from inflammatory diseases: Extra vitamin A given to children with measles reduces the likelihood of complications as well as their chances of dying.[42] Adequate amounts of B_6 and zinc prevent recurrent middle ear infections,[43] and high doses of B vitamins can apparently prevent the paralysis of polio.[44] Even undulant fever, which is supposed to be caused by unpasteurized milk, is symptomatic of a trace mineral deficiency and can be cleared up if above-adequate amounts of manganese and magnesium are given.[45]

Once we begin thinking about disease in simpler, more self-empowering ways and looking in other (nondrug, nonvaccine) directions for answers, we will begin to develop immunity to "diseasescare," the fear that fuels public acceptance of mass vaccination programs.

SOCIETY "IN JEOPARDY"?

Are unvaccinated persons a danger to others? At this point, the question is rhetorical, and I ask it only because parents who choose not to have their children vaccinated will likely be confronted by people who think their decision a selfish one and their children a public health threat. This happened to my daughter, Tanya, when she refused to have her son vaccinated. One of the arguments of the prosecuting attorney was that "society has rights."

To a person whose understanding of the nature of bacteria and their relation to disease consists of a world inhabited by unseen "enemies" who "attack" "unprotected" persons, this fear of contamination by the "unprotected" is quite real. However, if they themselves are "protected," what have they to fear? As Clarence Darrow said, "If vaccination does what its advocates claim for it, the person who is vaccinated ought to be safe no matter whether anybody else is vaccinated or not." "There is no rationale for forcing immunization," says Dr. J. Anthony Morris, former chief vaccine control officer of the FDA, who was fired for blowing the whistle on the swine flu vaccine program.[46]

Do the "protected" ever stop to think that there are probably hundreds of thousands of unvaccinated "threats" living among them? Besides an increasing number of families like ours who simply don't buy into the paradigm, there are those who object on religious grounds, for example, Christian Scientists, Church of Life Science in Texas, Lord's Covenant Church in Arizona, and others. No one seems to think that people who refuse vaccination for religious reasons pose a threat to the community. In fact, Dr. Mendelsohn says that the life expectancy records of the Christian Scientists are one of the best in the country.[47]

We are living in an age of alternatives, of energies and images that liberate us from cultural monoliths. We speak of alternative schooling, alternative lifestyles, alternative health care. We speak of becoming "conscious." To become conscious we must become aware of our viewing lenses and the assumptions that have shaped and colored them. We can't really become aware of our assumptions until we expose ourselves to realities based on different assumptions.

Let's begin our journey into greater consciousness by going "through the looking glass" and exploring a world that is almost a mirror image of our present world, a world in which the understanding of our relationship to disease, health, and microorganisms is the reverse of our present one, a world in which the villain becomes the hero, the mischief maker the teacher, and the sickness the process by which the body—and society—heals itself.

But first we must turn back the pages of time and find a chapter in the history of biology that was lost.

NOTES

1. Walene James, "Immunization Law Based on Myth," *Health Freedom News*, October 1983.

2. William Frederick Koch, *The Chemistry of Natural Immunity* (Boston: Christopher Publishing House, 1939), p. 105.

3. As a child, I had hayfever for which I was treated by the usual "shots." This eventually resulted in asthma, which became incapacitating and which I corrected by changing my diet to one of "natural" foods—whole grains, raw milk, fresh fruits and vegetables, fertile eggs, and occasionally fresh fish, fowl, and organ meats. Because this treatment was not "holistic"—meaning the mind and emotions were not addressed—a sufficiently stressful experience could trigger an "episode" of asthma.

4. Gary Null Show, WNIS, August 8, 1993. Aside from statistical artifact (discussed in Chapter 3), could the increased use of alternative sweeteners, both natural and synthetic (this last has its own health risks) and the increased sedentariness of our TV generation have something to do with the *apparent* decline in polio?

5. Benjamin P. Sandler, *Diet Prevents Polio* (Milwaukee: Lee Foundation for Nutritional Research, 1951), p. 43.

6. Royal Lee, "Food Integrity—the Foundation of Health" (address to the Organic Health Foundation of America, January 20, 1955).

7. Morton S. Biskind, "Public Health Aspects of the New Insecticides," *American Journal of Digestive Diseases*, November 1953, p. 334.

8. Sandler, *Diet Prevents Polio*, 68–73. Other articles that support the above line of reasoning are: W. J. McCormick, "Poliomyelitis, Infectious or Metabolic?" *Archives of Pediatrics* 67 (February 1950): 56–73; R. H. Scobey, "The Poison Cause of Poliomyelitis and Obstructions to Its Investigation," *Archives of Pediatrics* 69 (April 1952): 172–193; idem, "Is the Public Health Law Responsible for the Poliomyelitis Mystery?" *Archives of Pediatrics* 68 (May 1951): 220–232.

9. Cash Asher, *Bacteria, Inc.* (Boston: Bruce Humphries, 1949), pp. 36–37.

10. Henry E. Sigerist, *Civilization and Disease* (Ithaca, NY: Cornell University Press, 1943), p. 14.

11. Lily Loat, *The Truth About Vaccination and Immunization* (London, England: Health for All, 1951), p. 7.

12. Rene Dubos, "Second Thoughts on the Germ Theory," *Scientific American*, May 1955, p. 34.

13. Asher, *Bacteria, Inc.*, p. 42.

14. Sandler, *Diet Prevents Polio*, pp. 35–36.

15. Weston A. Price, *Nutrition and Physical Degeneration* (Los Angeles, CA: American Academy of Applied Nutrition, 1939).

16. Archie Kalokerinos and Glen Dettman, "A Supportive Submission," *The Dangers of Immunization* (Australian edition of *The Dangers of Immunization* by Harold Buttram et al., Quakertown, PA, 1979), Warburton, Victoria, Australia, 1979, p. 68.

17. J. C. de Wit, abstract, *Journal of the American Medical Association* 144 (November 4, 1950): 879.

18. Adelle Davis, *Let's Eat Right to Keep Fit* (New York: Harcourt, Brace, 1954), pp. 145–146.

19. Adelle Davis, *Let's Have Healthy Children*, rev. Marshall Mandell (New York: Signet, 1981), p. 272.

20. Davis, *Let's Eat Right to Keep Fit*, pp. 146–147.

21. Ibid., p. 143.

22. Daniel Q. Haney, "Wave of Infant Measles Stems from '60s Vaccinations," *Albuquerque Journal*, November 23, 1992, p. B3; reported by Neil Z. Miller, *Vaccines: Are They Really Safe and Effective?* (Santa Fe, NM: New Atlantean Press, 1993).

23. Adelle Davis, *Let's Get Well* (New York: Harcourt, Brace & World, 1965), pp. 141–142.

24. P. A. Skudder and J. R. McCarrol, "Current Status of Tetanus Control," *Journal of the American Medical Association 188* (1964): 625–627; cited by Randall Neustaedter, *The Immunization Decision* (Berkeley, CA: North Atlantic Books, 1990), p. 36.

25. Clinton Miller, phone conversation, latter part of 1981.

26. Richard Moskowitz, "Immunizations: The Other Side," *Mothering*, spring 1984; reported by Miller, *Vaccines*, p. 32.

27. *Science*, May 26, 1978, p. 905; reported by Miller, *Vaccines*, p. 32. Also, "Tetanus—United States, 1987 and 1988," *Morbidity and Mortality Weekly Report* 39 (January 26, 1990): 37–41; reported by Cynthia Cournoyer, *What About Immunizations? Exposing the Vaccine Philosophy* (Santa Cruz, CA: Nelson Books, 1991), p. 55.

28. "Tetanus—United States, 1987 and 1988" reported by Cournoyer, *What About Immunizations?* pp. 53–54.

29. *Statistical Abstracts of the United States* (Washington, D.C.: GPO, 1992).

30. "Tetanus—United States, 1987 and 1988" reported by Cournoyer, *What About Immunizations?* p. 54. These figures vary according to source. For instance, the *Vital Statistics of the United States* Vol. 2, P.A (Washington, D.C.: GPO, 1988), lists 17 deaths from tetanus for the year 1988.

31. Literature distributed by the *Polio Foundation of California* during the late 1950s and early 1960s. Leaflet called "Conquering Paralytic Polio."

32. J. I. Rodale, *The Road to Polio Prevention* (Emmaus, PA: Rodale Press, 1954), p. 7.

33. J. F. Edward, "Iodine, Its Use in the Treatment and Prevention of Poliomyelitis and Allied Diseases," *Manitoba Medical Review* 34, no. 6 (June–July 1954): 337–339.

34. J. F. Edward, *Canadian Medical Journal*, September 1, 1955, *Prevention* flier, undated.

35. D. C. Jarvis, "The Use of Honey in the Prevention of Polio," *American Bee Journal* 91, no. 8 (August 1951): 336–337.

36. Linda Clark, *Get Well Naturally* (New York: ARC Books, 1972), pp. 120–121.

37. Moskowitz, "Immunizations," p. 36; reported by Miller, *Vaccines*, p. 18.

38. Edgar Cayce, Reading #480–19. Cayce specified in a number of readings that if one would avoid colds and flu, he must "keep the body alkaline." The Cayce readings are filed numerically in the library of the Association for Research and Enlightenment at Virginia Beach.

39. Alkalinity and acidity refer to the final metabolic residue of a food after it is "burned" or digested. Too keep our bodies alkaline, 80 percent of our diets should consist of fresh fruits and vegetables. This figure varies somewhat with age and lifestyle of the person as well as the season and climate.

40. John Christopher, *Childhood Diseases* (Springville, UT: Christopher Publications, 1978), discusses herbal remedies helpful in treating childhood diseases.

41. From a flier distributed by Shaklee supervisor Irma Ahola, "Alfalfa," John W. Shenton, Johannesburg, South Africa, n.d.

42. Gerald T. Keusch, "Vitamin A Supplements—Too Good Not to Be True," *New England Journal of Medicine*, October 4, 1990, pp. 985–987, reported by Miller, *Vaccines*, p. 27.

43. Leon Chaitow, *Vaccination and Immunization: Dangers, Delusions and Alternatives* (Essex, England: C. W. Daniel Company Limited, 1987), p. 134. Dr. Chaitow points out that this is just one example of the interacting dependency that nutrients have with each other.

44. Davis, *Let's Get Well*, p. 149.

45. Ed Rupp, "What About Trace Minerals?" *Missouri Ruralist*, April 9, 1949; "Are We Starving at Full Tables?" Ira Allison, *Steel Horizons* 12, no. 3; Davis, *Let's Get Well*, p. 149.

46. Reported by a reader in *Organic Consumer Report*, April 25, 1978.

47. Robert S. Mendelsohn, *The Risks of Immunizations and How to Avoid Them* (Evanston, IL: The People's Doctor Newsletter, Inc., 1988), p. 7.

PART II   Beyond Disease Wars

Either war is obsolete or men are.

—R. Buckminster Fuller

5   Do Germs Cause Disease or Does Disease Cause Germs?

Two roads diverged in a wood, and I—
I took the one less traveled by
And that has made all the difference.

> —Robert Frost,
> "The Road Not Taken"

A LOST CHAPTER IN THE HISTORY OF BIOLOGY[1]

Are there forks in the roads of history and choices that make "all the difference"? Is our way of thinking about disease—particularly infectious disease—largely the result of a choice that was made around the middle of the last century? Was this choice the result of a fork in the road in which we took one path and not the other? Is the road we didn't take more salutary, less conductive to commercial exploitation, and therefore "the road not taken"?

Let's go back to the scientific world of about 130 years ago. Scientists were arguing about the origin and nature of living matter and were asking such questions as, What is the "thing" that causes milk to sour, meat to spoil, and wine to ferment? Where does it come from? Does it come from the air? Does it grow from other matter? Or does it just appear from nowhere?

Most scientists believed the "thing" (living matter) that caused fermentation appeared from nowhere. This theory was called "spontaneous generation." One French scientist, however, proved through experiments in his laboratory that fermentation was the result of living organisms and that these organisms are imported by the air, which in turn grow in the food and ferment it by a process of their own digestion, assimilation, and excretion.

Does this sound like I am talking about Louis Pasteur? Read on.

This same scientist also discovered that living organisms exist within cells as well as on external surfaces and that these organisms can cause fermentation as well as airborne organisms.

Meanwhile, another scientist, a sponteparist (one who believes in the spontaneous generation of matter) seized upon this first scientist's ideas and claimed them as his own. Being an extraordinarily ambitious man with a genius for self-promotion, he popularized as well as plagiarized the original scientist's ideas when he found that his own observations and explanations would not stand up to scrutiny. This plagiarism—the first of many such plagiarisms—would not be so devastating had the ideas not been oversimplified and distorted. For instance, having realized that airborne microorganisms (later known as bacteria) caused fermentation, he became fixated and sought to explain by "germs [microorganisms] of the air all that he had explained before by spontaneous generation."[2] He ignored those microorganisms within the cells of a body that can not only cause fermentation but perform other important biological functions as well.

He also taught that these minute organisms were fixed—monomorphic—entities, and he divided them into different classes, claiming that each group fermented one kind of food and another fermented another, and so on. This eventually led to the theory that different bacteria caused different diseases.

This is the familiar *germ theory of disease*, of course, and the opportunist and plagiarist was none other than the hallowed Louis Pasteur! This is a heretical idea and easy to say at this distance in time, but the facts as set forth by Ethyl Douglas Hume in her book *Bechamp or Pasteur?* are extraordinarily well documented. Hume spent years, apparently, poring over every scientific paper presented by chemist Louis Pasteur and chemist, physician, naturalist, and biologist Professor Pierre Jacque Antoine Bechamp. As she noted their dates, it became clear that Pasteur, who in many instances first ridiculed Bechamp's theories, later appropriated them and took full credit for their discovery. Bechamp, on the other hand, was a brilliant scientist whose painstaking experiments and astute observations forged a theory of the nature of living bodies and their relationship to their environment that is far more salutary and, yes, holistic than Pasteur's. Heresy, again, but again, it is well documented. (For those interested in exploring the details and more technical aspects of the experiments, observations, and arguments of these two men, I refer them to Hume's book.)

The Germ Theory

Let's look first at Pasteur's ideas and see why they were so readily accepted. Aside from self-promotion, the ideas themselves were simple and easy to understand. To quote Rene Dubos of the Rockefeller Institute: "The germ theory of disease has a quality of obviousness and lucidity which makes it equally satisfying to a schoolboy and to a trained physician. A virulent microbe reaches a susceptible host, multiplies in its tissues and thereby causes symptoms, lesions and at times death. What concept could be more reasonable and easier to grasp?"[3] Or to use J. I. Rodale's summation of Pasteur's germ theory: "Germs live in the air, every once in a while get into a human body, multiply and cause illness. Nothing to it at all. All you have to do is kill the germs and disease is licked."[4]

Other reasons why the germ theory became popular are: First, it fit neatly into the mechanistic theories of the universe that were popular in the nineteenth century. Second, it fit "human nature." Man, apparently, ever ready to avoid responsibility and place causation outside himself, found an easy scapegoat in the bad little organisms that flew about and attacked him. After all, it wasn't too long ago that evil spirits had been responsible for man's ills. Third, it fit "commercial nature." When we place causation outside ourselves, we create vast armies of attackers and defenders, assailants and protectors. In the case of disease causation, our protectors are such things as vaccines, drugs, X rays, and the like, and their administrators, medical practitioners. The possibilities for commercial exploitation are endless. Is it any wonder that the "powers that be"—conservative, well-established scientific authorities—were behind Pasteur?

Nevertheless, the flaws in the fabric of the germ theory are becoming more apparent with time. Not only are they apparent with respect to vaccination—a practice based on the germ theory, which we discussed earlier—but with respect to other practices based on it that we will discuss later. Dubos suggests these flaws when, after the summary statements of the theory quoted earlier, he goes on to say, "In reality, however, this view of the relation between patient and microbe is so oversimplified that it rarely fits the facts of disease. Indeed, it corresponds almost to a cult—generated by a few miracles, undisturbed by inconsistencies and not too exacting about evidence."[5]

The Cellular Theory[6]

Now let us turn to Bechamp and his theories. As we proceed, you will notice that Bechamp's ideas are almost the inverse of Pasteur's. In essence, Bechamp's theories are as follows:

The smallest units of living matter are what cytologists have called *cell granules*, which Bechamp sometimes referred to as *granulations of the protoplasm*. *Molecular granulations* and *scintillating corpuscles* are some of the names earlier researchers gave them. Bechamp called these organisms *microzymas*, from the Greek meaning "small ferment," because they induce fermentation. Not all cell granules are microzymas, however. Microzymas are identifiable because they have some structure and are autonomous, having independent individuality and life. They are the antecedents of cells and "the fundamental unit of the corporate organism."[7] Every living being has arisen from the microzyma, and "every living being is reducible to the microzyma."[8] To get an idea of their size, we might say that they are to the cell what an electron is to an atom.

Microzymas are constantly developing into bacteria. In fact, bacteria are an evolutionary form of microzymas—actually microzymas fully grown. They develop from the cells of the host organism when that organism dies. So-called virulent or pathogenic bacteria are generated by decaying matter, their function being to reduce (decompose) matter back to its constituent elements. When their job is finished, they become microzymas again. Pathogenic bacteria could be thought of as nature's undertakers or clean-up crew.

The microorganisms known as *disease germs* are either "diseased" microzymas, as Bechamp called them, or their evolutionary bacterial forms. "In a diseased body a change of function in the microzymas may lead to a morbid bacterial evolution."[9] If tissue is healthy, the microzymas will function to support the life and integrity of the cells; if the cells have been damaged, they will produce morbid or diseased microzymas that may evolve into pathogenic (disease-producing) bacteria. In short, the microzyma has two functions: to build or to disintegrate tissue.[10] Another way of thinking about the function of microzymas is: They secrete ferments that aid digestion, and when they encounter dead or damaged cells, they evolve into bacteria.

Bechamp found microzymas everywhere—innumerable in healthy tissues and associated with various kinds of bacteria in diseased tissues. Whether microzymas become healthy and evolve into "friendly" (aiding constructive metabolism) bacteria or diseased and evolve into pathogenic bacteria depends on the character of the medium—cellular fluids—upon which they feed. That is, the character of the "soil"—health or unhealth of the host organism—determines the character of the microorganismic life within it. Bodies in which pathogenic bacteria form are not healthy; merely fighting and killing bacteria will not bring health, for the condition that gave rise to the bacteria will do so again.

Bechamp showed that bacteria function in whatever medium they find themselves, even changing their shapes as well as their function to accord with that medium. In comparing Pasteur's understanding of bacteria with Bechamp's, J. I. Rodale gives us this illustration: "Pasteur might have commented, while looking into a microscope 'Ah, here is the bacteria that ferments beer and this is its shape.' Bechamp might have commented, 'Here is a bacteria fermenting beer. In beer it takes on this shape.' "[11] In other words, bacteria are pleomorphic (form changing) rather than monomorphic (form fixed). They *reflect* the conditions in which they find themselves rather than create those conditions.

Modern medicine, under the spell of the germ theory, tells us that for every disease there is a disease entity—an individual bacteria shaped in a particular way—that causes a particular disease. Bechamp showed through innumerable experiments not only that the germ we associate with a particular disease is a product and not the cause of the disease but also that what some researchers would call different species of bacteria are really different stages of microzymian evolution into their bacterial forms. Let's look at a few of Bechamp's experiments that illustrate some of the ideas we have been discussing.

Working in a laboratory where he could get material from the nearby hospital of the Medical University of Montpellier, Bechamp and his colleagues examined a cyst that had been exised from a liver. They found microzymas in all stages of development; isolated, associated, elongated—in short, bacteria. One of Bechamp's medical pupils, for instance, demonstrated that the contents of a blister included microzymas and that these evolve into bacteria. They consistently found microzymas and many forms of bacteria in various phases of development in diseased tissue.

One day, an accident victim was brought to the hospital, where his arm was subsequently amputated. The amputation was performed between seven and eight hours after the accident and the amputated arm was carried immediately to the laboratory of one of Bechamp's colleagues, Dr. Estor. When Drs. Bechamp and Estor examined the arm, they found all the signs of gangrene. Under the microscope, they saw microzymas associated and in chaplets (strung like beads) but no actual bacteria. Because the changes brought about by the injury had progressed so rapidly, bacteria did not have time to develop. They were merely in the process of formation. "This evidence against bacteria as the origin of the mortification was so convincing that Professor Estor at once exclaimed: 'Bacteria cannot be the cause of gangrene; they are the effects of it.' "[12] We might say that while Pasteur taught that germs cause disease, Bechamp taught that disease generates germs.

Years earlier when Bechamp was developing his theories, he performed a number of experiments that proved that bacteria are indigenous to the organism and that airborne organisms need have nothing to do with their appearance in the tissues. In one experiment, he preserved the carcass of a cat in a bed of pure chalk (carbonate of lime) prepared in such a way that air would continually be renewed without permitting the intrusion of dust or microorganisms. At the end of six and half years, he removed the chalk and found nothing but fragments of bone and dry matter. There was no odor, nor was the artificial chalk discolored. Under the microscope, Bechamp found microzymas swarming by the thousands in that portion of the lime where the cat's body had rested.

Repeating the experiment, he buried, in addition to the carcass of a kitten, a case containing the kitten's liver and another case containing the heart, lungs, and kidneys, taking even greater precaution to exclude airborne organisms. At the end of seven years, he found in the bed of artificial chalk near the remains of the organs not only microzymas swarming but also well-formed bacteria. Because this second experiment had to be transported from the warmer climate of Montpellier to the colder climate of Lille a little over a year after it was commenced, the destruction of the carcass was less advanced than in the previous experiment. Hence, the bacteria had not yet reverted back to microzymas as they had in the previous experiment.[13]

These two experiments confirmed the ideas suggested to Bechamp by many earlier experiments and observations. Some of the lessons learned from these as well as the earlier experiments and observations are: First, after the death of an organ, its cells disappear, but in their place remain myriads of microzymas. Second, microzymas can live on indefinitely after the decay of the plant or animal bodies they originally built up. Microzymas are the only nontransitory elements of the organism. Third, microzymas are the builders of plant and animal cells, which evolve into bacteria upon the death of the plant or animal. By their nutritive processes, bacteria bring about the decomposition of plant and animal bodies and, when completed, revert back to microzymas. Fourth, airborne organisms, so-called atmospheric germs, are simply microzymas or their evolutionary forms (bacteria) set free by decomposition of the plant or animal body in which they lived. And fifth, the microzymas Bechamp had found earlier in natural chalk buried in limestone—but not in the artificial chalk produced in his laboratory—are the survivors of the constructive cellular elements of living forms of past ages. No wonder Bechamp would say, "Nothing is the prey of death; everything is the prey of life."[14]

One of his most seminal discoveries was: There are functional but not necessarily morphological (form) differences between the microzymas of different organs of the same animal. Later Bechamp would find that there are functional differences in the microzymas of (1) the same organs and tissues of the same animal at different ages, (2) the blood and tissues of different species, and (3) the blood and tissues of different individuals of the same species. Because microzymas of different species are functionally different, each species has diseases peculiar to it. Certain diseases are not transmissible from one species to another and often not from one individual to another, even of the same species. Microzymas, then, are species and organ specific and even person and age specific.

Implications

What implications do these ideas have for the theory and practice of vaccination? If, as we have already suggested, germs are the result—one of the symptoms—of disease and not its cause, then killing, weakening, or otherwise "treating" germs will not prevent or cure disease. It is true, however, that inoculation with a specific disease germ can produce a specific disease, sometimes one associated with the specific bacteria that was injected. In one of Bechamp's experiments, he inoculated plants with bacteria and studied the results of this foreign intrusion. He observed increasing swarms of bacteria in the plant interiors, but he "had cause to believe that these were not direct descendants of the invaders. He became convinced," according to Hume, "that the invasion from without disturbed the inherent microzymas and that the multiplying bacteria he noted in the interior of the plants were, in his words, 'the abnormal development of constant and normal organisms.' "[15] In modern terminology, the introduction of foreign organisms disturbed the homeostasis of the plant by disrupting the normal functioning of its intracellular organisms (microzymas), thus causing them to mutate into bacteria. Another way of thinking about this would be to say that the introduction of foreign matter into the body of a plant or animal constitutes an injury, and the symptoms of that injury will accord with the nature of the injury as it interacts with the nature and condition of the organism.

If germs do not cause disease, why is it that cleanliness and aseptic surgery (essentially clean surgery) brought about such dramatic reductions in hospital fatalities resulting from such complications as puerperal (childbed) fever and wound infection? Simply, when unclean or putrefying matter—conveyed by hands, dressings, or other means—contacts fresh wounds, it introduces morbid microzymas that alter the normal function of the inherent microzymas of the body.

Pasteur talked of "invaded patients" and declared the danger of morbidity and infection to arise from atmospheric particles that he later called "microbes." In puerperal fever, for instance, the culprit was a chainlike organism he called the germ of puerperal fever. Bechamp, on the other hand, "maintained that in free air even morbid microzymas and bacteria soon lose their morbidity, and that inherent organisms are the starting point of septic and other troubles."[16]

Perhaps the best summation of the teachings of Bechamp is given by Dr. Henry Lindlahr in the 1918 edition of his book *Philosophy of Natural Therapeutics*. In his discussion of Bechamp, Dr. Lindlahr says:

The physical characteristics and vital activities of cells and germs depend upon the soil in which their microzymas feed, grow and multiply. Thus microzymas, growing in the soil of procreative germ plasm, develop into normal, permanent, specialized cells of the living vegetable, animal or human organism. The same microzymas feeding on morbid materials and systemic poisons in these living bodies develop into bacteria and parasites.

Dr. Lindlahr adds that he was delighted to find this scientific confirmation of the philosophy of Nature Cure, which claims that "bacteria and parasites cannot cause and instigate inflammation and other disease processes unless they find their own peculiar morbid soil in which to feed, grow and multiply!"[17]

Dr. Lindlahr compares cells to atoms and microzymas to electrons: "As the electrons, according to their numbers in the atom and their modes of vibration, produce upon our sensory organs the effects of various elements of matter, so the microzymas, according to the medium or soil in which they live, develop into various cells and germs, exhibiting distinctive structure and vital activities." He suggests that the mysteries of heredity are explainable by Bechamp's theory: "If the microzymas are the spores, or seeds of cells, it is possible to conceive that these infinitesimal, minute living organisms may bear the impress of the species and of racial and family characteristics and tendencies, finally to reappear in the cells, organs and nervous system of the adult body."[18]

Florence Nightingale, the great pioneer of nursing, noted along with Drs. Creighton, Farr, and others that infectious diseases replace each other according to the varying degrees of unhealthiness of the living conditions of the people. For instance, in his *History of Epidemics in Britain*, Dr. Creighton suggests that plague was replaced by typhus and smallpox; and later on, measles—insignificant before the middle of the seventeenth century—began to replace smallpox.

Regarding the germ theory, Florence Nightingale remarked:

Is it not living in a continual mistake to look upon diseases, as we do now, as separate entities, which must exist, like cats and dogs, instead of looking upon them as conditions, like a dirty and clean condition, and just as much under our own control . . . ? I was brought up to believe . . . that smallpox was a thing of which there was once a specimen in the world, which went on propagating itself in a perpetual chain of descent, just as much as that there was a first dog (or pair of dogs), and that smallpox would not begin itself anymore than a new dog would begin without there having been a parent dog. Since then I have seen with my eyes and smelt with my nose smallpox growing up in first specimens, either in close rooms or in overcrowded wards, where it could not by any possibility have been "caught," but must have begun. Nay, more, I have seen diseases begin, grow up and pass into one another. Now dogs do not pass into cats. I have seen, for instance, with a little overcrowding, continued fever grow up, and with a little more, typhoid fever, and with a little more, typhus, and all in the same ward or hut. For diseases, as all experience shows, are adjectives, not noun substantives. . . . There are no specific diseases: there are specific disease conditions.[19]

MORE LOST CHAPTERS

Is there any recent research that supports Bechamp's theory (1) that life is based on some elementary organizing energy and while this energy may take many different forms—humans, animals, insects, plants, microorganisms—the basic material is the same and (2) that disease arises from a disturbance of the normal functioning of these primal units of energy within the organism? (Compare the germ theory and the cellular theory of disease in Table 1.) And what about the idea that this organizing energy is contained in the "spores" or seeds of cells—to use Dr. Lindlahr's terms—that are functionally programmed for the specific organ, person, and species of which they are a part and which they helped build? What implications does this have for our practice of injecting material (microzymas) from one species into the bloodstream of another as in vaccination?

Let's begin with the idea that bacteria are not fixed—monomorphic—entities, as the germ theory insists they are, but are in fact form changing or pleomorphic. The work of Dr. E. C. Rosenow is, as far as I know, the earliest record we have of the corroboration of Bechamp's theories. In 1910, at the Mayo Biological Laboratories, Dr. Rosenow began a series of experiments in which he took bacterial strains from many different disease sources, such as puerperal sepsis, arthritis, tonsillitis, and cow's milk and put them into one culture of uniform media. "After a while, there was no difference between the germs; they became all one class. Dr. Rosenow therefore concluded there was no particularly fixed

TABLE 1. TWO THEORIES OF DISEASE

GERM THEORY	CELLULAR THEORY
1. Disease arises from micro-organisms outside the body.	1. Disease arises from micro-organisms within the cells of the body.
2. Microorganisms are generally to be guarded against.	2. These intracellular micro-organisms normally function to build tissue and assist in the metabolic processes of the body.
3. The function of microorganisms is constant.	3. The function of these microorganisms changes to assist in the catabolic (disintegration) processes of the host organism when that organism dies or is injured, which injury may be chemical as well as mechanical.
4. The shapes and colors of microorganisms are constant.	4. Microorganisms change their shapes and colors to reflect the medium upon which they feed.
5. Every disease is associated with a particular microorganism.	5. Every disease is associated with a particular condition.
6. Microorganisms are primary causal agents.	6. Microorganisms become "pathogenic" as the health of the host organism deteriorates. Hence, the condition of the host organism is the primary causal agent.
7. Disease can "strike" anybody.	7. Disease is built by unhealthy conditions.
8. To prevent disease we have to "build defenses."	8. To prevent disease we have to create health.

species of different germs and they all had the capacity to change their structure with the changes in their nutriments."[20]

The results of his studies were published in 1914 in the *Journal of Infectious Diseases* 14: 1–32. Rosenow demonstrated

that simple bacterial forms like streptococci (pus germs) could be made to assume all of the characteristics of pneumococci (pneumonia germs) simply by feeding them on pneumonia virus and making other minor modifications in their environment. And when Rosenow reversed the procedure and fed pneumonia germs on pus, they quickly changed into streptococci. Many other experiments were carried on, and, in every instance, the germs, regardless of type, changed into other types when their food and environment were altered.[21]

In other words, Rosenow found that various strains of bacteria "or what one might call sub-sub species of them, could when suitably treated, become any of the other strains."[22]

Dr. Rosenow wrote in his 1914 article, "It would seem, therefore, that focal infections are no longer to be looked upon merely as a place of entrance of bacteria but as a place where conditions are favorable for them to acquire the properties which give them a wide range of affinities for various structures."[23]

"The truth of this idea has been demonstrated in countless instances in sanitary practices," William Miller tells us. "When typhoid fever was discovered to come with contaminated water, pure water quickly eliminated typhoid. The same is true of puerperal fever which killed so many women in childbirth. Though Semmelweiss had a hard time convincing physicians they were spreading the disease with their contaminated hands and instruments, puerperal fever was eliminated as soon as such sources of infection were removed."[24]

Cash Asher tells us that other bacteriologists have verified Rosenow's findings and mentions "two New York researchers who reported transforming cocci, the round berry-shaped type of bacteria, into bacilli, the long, rod-shaped species." In the course of their experiments, they discovered that

bacteria found in the primary stages of pus formation are invariably the streptococci, while in the later stages as the blood cells undergo more and more disintegration and the chemistry is altered, the "streps" change into staphylococcus. These germs do not maintain their structural identity in an alien medium. . . . Denied their exclusive type of food, moved from their natural habitat, and fed on other kinds of food, they quickly change into forms native to their new surroundings.[25]

Asher likens this transformation of germs from one type to another to a mouse slowly changing into an opossum, this adaptability being characteristic of life in the microscopic world.

In the latter third of her book, particularly in chapter 14, Hume describes later researchers who have confirmed Bechamp's theories. A few examples are the following.

On April 8, 1914, the *Daily News* of London carried this story:

Mme. Victor Henri, the lady bacteriologist, has made one of the most important discoveries in the branch of research for many years. She has, by subjecting bacteria to the action of ultra-violet rays, succeeded in creating a new species of bacteria from a species already known. The experiment was made with the anthrax bacillus, which from a rod-shape was transformed into a spherical coccus.[26]

A Frenchman, M. V. Galippe, carried out experiments on fruit and animal tissues that were reported in the *Bulletin de l'Academie de Médicine* (Paris, July 1917, no. 29). In experimenting with apples, he found that he could induce the appearance of microorganisms from the biological activity of the microzymas by subjecting the apples to mechanical trauma such as contusions. In the case of wounds—specifically war wounds—he found not only that the crushed tissues of the wound favor the appearance and evolution of certain intracellular elements (bacteria and microzymas) but that the crushed tissues and extravasated blood "may give birth directly without foreign collaboration, to infectious elements, so that an absolutely aseptic projectile is capable of infecting a wound solely by its mechanical action in starting the abnormal evolution of the living intracellular elements already present."[27]

Again we see that microorganisms from the outside are not necessary to initiate the disease process, only injury of some sort. "[I]n Pidoux' happy words: 'Disease is born of us and in us,' "[28] Bechamp reminds us. And like Bechamp, Galippe pointed out that microzymas are indestructible: "Neither glycerine, nor alcohol, nor time destroy the microzymas of the tissues. These different agents can only diminish or suspend their activity. They are endowed with perennial life."[29]

A reprint of speeches in the House of Lords (February 2, 1944) records a moving and interesting tribute to the work of Bechamp, given by Lord Geddes. Among other things, Lord Geddes said that he had seen and examined the little bodies under a microscope and had observed the "most extraordinary differences between people fed in different ways and in different states of health."[30]

But perhaps the most remarkable confirmation of Bechamp's ideas comes from the research of Dr. Royal Raymond Rife of San Diego, California, who for many years built and worked with light microscopes that possessed "superior ability to attain high magnification with accompanying high resolution."[31] "With his 150,000 power microscope that made live germs visible (and) as clear as a cat in your lap, Rife showed that . . . by altering the environment and food supply, friendly germs such as colon bacillus can be converted into pathogenic germs such as typhoid."[32] (This process is reversible.) Experiments conducted in the Rife Laboratories established the fact that the virus of cancer, like the viruses of other diseases, can be easily changed from one form to another by means of altering the media upon which it is grown. With the first change in media, the B.X. virus becomes considerably enlarged although its purplish-red color remains unchanged. Observation of the organism with an ordinary microscope is made possible by a second alteration of the media. A third change is undergone upon asparagus base media where the B.X. virus is transformed from its filterable state into cryptomyces pleomorphia fungi, these fungi being identical morphologically both mac-roscopically and microscopically to that of the orchid and of the mushroom. And yet a fourth change may be said to take place when this cryptomyces pleomorphia, permitted to stand as a stock culture for the period of metastasis, becomes the well-known ma-hogany-colored Bacillus Coli. . . . By altering the media—four parts per million per vol-ume—the pure culture of mahogany-colored Bacillus Coli becomes the turquoise-blue Bacillus Typhosus.[33]

Simply stated, this means that the virus of cancer can be easily changed into the type of bacteria that normally inhabits the colon, and it can also be changed into the destructive bacteria of typhoid simply by slightly altering the media in which it is grown.

It is Dr. Rife's belief that all microorganisms fall into one of not more than ten individual groups . . . and that any alteration of artificial media or slight metabolic variation in tis-sues will induce an organism of one group to change over into any other organism included in that same group, it being possible, incidentally, to carry such changes in media to tissues to the point where the organisms fail to respond to standard laboratory methods of diagnosis. These changes can be made to take place in as short a period of time as forty-eight hours.[34]

Dr. Rife, himself, said: "In reality, it is not the bacteria themselves that produce the disease, but we believe it is the chemical constituents of these micro-organisms enacting upon the unbalanced cell metabolism of the human body that in actuality produce the disease. We also believe if the metabolism of the human body is perfectly balanced or poised, it is susceptible to no disease."[35] Before he died, Rife stated: "We have in many instances produced all the symp-toms of a disease chemically in experimental animals without the inoculation of any virus or bacteria into their tissues."[36] Again, "germs" are part of the disease process rather than the instigator of this process.

What about microzymas? The Universal Microscope, the most powerful Rife scope, made it possible to view the

interior of the "pin point" cells, those cells situated between the normal tissue cells and just visible under the ordinary microscope, and to observe the smaller cells which com-pose the interior of these pin point cells. When one of these smaller cells is magnified, still smaller cells are seen within its structure, and when one of the still smaller cells, in its turn, is magnified, it, too, is seen to be composed of smaller cells. Each of the sixteen times this process of magnification and resolution can be repeated, it is demonstrated that there are smaller cells within the smaller cells, a fact which amply testifies as to the magnification and resolving power obtainable with the Universal Microscope.[37]

Are these cells within cells the microzymas of Bechamp?

When Bechamp and Estor were working together, they observed that cell granules (microzymas) associate and develop into threadlike forms. They were no doubt observing different stages of mitosis or cell division and the development of chromatin threads. Bechamp earlier had observed these rodlike groupings of microzymas, which now go by the name of chromosomes, and in his book *Blood and Its Elements* he noted that the coming together of the microzymas forms a figure eight (double-helix formation). What he saw was not fully described until the 1960s when Wilkins, Watson, and Crick won the Nobel Prize for their discovery of the DNA/RNA molecule, the basic unit of heredity.[38] Indeed, according to Drs. Dettman and Kalokerinos, Bechamp's microzymas were actually living genes.[39]

And what about viruses? We now know that a virus consists of simply a core of genetic material—either a DNA or an RNA molecule—and a protective envelope made of proteins. *Time* magazine (November 3, 1986) calls them "models of biological minimalism." Unlike all life forms as we know them, the virus lacks a cell structure. It does not need and cannot metabolize nutrients, does not grow, and cannot replicate without the help of its host. Put a virus in a test tube and it cannot do anything.[40] In other words, a virus is completely dependent on its host (organismic environment), which gives it its character—harmful or harmless—and its ability to reproduce.

According to Dettman, Kalokerinos, and Chaitow, microzymas can evolve into viruses or bacteria, harmless or harmful depending on their nutritional environment.[41] Microzymas, then, are incipient viruses and bacteria.

Dr. Salvador E. Luria, writing in *Scientific American*, points out that "a new view of the nature of viruses is emerging. They used to be thought of solely as foreign intruders—strangers to the cells they invade and parasitize. But recent findings, including the discovery of a *host-induced modification of viruses* [italics mine], emphasize more and more the similarity of viruses to hereditary units such as genes. Indeed, some viruses are being considered as bits of heredity in search of chromosomes."[42]

Dr. Lewis Thomas reaffirms this idea: "The viruses, instead of being single minded agents of disease and death, now being to look more like mobile genes."[43] In commenting on Dr. Luria's article, Dr. Morton Biskind says, "I would carry this thought one step further to describe viruses as aberrant nucleoproteins which may arise in the chemically or physically damaged cell, or when introduced from without, are capable of displacing normal nucleoproteins. Just as the cell can produce its normal nucleoproteins, it now reproduces the aberrant molecules."[44] Bechamp believed that damaged cells produced morbid or diseased microzymas. Dr. Biskind calls these "aberrant nucleoproteins."

But are mutated forms of microzymas—bacteria and viruses—necessarily harmful or merely harmless? We know that certain bacteria are necessary participants in the metabolic processes of the body; for example, certain bacteria in the colon synthesize vitamins B and K but when improperly fed can produce abnormal or even virulent strains, that generate disease.[45] Could viruses have a similar function?

If we think of microzymas, bacteria (single-cell microorganisms), and viruses as carriers of genetic material—DNA and RNA—it becomes apparent that they can have important metabolic functions in the body. DNA, for instance, not only makes the enzymes that build the structures of the body and regulate cell metabolism, but it regenerates the body.[46] According to an article in the *New York Times*, RNA not only carries genetic instructions and helps assemble proteins for the vital processes of life, but it also "serves as an enzyme, or biological catalyst, that governs some of the chemical reactions necessary for those life processes." In fact, RNA acts as a class of enzymes, those "substances that regulate the chemical activities of every living cell." Moreover, some scientists believe these findings "eventually might help them better understand the origin of life."[47]

Enzymes, small ferments (microzymas), architects of biological structures, origins of life. Shades of Bechamp! It seems clear that Bechamp's microzymas were, in all likelihood, what we now call genes that form particles of the DNA molecule contained in the bacteria and viruses into which microzymas evolve. But Bechamp saw them living. And that made all the difference.

Vaccination Revisited 1

Besides obvious chemical or physical injury, for example, malnutrition and accidents, are there other ways nucleoproteins or microzymas can be damaged? Earlier we saw that one way of damaging a cell is to introduce microzymas from one species into the blood of another species, or even one organ of an animal into another organ of that animal. In the words of Bechamp:

The most serious, even fatal, disorders may be provoked by the injection of living organisms into the blood; organisms which, existing in the organs proper to them, fulfill necessary and beneficial functions—chemical and physiological—but injected into the blood, into a medium not intended for them, provoke redoubtable manifestations of the gravest morbid phenomena. . . . Microzymas, morphologically identical, may differ functionally, and those proper to one species or to one centre of activity cannot be introduced into an animal of another species, nor even into another centre of activity in the same animal, without serious danger.[48]

If the injection of microzymas from one species to another or from one organ to another is hazardous, how much more hazardous it must be to inject foreign species of microzymas that are in diseased or morbid condition. We are talking, of course, about some of the "foreign proteins" referred to in Chapters 2 and 3, which are primary constituents of vaccines.

Bechamp wasn't the first person to warn about the dangers of vaccines. During the last century and early part of this one, many doctors and researchers were opposed to vaccination, citing the folly of attempting to eradicate disease by altering the blood with "disease taints" and "filthy bacterial extracts" instead of correcting the unsanitary, unhygienic conditions which were the real cause of the problem.[49] But the danger of genetic transfer from foreign RNA and DNA, which was fully articulated later in this century (see Chapter 2), wasn't, as far as I know, expressed until 1929, when Dr. W. H. Manwaring, professor of bacteriology and experimental pathology at Stanford University, warned against the injection of biological substances directly into the bloodstream:

... There is ground for believing that the injected germ proteins hybridize with the body proteins to form new tribes, half animal and half human, whose characteristics and effects cannot be predicted.... Even non-toxic bacterial substances sometimes hybridize with serum albumins to form specific poisons which continue to multiply, breed and crossbreed ad infinitum, doing untold harm as its reproductivity may continue while life lasts.[50]

Although the language clearly marks this as belonging to another era, it suggests that one reason for the lack of scientific precision in this statement might be that the author didn't have the technological tools available to later researchers. I refer specifically to the light microscopes of which Rife's scope was one. How then did Bechamp manage not only to see the infinitesimally small microzymas but also to observe them metamorphosing into other forms as part of a cycle of evolution/devolution? Bechamp's method of enhancing visualization was to use polarized light, produced by a Nicol prism, which vibrated in one plane and which was then viewed through a second prism.[51] Later in this century a compatriot of his was to build a light microscope of such resolution and magnifying power that he not only could see what he believed to be the precursors of DNA but was able to observe their full cycle of evolution/devolution. Of even greater interest, perhaps, he was able to use his discoveries to develop cures for some of the most "intractable" diseases of our time. And he paid a terrible price, as we shall see in Chapter 7.

NOTES

1. Subtitle of Hume's book. Ethyl Douglas Hume, *Bechamp or Pasteur? A Lost Chapter in the History of Biology* (Essex, England: C.W. Daniel Company Limited, 1947).

2. Ibid., p. 60.

3. Rene Dubos, "Second Thoughts on the Germ Theory," *Scientific American*, May 1955, p. 31.

4. J. I. Rodale, "*Bechamp or Pasteur*," *Prevention*, August 1956, p. 69.

5. Dubos, "Second Thoughts," p. 31.

6. My Term.

7. Hume, *Bechamp or Pasteur?*, p. 148.

8. Ibid., p. 112.

9. Ibid., p. 148.

10. The physiological analog is *anabolism*, which refers to constructive metabolism, and *catabolism*, which refers to destructive metabolism. *Constructive* or *anabolic metabolism* refers to the process of converting substances into complex compounds; *catabolic metabolism* refers to the process of converting tissue from a higher to a lower level of complexity or specialization. The former is constructive and proliferative; the latter releases energy from stored resources. Both processes are necessary to life; good health results from a balance of these two processes.

We might carry this further and parallel these processes with the yin and yang of Taosim. Anabolic metabolism would be yang because it consolidates energy into matter. Catabolic metabolism would be yin because it releases energy from matter.

11. Rodale, *"Bechamp or Pasteur,"* p. 61.

12. Hume, *Bechamp or Pasteur?*, p. 118.

13. Ibid., pp. 109–111.

14. Ibid., p. 78.

15. Ibid., p. 122.

16. Ibid., p. 167.

17. Ibid., p. 161.

18. Ibid., p. 162.

19. Ibid., pp. 149–150.

20. William Miller, "Germs . . . Cause of Disease?" *Health Culture*, June 1955, p. 2.

21. Cash Asher, *Bacteria, Inc.* (Boston, MA: Bruce Humphries, 1949), p. 14.

22. Christopher Bird, "What Has Become of the Rife Microscope?" *New Age*, March 1976, p. 43.

23. Ibid., p. 45.

24. Miller, "Germs," p. 2.

25. Asher, *Bacteria, Inc.*, pp. 14–15.

26. Hume, *Bechamp or Pasteur?*, p. 158.

27. Ibid., p. 159.

28. Ibid., p. 124.

29. Ibid., pp. 159–160.

30. Ibid., p. 164.

31. R. E. Seidel and M. Elizabeth Winter, "The New Microscopes," *Journal of the Franklin Institute*, February 1944, p. 117.

32. Royal Lee, "The Rife Microscope or 'Facts and Their Fate,' " (reprint no. 47, Lee Foundation for Nutritional Research, Milwaukee, WI). (Cover article for ibid.)

In the 1920s, Rife designed and built five microscopes with a range of magnification from 5,000 to 50,000 diameters at a time when the best laboratory microscopes in use could achieve no more than 2,000 diameters of magnification. The most powerful of the Rife microscopes was the Universal Microscope with a magnification of 60,000 diameters and a resolution of 31,000 diameters, as against 2,000 to 2,500 diameters in common use in that day.

The new electron microscopes have resolutions up to 20,000 or 25,000 diameters and magnifications up to 100,000 to even 200,000 diameters; however, the disadvantage of the electron microscope is that because the tiny living organisms put in it are in a vacuum and are bombarded by a virtual hailstorm of electrons, they undergo protoplasmic changes and cannot be seen in their living state. The Rife microscope did not have this disadvantage; Rife was able to look at organisms in their living state. (See notes 22 and 31, referring to articles by Christopher Bird, and Seidel and Winter.)

33. Seidel and Winter, "The New Microscopes," pp. 124–125.

34. Ibid.

35. Ibid., p. 126.

36. Bird, "What Has Become," p. 47.

37. Seidel and Winter, "The New Microscopes," pp. 123–124.

38. Leon Chaitow, *Vaccination and Immunization: Dangers, Delusions and Alternatives* (Essex, England: C.W. Daniel Company Limited, 1987), p. 12.

39. Drs. Archie Kalokerinos and Glen Dettman described this at the International Academy of Preventive Medicine Seminar in Phoenix, AZ, August 28, 1977. Reported in ibid.

40. "Viruses," *Time*, November 3, 1986, p. 68.

41. Chaitow, *Vaccination*, p. 10.

42. Italics added. See Salvador E. Luria, "The T2 Mystery," *Scientific American*, April 1955, p. 98.

43. Lewis Thomas, *The Lives of a Cell* (New York: Bantam Books, 1974), p. 3.

44. Morton Biskind, *American Journal of Digestive Diseases*, quoted by Rodale, "*Bechamp or Pasteur*," p. 70.

45. Miles Robinson, "On Sugar and White Flour . . . the Dangerous Twins!" *Executive Health* 11, no. 6, referred to in the article "Don't Eat Sugar!" *Better Nutrition*, April 1980, pp. 19, 38.

46. Richard Passwater, *The New Superantioxidant—Plus* (New Canaan, CT: Keats, 1992), pp. 8, 17.

47. "A Function of RNA Discovered," New York Times News Service, *Virginian-Pilot*, December 17, 1983, p. A3.

48. Hume, *Bechamp or Pasteur?*, p. 242.

49. Literature from the Anti-Vaccination League of Great Britain; also Chaitow, *Vaccination*, p. 115.

50. Asher, *Bacteria, Inc.*, p. 19.

51. Chaitow, *Vaccination*, p. 12.

6   Germ Fallout: Rabies, Pasteurization, and Vaccines

> Theories imprint a whole view of the universe and make you look at everything through blinders.
>
> —William Corliss,
> *Brain/Mind Bulletin*, January 24, 1983

TWO LEGACIES

Theories come and theories go. Many of yesterday's theories and practices in medicine are now regarded as superstition, for example, bloodletting and the theory of humours. What will tomorrow's savants think of our preoccupation with vaccination and fighting germs? Indeed, yesterday's knowledge frequently becomes today's superstition, and today's knowledge tomorrow's superstition. John Stuart Mill once said, "It often happens that the universal belief of one age—a belief from which no one was free, nor without an extraordinary effort of genius could, at that time, be free—becomes to a subsequent age so palpable an absurdity that the only difficulty is to imagine how such a thing can ever have appeared credible."[1]

Let's look at a few of the legacies of the germ theory, beginning with some of Pasteur's greatest "triumphs"—the supposed eradication of such diseases as rabies, anthrax (sheep and cattle disease), pebrine (silkworm disease), and indirectly, undulent fever (brucellosis) by the pasteurization of milk. Since anthrax and pebrine are somewhat afield of our concern here, we shall not explore the chicanery involved in the promotion of the idea that Pasteur saved the livestock and silk industries. It is largely a repeat of the opportunism mentioned in Chapter 5, and anyone wishing more details on the subject may consult Hume's book. Consideration of the other two diseases, rabies and undulant fever, has important lessons for us since many people believe Pasteur saved the world from the ravages of milk-borne diseases and the bite of mad dogs. Let's begin with rabies.

RABIES

Rabies, according to one medical dictionary, is an infectious disease caused by a filterable virus that is communicated to man by the bite of an infected animal. Some of the symptoms listed are choking; tetanic spasms, especially of respiration and deglutition (act of swallowing), that are increased by the attempts to drink water or even the sight of water; mental derangement; vomiting; and profuse secretion of sticky saliva. And the disease is usually fatal. No wonder Pasteur, with his antirabies vaccine, was so readily hailed as the savior of humanity from this frightening scourge!

Much has been made of the startling cure of 9-year-old Joseph Meister, whom Pasteur "saved" from hydrophobia (rabies). The cure seems less than miraculous when we discover that several other persons, including the dog's owner, were bitten by that same dog on the same day and continued in good health without receiving Pasteur's inoculations. Other children were not so fortunate. Mathieu Vidau died seven months after being personally treated by Pasteur. Also, another child, Louise Pelletier, died after receiving the Pasteur treatment. Dr. Charles Bell Taylor, in the *National Review* for July 1890, gave a list of cases in which patients of Pasteur's had died, while the dogs that had bitten them remained well.[2]

Apparently, then as now, organized medicine was using the police powers of the state to enforce obedience to its doctrines: A French postman, Pierre Rascol, along with another man was attacked by a dog supposed to be mad, but he was not actually bitten, for the dog's teeth did not penetrate his clothing. Pierre Rascol's companion, however, received severe bites. Rascol was forced by the postal authorities to undergo the Pasteur treatment, which he did from March 9 to March 14. On April 12, severe symptoms set in, with pain at the points of inoculation. "On the 14th of April he died of paralytic hydrophobia, the new disease brought into the world by Pasteur. What wonder that Professor Michel Peter complained: 'M. Pasteur does not cure hydrophobia: he gives it!' "[3] What happened to Rascol's companion who was severely bitten? He refused to go to the Pasteur Institute and remained in perfect health!

These stories could easily be dismissed as anecdotal except that there are a great many of them. An article in the *Archives of Neurology and Psychiatry* (January 1951) gives an account of two patients who became paralyzed after they had been treated by the Pasteur vaccine. A report in the *Journal of the American Medical Association* (January 14, 1956) relates that at a meeting of the Academy of Medicine in France it was pointed out that the use of the Pasteur vaccination for rabies may be followed as long as 20 years later by a disorder called Korsakoff's psychosis, which is a state of delirium. Twenty years later! It was also brought out at that same meeting that in a study of 460 patients treated with the Pasteur injection, 20 died.[4]

The *Indiana State Medical Journal* (December 1950) reports the case of a man of 25 who received the Pasteur rabies treatment and became paralyzed from the waist down and died shortly thereafter. ''The authors say that no one knows what causes these paralytic reactions. However, it has been definitely established, they say, that they are not caused by the rabies virus. In other words, vaccination, not rabies, is the danger here. The authors go on to quote Sellers, another authority, who believes that 'not hydrophobia but rather rabiophobia is the most troublesome problem.' Fear of rabies, then, is what we have to fear most.''[5]

A story illustrating the power of suggestion to create sickness or health is told by Millicent Morden:

A ten year old boy in town had been bitten by a dog, supposedly mad. Local newspapers reported he was dying of hydrophobia. Flocks of curious people were going to the house to enjoy the horrifying spectacle. The offer of a drink of water would throw the boy into a convulsion. If any object like a handkerchief or pencil were held near his head, he would growl, snapping at it savagely with his teeth and frothing at the mouth. He frequently uttered menacing growls like those of a vicious dog.

The student doctor hypnotized him and suggested that at 5 P.M. he would suddenly get well. He left asking that a swarm of visitors be kept out.

At 5 o'clock the boy announced that he was well and wanted supper. The crowd now wanted to see the one who had wrought the miracle in curing hydrophobia. All wanted to be treated by him.[6]

This story, along with many others, tends to support statements made by some doctors and kennel owners that rabies is an imaginary disease. In the same radio address (quoted above), Dr. Morden mentioned other occasions when she entered a room where the patient was strapped down and even held during convulsions by one or more attendants. When she unstrapped the patient, dismissed the attendants, and assured the patient there was no such disease, she said rapid recovery followed.

Dr. Robert Mendelsohn, who was unconditionally opposed to the rabies vaccine because of well-documented neurologic damage and death from it, tells of a medical officer in Canada, Dr. Peter Cole, who points to inferential evidence that the disease is not as readily communicable to humans as is commonly thought.[7]

Many kennel owners report that in 30, 40, and even 50 years of working with dogs, they have never seen a case of rabies and that they and their coworkers have been repeatedly bitten by dogs and have simply washed the wound thoroughly with soap and water and that was the end of it.[8]

Time magazine (November 19, 1951) gives some advice on what to do if you are bitten by a dog. "It was proved eight years ago that rabies virus can be removed from a wound more thoroughly by soap and water than by nitric acid or any other cauterizing agents." Rabies virus can be inactivated by (1) interferon, a protein substance produced by the body and activated by parts of the B complex, and (2) vitamin C. As we discussed in Chapter 4, vitamin C in sufficient quantities will prevent the development of infectious disease. Fred Klenner found that nerve-type diseases such as polio and tetanus could be successfully treated with the proper amount of vitamin C.[9] Rabies virus can be inactivated in a test tube by the addition of vitamin C, and in 1967, a veterinarian proved he could cure distemper with vitamin C.[10]

What is the rabies virus? The identifying bacteria are called "Negri bodies" and are found in the brain of the dead animal. However, these bodies are found in the brains of animals and people who have died of causes having nothing to do with rabies. Frequently, they are not found in the brains of animals that the experts were sure had rabies. No wonder Dr. William Brady wrote as follows in the *Berkeley Gazette* for September 1, 1954:

I have never seen a case of rabies in man and I have never met a doctor who has seen a case, yet we know that the preventive inoculation of Pasteur virus sometimes causes death. . . . The Pasteur treatment for rabies is a blind treatment and no one knows whether Pasteur treatment confers any protection against rabies. I'd never willingly receive Pasteur treatment or give it to anyone under any conceivable circumstances, because I fear the material so injected has a disastrous effect in some instances. It is not always successful and occasionally paralysis follows its use.[11]

What is rabies? T. D. Dillon, proprietor and kennel owner, said that most cases of supposed rabies are really running fits, teething fits, worm fits, sunstroke from heat exposure, or hysteria caused by the dog finding itself in a strange environment such as a hostile, bustling, crowded city. Other kennel owners have suggested that the so-called rabid dog can be suffering from poor treatment, hunger, thirst, fear. At any rate, the Pasteur treatment is as unhealthy and risky for dogs as it is for humans. Dillon goes on to say that most dogs that he has known to be inoculated with the rabies serum have died from its aftereffects.[12]

Did, in fact, the incidence of hydrophobia decrease after the introduction of the Pasteur treatment? Dr. Charles W. Dulles, former lecturer at the University of Pennsylvania, said, "It has been shown by statistics that in countries where that method [the Pasteur treatment] is employed the number of deaths from hydrophobia has increased and not diminished."[13] Ethyl Douglas Hume points out that prior to the Pasteur treatment the average number of deaths per year from hydrophobia in France was 30. After the Pasteur treatment, the number jumped to 45. She also discusses at length how the figures were manipulated to give the impression of "success."[14] Does this sound familiar?

What we said about the rabies virus is true for other viruses as well. The

TABLE 2. THE GERM THEORY VERSUS EXPERIMENTAL DATA

KOCH'S POSTULATES*	CONTRAINDICATIONS FROM EXPERIMENTAL DATA

To be the causative agent a particular disease germ:

1. Must be found in every case of the disease.	1. May not be found in every case of the disease.
2. Must never be found apart from the disease.	2. May frequently be found apart from the disease.
3. Must be capable of culture outside the body.	3. May be capable of culture outside the body. However, the original disease germ must be obtained from diseased tissue.
4. Must be capable of producing by injection the same disease as that undergone by the body from which the disease germs were taken.	4. May or may not produce the same disease as the body from which the disease germs were taken. For instance, the pneumococcus of pneumonia introduced into the lung of a rabbit results not in pneumonia but septicemia.**

*The germ theory is based upon these formulations by a 19th-century German doctor, Robert Koch.

**Ethyl Douglas Hume, *Bechamp or Pasteur? A Lost Chapter in the History of Biology* (Essex, England: C.W. Daniel Company Limited, 1947) p. 208.

disease with which a particular virus is associated is sometimes present and sometimes not; people who have a particular virus may or may not have the disease associated with it. (See Table 2.) Several years ago, I heard psychiatrist Dr. George Ritchie describe in a public lecture the ubiquitousness of the polio virus. He told of a small town in Virginia (I've forgotten the name) in which doctors took a throat culture of everyone in town. Everyone had polio virus, yet less than 10 percent of the population showed any symptoms. Of these, one third had a slight cold, one third had stiffness in limbs, and one third died of bulbar polio.[15]

All in all, a new look at the biological formulation of the germ theory seems warranted," Rene Dubos tells us. "We need to account for the peculiar fact that pathogenic agents sometimes can persist in the tissues without causing disease and at other times can cause disease even in the presence of specific antibodies. We need also to explain why microbes supposed to be nonpathogenic often start proliferating in an unrestrained manner if the body's normal physiology is upset. . . .

During the first phase of the germ theory the property of virulence was regarded as lying solely within the microbes themselves. Now virulence is coming to be thought of as ecological. Whether man lives in equilibrium with microbes or becomes their victim depends upon the circumstances under which he encounters them. This ecological concept is not merely an intellectual game; it is essential to a proper formulation of the problem of microbial diseases and even to their control.[16]

The narrow focus on ridding ourselves and our world of harmful bacteria without considering the ecological relationships within the milieu in which they function has been disastrous in many instances. For example, antibiotics can unbalance the ecology of the body to the point where protective or beneficial bacteria are destroyed and fungus infestations, such as the recent "epidemic" of *Candida albicans*, can result. Inflammations and increased susceptibility to infections are also possible side effects. Other serious problems can occur as well. For instance, streptomycin destroys the innervation to the balancing mechanism of the inner ear. Sulfa drugs—effective because they mobilize vitamin C from the tissues into the blood—can damage the kidneys.[17] Sulfa drugs can also cause anemia, allergies, and inflammation of the heart.[18]

Now let's take a look at milk and see what effect the narrow focus of just destroying "harmful" bacteria has had on the nutritional value and even the safety of milk.

MILK PASTEURIZATION

Pasteurization, named in honor of its founder, Louis Pasteur, is the process of heating milk, or other substances, to 130° to 158° Fahrenheit for 20 or 30 minutes. The new "flash" methods of pasteurizing heat the milk to 150° to 170° for 15 to 22 seconds. This is done to kill pathogenic bacteria and delay the development of other bacteria. However, according to Norman Walker, temperatures from 190° to 230° Fahrenheit are required to kill pathogenic organisms such as typhoid, bacilli coli, tuberculosis, and undulant fever. This, of course, would damage the milk to such an extent that no cream would rise—a drawback from a commercial standpoint.[19]

The heat of pasteurization is enough, however, to kill the beneficial lactic acid or souring bacteria—*lactobacillus acidophilus*—which help to synthesize B vitamins in the colon and hold the putrefactive bacteria in check. Raw milk will eventually curdle and clabber if allowed to sit at room temperature because of the lactic acid bacteria, which, as mentioned, hold down the putrefactive bacteria population. Pasteurized milk, having no such protection, will rot. Hence, the irony of pasteurization is that it destroys the germicidal properties of milk. While pasteurization cuts down the bacterial count temporarily, the count soon exceeds the figure prior to pasteurization because bacteria multiply more rapidly in pasteurized milk than in raw milk. Royal Lee claims many cases of undulant fever can be found in communities where all milk is pasteurized.[20] Salmonella food poisoning, which affected over 500 people in Illinois and Iowa (March–April 1985), was traced to pasteurized milk.[21]

What causes undulant fever? As we said in Chapter 4, it has been shown to be a deficiency disease curable in both man and animal by the administration of trace minerals.[22] Particularly important are manganese and magnesium.[23]

The primary commercial advantages of pasteurizing milk are: First, it enables the farmer to be dirty. Standards for certified dairy herds and milk handlers are considerably higher than those for herds whose milk is to be pasteurized; hence, it costs more to make clean, raw dairy products. Second, it is a convenience for the grocer as well as the farmer. Although raw milk will generally keep longer than pasteurized milk, if it is not produced under sanitary conditions, it will begin to curdle sooner than pasteurized milk and will begin to smell rotten. Hence, pasteurization can hide staleness and give milk a longer shelf life.

How does the heat of pasteurization affect the nutritional value of milk? Heating any food above 122° Fahrenheit destroys enzymes, those biochemical transformers that trigger the thousands of chemical processes going on in our bodies all the time. One of the functions of enzymes is to release nutrients in the foods we eat. The heat of pasteurization destroys the enzyme phosphatase, which is necessary for the assimilation of calcium. Some researchers claim that as much as 50 percent of the calcium in pasteurized milk is not utilized by the body.[24] (A number of studies have pointed to widespread symptoms of calcium deficiency among Americans, and yet, according to Harvey Diamond, we consume more dairy products than any other country in the world—300 pounds a year per person![25] Could pasteurization of milk and other dairy products have something to do with this?)

Other food factors and skeletal structures adversely affected by pasteurization as well as diseases promoted by this practice are:

1. *Vitamins.* The loss of fat-soluble vitamins such as A and E may run as high as two thirds. The loss of water-soluble vitamins such as B and C can run from 38 percent to 80 percent. The vitamin C loss usually exceeds 50 percent.[26]

2. *Minerals.* Twenty percent of available iodine is lost by volatilization. Loss of availability of other minerals occurs in varying degrees.[27]

3. *Thirty-eight or more food factors* are changed or destroyed, including protein and hormones as well as the vitamins and minerals discussed. Fats are also altered by heat as well as the whole protein complex, which is rendered less available for tissue repair and rebuilding.[28]

4. *Antistiffness and antianemia factors.* Pasteurization destroys the guinea pig antistiffness (Wulzen factor) and antianemia factor in milk.[29]

5. *X factor.* The X factor in tissue repair is destroyed.[30]

6. *Teeth and bones.* Children's teeth are less likely to decay on a diet supplemented with raw milk than with pasteurized milk.[31] Dr. F. M. Pottenger, Jr., who has studied the effects of raw milk on both experimental animals and people, reported that raw milk produced better bones and teeth than pasteurized milk and that it protected against or prevented dental problems, deafness, arthritis (due to presence of the Wulzen factor), rheumatic fever, and asthma.[32]

7. *Coronary thrombosis and arteriosclerosis.* "Dairy products fed [eaten] in large amounts, including raw cream and raw butter, do not produce atheroma, do not raise the blood cholesterol, while the highest grade pasteurized produce does."[33] "Pasteurization, or the heating of milk which changes the structure of protein, is a major cause of coronary thrombosis," declared Dr. J. C. Annand from Dundee, Scotland. "The consumption of heated milk protein . . . not milk fat . . . has been found to correlate historically to the high incidence of thrombosis," he added.[34]

8. *Skeletal deformities and degenerative diseases.* Experimental animals deteriorate rapidly on pasteurized milk. For instance, calves fed pasteurized milk die within 60 days, as shown by numerous experiments.[35] Perhaps the most famous and, by now, classical experiment is the one of Dr. Francis M. Pottenger's, which was reported at the Second Annual Seminar for the Study and Practice of Dental Medicine in Palm Springs, California, in October 1945. The report outlined the results of 10 years of careful study of approximately 900 cats that were bred and studied for four and five generations. The cats were divided into six groups. The first group was fed raw meat, raw milk, and cod liver oil. The second group was fed the same except the meat was cooked. The other groups were fed raw meat and various kinds of cooked milk, that is, pasteurized milk, evaporated milk, and sweetened condensed milk. Only the cats in the first group remained healthy throughout the experiment. The cats in the other groups suffered every kind of abnormality including skeletal deformities, parasititic infestations, allergies, arthritis, reproductive failure, skin lesions, cardiac lesions, and many other degenerative conditions familiar in the literature of human medicine.

One of the more interesting features of the experiment was observing what happened in each of the pens that housed the cats after the experiment was over. The pens lay fallow for several months. Weeds sprang up in each pen, but only the pen that housed the raw meat, raw milk–fed cats supported luxuriant growth. This led the experimenters to perform a further experiment. They planted beans in each pen, and again, only the pen of the raw milk, raw meat–fed cats supported the growth of the bean plants to any real degree. Vegetation in the other pens was sparse and scraggly, being the most sparse in the pen of the sweetened condensed milk–fed cats. These cats were the ones that showed the most marked deficiencies and degenerative changes during the experiment. (I couldn't help thinking as I read this, "This is the kind of milk, essentially, that many people feed their babies!")

The experimenters concluded: "The principles of growth and development are easily altered by heat and oxidation, which kill living cells at every stage of the life process, from the soil through the animal. Change is not only shown in the immediate generation, but as a germ plasm injury which manifests itself in subsequent generations of plants and animals."[36]

Fresh, raw milk has been successfully used as a therapeutic agent since Hippocrates, who prescribed it for tuberculosis, Dr. William Campbell Douglass reminds us. In his informative and humorous book *The Milk of Human Kindness Is Not Pasteurized*,[37] he describes many other ailments that have been successfully treated with fresh, whole, clean, raw milk. Some of these are (1) edema, (2) obesity, (3) allergies, (4) high blood pressure, (5) psoriasis, (6) diabetes, (7) diseases of the prostate gland, (8) urinary tract infections, (9) heart and kidney disease, (10) hardening of the arteries, (11) neurasthenia, (12) arthritis, (13) gastric and duodenal ulcers, and (14) muscle cramps during pregnancy. Pasteurized milk will not work. It must be raw.

Caveat: Because the modern factory dairy cow is so inhumanely treated, including being fed a mash full of drugs, waste products (yes, cooked manure), and meat from infected animals (the cow is herbivorous), its milk can be seriously contaminated.[38] Unless you are thoroughly familiar with the way the animal is treated and what it eats, avoid milk and milk products.

FROM FRAGMENTATION TO HOLISM

The primary legacy of the germ theory is its fragmentation and narrow focus—its focus on microorganisms rather than on milieu, on symptoms rather than on causes, on parts rather than on wholes. Our discussion of milk pasteurization is particularly illustrative of the counterproductivity of focusing on destroying the "bad guys" or life forms that appear inimical to health. When we ignore the ecological web that sustains both the "good guys" and the "bad," we destroy "friends" along with "enemies." We can clearly see this principle operating in the field of agriculture in which the same kind of tunnel vision is responsible for ever-more potent pesticides that destroy not only the "bad" bugs but their natural predators as well, to say nothing of the toxic residues of the pesticides that enter the food chain and eventually the human digestive tract.

The germ theory is at least partly responsible for our obsession with pathology and our sense of alienation from the natural world, an alienation so profound we feel justified in inflicting pain and suffering upon animals to measure the course of some pathology or to obtain a new medicine or vaccine. For instance, this is how the rabies vaccine was made. I say "was" because now, I hear, there is a new vaccine, but this is how it was made until at least 1947:

1. A rabbit, dog, or goat is strapped and its head held.

2. With no anesthetic, a cut is made through the skin on top of the head.

3. Skin is separated from the skull.

4. A circular saw then removes some bone.

5. A piece of the brain of a so-called rabid dog is then inserted and the skin sewed up; the animal is then placed in a cage to die a slow and horrible death.

6. In from 13 to 27 days, death occurs from inflammation of the brain. At death, the

brain and spinal cord are removed, dried, and later mashed up in a distilled water and salt solution to which carbolic acid or chloroform is added.

7. After straining, it is ready for animal or human use.[39]

Could man's proverbial inhumanity to man have at least some of its genesis in the license he takes with his fellow creatures?

Because many early opponents of vaccination, including some doctors I've already mentioned, referred to vaccinations as injecting pus into the body, let's look at the production of the vaccine to which they referred. This is the smallpox vaccine that today is used for research on AIDS and the new genetically engineered recombinant vaccines.[40]

1. A young calf has his belly shaved.

2. Many slashes are made in the skin.

3. A prior batch of smallpox vaccine is dropped into the slashes and allowed to fester over a period of days.

4. During this time, the calf stands in a headstock so that he can't lick his belly. The calf then is led out of the stock to a table where he is strapped down.

5. His belly scabs and pus are scraped off and ground into a powder.

6. That powder is the next batch of smallpox vaccine.

Besides dried pus and scabs in the smallpox vaccine, incidental viruses that the calf was carrying could be contained in this preparation.[41]

Other animals have similarly been used for the production of vaccines. For the production of diphtheria antitoxin, a horse is generally used and the process is similar. The animal is injected with incremental amounts of putrified beef broth, containing the diphtheria bacillus, until it has the symptoms of blood poisoning—elevated temperature, no appetite, and frequently diarrhea and shivering fits. The injections are continued until the animal—if it does not die—ceases to react. It is then said to be immune. The bleeding process then begins, usually on the third day after the last injection. Two or three gallons of blood are drawn off over 6 to 7 weeks until the animal is exhausted or dies. The blood coagulates, and the clear fluid that rises to the surface—called serum—is put into tubes and sold under the name of diphtheria antitoxin.[42]

As you can see, vaccines are not cruelty-free products, nor are they vegetarian. Cruelty to animals and the ingestion of putrid matter for therapeutic purposes did not begin with the germ theory, of course. Three hundred years ago, to restore health we swallowed such "therapeutic" agents as bat's blood, afterbirth, powdered mummy, hair, earwax, finger- and toenails, animal intestines, human saliva, lice, spiders, snakes, mice, brains, and excrement and urine—both human and animal.[43] We're still doing it today (see next section). Technology merely camouflages this reality.

What the germ theory has done is to systematize and legitimize the mind-set that sees disease as a treacherous foe, "a thief in the night" who strikes without warning, and man as a warrior who must build defenses and destroy enemies (germs). This reduction of the universe to a battlefield and man to a warrior in a perpetual state of seige not only erodes man's sense of harmony and relatedness to the natural world but belittles the human spirit. Sri Aurobindo, the great Hindu sage, poet, and philosopher, states the case succinctly: "I would rather die and have done with it than spend life in defending myself against a phantasmal siege of microbes. If that is to be barbarous, unenlightened, I embrace gladly my Cimmerian darkness."[44]

What would medicine be like if Bechamp's ideas had been accepted instead of Pasteur's? First, it would be health rather than disease oriented. Rather than focusing on disease symptoms, it would focus on the patient—his lifestyle, his temperament, his body type; his habits of eating, exercising, thinking, and feeling. Instead of classifying microorganisms and disease entities, it would classify environments and lifestyles; instead of fighting germs, it would focus on building healthy bodies; and in agriculture, it would focus not on killing pests but on building a balanced, healthy soil that in turn produces healthy plants that don't "attract pests." (See Chapter 13.)

Does any of this sound familiar? Yes, we are talking about holistic health, natural healing, and organic gardening—ideas whose time has come.

Vaccination Revisited 2

> Fillet of a fenny snake,
> In the cauldron boil and bake;
> Eye of newt and toe of frog,
> Wool of bat and tongue of dog,
> Adder's fork and blind-worm's sting,
> Lizard's leg and howlet's wing,
> For a charm of pow'rful trouble,
> Like a hell-broth boil and bubble.
>
> Second witch, *Macbeth* 4.1

Besides microorganisms that are foreign to the body, vaccines also contain other ingredients. Public health worker Carol Horowitz points out, "most parents who are trying to feed their children properly would not let them eat a food which contained any of the many ingredients of immunizations."[45] In Chapter 2 we mentioned some of these ingredients, such as formaldehyde, mercury, and aluminum phosphate. Formaldehyde, which is commonly used to embalm corpses, is a known carcinogen. Mercury is a toxic heavy metal, and aluminum phosphate is a toxin used in deodorants. Some of the other toxic ingredients Horowitz lists are phenol (carbolic acid), alum (a preservative), and acetone (a volatile solvent used in fingernail polish remover that can easily cross the placental barrier). Other decomposing animal proteins besides those mentioned in

Chapter 2 are (1) pig or horse blood, (2) cowpox pus, (3) rabbit brain tissue, (4) dog kidney tissue, and (5) duck egg protein.

A more graphic description of some of the more noxious materials in specific vaccines can be found in the literature of the British National Anti-Vaccination League: "Materials from which vaccines and serums are produced: (1) rotten horse blood, for diphtheria toxin and antitoxin; (2) pulverized felt hats for tetanus serum; (3) sweepings from vacuum cleaners, for asthma and hayfever serums; (4) pus from sores on diseased cows for smallpox serums; (5) mucous from the throats of children with colds and whooping cough, for whooping cough serum; (6) decomposed fecal matter from typhoid patients for typhoid serum."[46]

Is it too impudent to suggest that man has long had a love affair with decomposing animal proteins, noxious potions that would ward off the demons of ill fortune? From the witches of old to modern medicine, man seems to be held captive by the notion that the ingestion of noxious substances protects him from the caprices of some threatening external agent. Is it too impertinent to suggest that the filth that once beset man from open sewers and unwashed bodies has returned in a new and different guise—the hypodermic needle?

NOTES

1. Quoted by Clinton Miller. House Committee on Interstate and Foreign Commerce, *Hearings on H.R. 10541*, 87th Cong., 2nd sess., May 1962, p. 86.

2. Ethyl Douglas Hume, *Bechamp or Pasteur? A Lost Chapter in the History of Biology* (Essex, England: C. W. Daniel Company Limited, 1947), pp. 196–198.

3. Ibid., p. 198.

4. J. I. Rodale, "Rabies, Fact or Fancy," *Prevention*, August 1956, p. 52.

5. Ibid., pp. 52–53.

6. Millicent Morden, radio address, WWRL, January 1947. (From a leaflet distributed by Health Research, Mokelumne Hill, CA.)

7. Robert Mendelsohn, *The Risks of Immunizations and How to Avoid Them* (Evanston, IL: The People's Doctor Newsletter, Inc., 1988), p. 92.

8. *The Fraud of Rabies*, collection of statements by medical doctors, veterinarians, and kennel owners distributed by the California Animal Defense and Anti-Vivisection League, Inc. (booklet, n.d.).

9. "The Vitamin and Massage Treatment for Acute Poliomyelitis," *Southern Medicine and Surgery*, August 1952, pp. 194–197, quoted by Marilyn Garvan, "Mandatory Rabies Shots Protested," *National Health Federation Bulletin*, 1974, p. 22.

10. Ibid.

11. Rodale, "Rabies," pp. 50–51.

12. *The Fraud of Rabies*.

13. Ibid.

14. Hume, *Bechamp or Pasteur?*, p. 200.

15. George Ritchie, "The Ego and the Holy Spirit" (lecture at Association for Research and Enlightenment, Virginia Beach, December 30, 1978).

16. Rene Dubos, "Second Thoughts on the Germ Theory," *Scientific American*, May 1955, pp. 34–35.

17. Royal Lee, "It Can Happen Here," *Nature's Path*, April 1951.

18. James Fuller and Peta Fuller, "The Other Side of the Wonder Drugs," *American Mercury*, Lee Foundation Reprint #46 (n.d.).

19. Norman Walker, *Diet and Salad Suggestion* (St. George, UT: Norwalk Laboratory, Publishing Department, 1947), p. 32.

20. Royal Lee, "The Battlefront for Better Nutrition," *Interpreter*, July 15, 1950.

21. "Food Poisoning Cases in Illinois," item in "Health Notes," *Health Freedom News*, May 1985, p. 31.

22. Ed Rupp, "What About Trace Minerals?" *Missouri Ruralist*, April 9, 1949; also see "Are We Starving at Full Tables?" Ira Allison *Steel Horizons* 12, no. 3.

23. Adelle Davis, *Let's Get Well* (New York: Harcourt, Brace & World, 1965), p. 149.

24. Elizabeth J. Broadston, "Hear Ye—Mothers!" *Let's Live*, February 1955, p. 12; also see Royal Lee, "Raw Food Vitamins" (address delivered before the Massachusetts Osteopathic Society Convention, Boston, MA, May 22, 1949).

25. Harvey Diamond and Marilyn Diamond, *Living Health* (New York: Warner Books, 1987), p. 243.

26. Linda Clark, *Stay Young Longer* (New York: Pyramid Books, 1971), p. 194; also see "Abstracts on the Effect of Pasteurization on the Nutritional Value of Milk," Lee Foundation for Nutritional Research, Reprint #7.

27. Jean Bullit Darlington, "Why Milk Pasteurization?" *Rural New-Yorker*, May 3, 1947, p. 4; also see Broadston, "Hear Ye—Mothers!" p. 12.

28. Broadston, "Hear Ye—Mothers!"p. 12.

29. Darlington, "Why Milk Pasteurization?" p. 5.

30. Ibid.

31. *Lancet*, May 8, 1937, p. 1142. (Taken from Lee Foundation for Nutritional Research, Reprint #7.)

32. Clark, *Stay Young Longer*, pp. 194–195.

33. Francis M. Pottenger, Jr., "A Fresh Look at Milk"; article first appeared in Mr. Kenan's report in the "History of Randleigh Farm." This reprint is undated, but an article by J. F. Wischhusen and N. O. Gunderson, "The Nutritional Approach to the Prevention of Disease," *Science Counselor*, September 1950, refers to the book, William R. Kenan, Jr., *The History of Randleigh Farm*, 4th ed. (Lockport, NY: Lee Foundation, 1942).

34. *Organic Consumer Report*, October 7, 1975, p. 1.

35. Henry G. Bieler, *Food Is Your Best Medicine* (New York: Random House, May 1969), p. 213.

36. Francis M. Pottenger, Jr., "The Effect of Heat-Processed Foods and Metabolized Vitamin D Milk on the Dentofacial Structures of Experimental Animals" (paper presented at the Second Annual Seminar for the Study and Practice of Dental Medicine, Palm Springs, CA, October 1945); *American Journal of Orthodontics and Oral Surgery* (August 1946): 467–485.

37. William Campbell Douglass, *The Milk of Human Kindness Is Not Pasteurized* (Marietta, GA: Last Laugh Publishers, 1985) chap. 11.

38. Harold Lyman, president of Pure Food, interviewed by Gary Null, WNIS-AM,

February 20, 1994. Also see John Robbins, *Diet for a New America* (Walpole, NH: Stillpoint, 1987).

39. Millicent Morden, "Rabies Vaccine," California Animal Defense and Anti-Vivisection League, Inc., Los Angles, CA. (This flier is not dated, but a radio address given by this same doctor and distributed by Health Research is dated January 25, 1947.)

40. Mendelsohn, *The Risks of Immunizations*, p. 78.

41. Ibid., p. 79. Also see *Strecker Memorandum*, 1988, video and literature from the California Animal Defense and Anti-Vivisection League (n.d.; but I picked it up in Los Angeles sometime in the early 1950s).

42. "Beware! The Danger of Vaccines and Serums," Citizens Medical Reference Bureau, distributed by the California Animal Defense and Anti-Vivisection League (n.d.; but I picked it up in Los Angeles in the early 1950s).

43. Diamond and Diamond, *Living Health*, pp. 47–48. Many other noxious substances used in vaccines, drugs, serums, cosmetic rejuvenators, and chemotherapy are also discussed.

44. Sri Aurobindo, "Natural Health—or 'Science'?" *Advent*, August 1953, p. 154 (reprinted by *Health Movement Review*, March 1955).

45. Carol Horowitz, "Immunizations and Informed Consent," *Mothering*, winter 1983, p. 39.

46. Leonard Jacobs, "Menage," *East West Journal*, September 1977, p. 15.

7   The New Biology, the New Immunology

> Every creative act in science, art, or religion involves a new innocence
> of perception liberated from the cataract of accepted beliefs.
> — Arthur Koestler,
> *The Sleepwalkers*

THE "NEW BIOLOGY"

"You see," the Rock Forest biologist told the journalist, "I've been able to establish a life-cycle of forms in the blood that add up to no less than a brand new understanding for the *very basis for life*. What we're talking about *is an entirely new biology.*" He went on to say that the ultramicroscopic entities that he had discovered in the blood of animals and humans—as well as in the saps of plants—were "precursors of DNA." This means that they supply a "missing link" to our understanding of the molecule that has been considered the irreducible building block of the life process.[1]

It is not only the missing link to our understanding of the molecule: it *is* the missing link between the living and the nonliving, according to Gaston Naessens, the Quebec biologist being interviewed.[2] These ultramicroscopic, subcellular, living and reproducing microorganisms, which Naessens calls *somatids* (tiny bodies), are autonomous and indestructible. They have survived 50,000 rems of nuclear radiation (far more than enough to kill any living thing), been totally unaffected by any acid, found impossible to cut with a diamond knife, and resisted carbonization temperatures of 200° C and more! Like other microorganisms, they are pleomorphic, evolving into different forms that reflect their nutrient ambience. These different forms are responsible for both building biological structures and disintegrating them (reducing them to their component elements).[3] Does this sound like Bechamp's microzymas?

When Naessens came across a description of Bechamp's work, he immediately recognized microzymas as "cousins" of somatids. I'm inclined to think they are the same, but Naessens's more technologically advanced microscope—which he invented himself—allowed him to see details that Bechamp's more primitive microscope couldn't. For instance, Naessens observed that the somatid goes through a 3-stage pleomorphic cycle necessary for its reproduction, and if the immune system of the host organism (animal, human, plant) is weakened or destabilized, it goes through an additional pleomorphic 13-stage pathological cycle.[4]

By studying the cycle, as seen in the blood of human beings suffering from various degenerative diseases such as rheumatoid arthritis, multiple sclerosis, lupus, cancer, and most recently, AIDS, Naessens has been able to associate the development of the forms of the pathological cycle with all of these diseases. Moreover, he has been able to predict the eventual onset of such diseases long before any clinical signs of them appear. In other words, he can "prediagnose" them.[5]

But early in his career Naessens made a costly "mistake." He applied what he had discovered to alleviate human suffering, developing highly effective biological treatments for various degenerative diseases, including, and perhaps most spectacularly, cancer and AIDS. At first, he treated only a relative and friends of friends who had terminal cancer, but word spread of their remarkable recoveries, and many others contacted Naessens, requesting his help. News of these successful treatments precipitated the attention of the French medical "authorities," which began for Naessens a life beset with harassment, emigrations, arrests, imprisonment, trials, hearings, and confiscation of most of his equipment (though he managed to preserve his precious microscope). His story is compellingly told by Christopher Bird in his book *The Persecution and Trial of Gaston Naessens*.[6] In spite of his difficulties with the medical establishment, Naessens's treatment has arrested or reversed over 1,000 cases of cancer (many of them considered terminal) as well as several dozen cases of AIDS.[7] This is particularly remarkable when we realize that the only way people had of learning about this treatment was "through the grapevine."

What are some of the implications of the "new biology" for the prevention and treatment of disease? Why are these ideas and their application so fiercely resisted by medical officialdom? This will become evident as we proceed.

1. *Disease is one.* This has been called the *unitary theory of disease* (as contrasted with the pluralistic theory of disease), meaning that all diseases are expressions of an underlying, common dysfunction. Naessens discovered that the degenerative diseases

he was treating had a *common functional principle*, Bird tells us, and were not separate, unrelated phenomena as orthodox medicine regards them.[8]

2. *Disease arises first from within.* A compromised immune system causes the somatid to enter the pathological cycle, sometimes called the macrocycle. The focus, then, is on the "whole terrain," that is, the health of the host organism, not just the microorganisms evolving within it. Therapy, therefore, is directed at restoring the health or integrity of the host organism, not destroying microorganisms which are merely "indicators" (Naessens's term) of its condition.

3. *The basis of life is electrical.* Somatids are essentially electrical in nature, concretizations of energy, Naessens said. During a 1991 symposium in Sherbrooke, Quebec, he said he believed somatids to be "a link between the material realm and the realm of cosmic energy . . . a primary manifestation."[9]

4. *Nature heals cyclically.* Naessens administers his treatments in a series of "shots." This product is derived from camphor, a natural substance produced by an East Asian tree of the same name. When properly injected—not intravenously nor intramuscularly but intralymphatically—into the lymph system (via a lymph node or ganglion in the groin), this product has "in over 75 percent of cases, restabilized, strengthened, or otherwise enhanced the powers of the immune system which then goes about its normal business of ridding the body of disease."[10] The new biology—and by implication, the new immunology—will focus on strengthening the immune system, not on strategies to destroy "enemy" microorganisms (or "enemy" cells).

5. *Health and healing are holistic.* They involve both lifestyle—for example, nutrition, exercise, recreation, rest—and "thinkstyle," which includes beliefs, attitudes, emotions. With respect to lifestyle, Naessens's treatment involves a dietary regime—fresh fruits and vegetables organically grown, whole grains, and some fresh fish and corn-fed chicken.[11] With respect to thinkstyle, the importance of mental and emotional health is implied in the discovery that the source of trauma that initiates the pathological somatid cycle may be physical (such as radiation), chemical (such as pollution), or psychological (such as depression).[12]

During the 1991 symposium in Quebec, referred to earlier, an erudite, articulate microbiologist/immunologist, Walter Clifford, spoke on his own work, which supported the somatid theory. He discovered, for instance, that killed bacteria were "recoverable" after exposure to extraordinarily high levels of radiation and heat. The suggestion was that they might be reverting back to their somatidian state, which Naessens has said can withstand such abuse and still be culturable. Again, even bacteria, which are altered forms of somatids, are apparently imperishable!

But of particular interest for us is what Clifford said about antibiotics, radiation, and cancer because this has a direct bearing on the probable effects of vaccination upon somatids, shedding still another light on the connection between vaccination and degenerative disease. He said that "antibiotics, rather than killing anything, cause form-changing behavior, probably driving the bacteria cell-wall deficient and then into the Somatid macro-cycle!" He called radiation "an absolute disaster." One reason for this statement is that, like

Naessens, he regards cancer as a general condition that localizes,[13] not a local condition that generalizes, as orthodox medicine regards it. Couldn't we say this for all diseases, that they are a general condition that localizes—or expresses—in different ways with different people and conditions?

This idea is not new, of course. It's a tenet of classical naturopathy. From Hippocrates to the Amerindian Medicine Man, the idea of the various manifestations of illness as expressions of an underlying disharmony or discord within the self and its relationships—including the self's relationship with the natural world—is perennial. What is new is the technology and terminology that allow greater focal clarity and verbal precision.

Is the new biology really new? If we think of the new biology as based on the idea of (1) an independent, indestructible living element that is the origin of all life, or biological organization, (2) this element taking different forms that have different functions, and (3) these forms and their functions indicating the condition of their ambience (environment), this idea is not strictly new. Bechamp discovered it a century ago. But if we take this idea one step further—as did Naessens—and say that it is a primary manifestation, a concretization of energy, and a link between the material realm and the realm of cosmic energy, then we have moved into a fundamental tenet of most of the world's great religions for example, Hinduism, Buddhism, Taoism, and esoteric Christianity, which maintain that there is a primordial, intelligent energy out of which arises the material world and into which it will return. This idea is also suggested by modern physics in both the law of conservation of energy and the equivalence of matter and energy. Again, this idea—intuited and experienced by sages and mystics down through the ages—is now being rediscovered by intuitive scientists of the nineteenth and twentieth centuries. It does apparently require some kind of intuitive development or, at least, special microscopic and perceptual skills to see this life particle because though many scientists are able to see it, not every scientist can.

OTHER INTUITIVE SCIENTISTS

Another great scientist who lived earlier in this century and whose discoveries closely parallel those of Naessens and Bechamp is Gunther Enderlein, former professor of zoology and microbiology at Berlin University. Like Naessens, he discovered the life particle, which he called the *protit*, as well as its pleomorphic nature. Using a powerful microscope to observe live blood samples, he discovered billions of colonies of bacteria coexisting in a natural mutually beneficial balance. "Illness occurs when this internal ecology becomes unbalanced, allowing blood microbes to become harmful and destroy tissue. Disease, therefore, is the initial stage of the body's decay, which is completed after death by the microbes," Dr. Eric Enby told a 1991 immune discoveries symposium in San Francisco. "To cure a sick person," Enby continued, "the destruction of the body's tissue must be stopped, and the internal milieu restored to proper balance.'' Using the Enderlein biological medications, the microbial attack can often be halted and diseases cured that orthodox medicine considers incurable, he explained.[14]

The biological medications (derived from plants or fungal extracts and given as a series of injections) are directed at the unhealthy organisms which then convert these organisms back to their healthy, harmless form. One of Enderlein's most profound discoveries is that ''there is a healthy and unhealthy form of every germ,'' Dr. Harvey Bigelsen points out. He goes on to say that the unhealthy form develops when the balance between the mineral salts (alkali) and acids in the blood is disturbed by prolonged wrong nutrition or other factors such as smoking, stress, or exposure to toxins. This results in loss of pH neutrality. Hence, Enderlein stressed the importance of diet in maintaining biochemical balance or neutrality. He strongly believed that a diet consisting of organically grown fruits and vegetables and little animal protein played an important role in preventing disease.[15]

How successful are the Enderlein remedies? Drs. Enby and Bigelson report between 70 and 80 percent success rate in reversing various types of cancer. Other diseases effectively treated with these remedies include AIDS, kidney disease, Crohn's disease, arthritis, lupus, ulcers, glaucoma, and mononucleosis.[16]

The Enderlein and Naessens therapies discussed here represent a model of health and disease processes that is almost the inverse of the current medical model. It is this latter model that forms the rationale for the practice of vaccination as well as the relatively ineffective treatments for degenerative diseases sanctioned by medical orthodoxy.

Two other twentieth-century scientists worth mentioning are (1) Austrian immigrant Dr. Wilhelm Reich, who named the life particle the *bion*, and (2) American Royal Raymond Rife (discussed in Chapter 5), who clearly demonstrated pleomorphism but never identified the life particle (or fundamental biological entity).

What happened to them and their discoveries? Wilhelm Reich died in 1957 in a federal prison after his books were burned by court order. Royal Raymond Rife saw his discoveries crushed and doctors forced to abandon them. He saw his microscope sabotaged, the mysterious death of a promoter (apparently by poisoning), and the confiscation and disappearance of his research.[17] Like Naessens, Reich and Rife had entered ''forbidden territory'' using their discoveries to develop treatments for serious diseases. I'm not familiar with how effective Reich's therapies were, but, from what I've read from various sources, Rife developed a remarkable treatment for serious diseases, particularly cancer. (Rife's cancer treatment is discussed in Chapter 9.)

As for Gunther Enderlein, he escaped this kind of persecution, but many doctors who use the Enderlein therapies have not been so fortunate. (Germany, apparently, has a more open, progressive medical system than most other countries.) Dr. Enby, who practices in Sweden, describes being shunned by colleagues, a few even threatening to ask the Swedish Medical Board to revoke his license.[18] Dr. Bigelsen was, as of this writing, involved in litigation with the federal government, whose indictment, he believes, is simply a continuation of 10 years of harassment and accusation for his research in pleomorphism, biological medicine, and successful European treatments for cancer, AIDS, arthritis, and other chronic diseases.[19]

Why the resistance to new ideas? Why the persecution of people with new ideas who use them to develop far less costly and more effective remedies for our ills? History has repeatedly shown that when ideas threaten powerful, entrenched interests, they are not welcome.

What are some of these ideas? First diseases—and the microorganisms associated with them—are not adversaries per se but part of a larger life process. Second, disease, like health, is contextual, or holistic, even on the microscopic level. Third, like health, disease is reversible by changing the context or terrain in which it develops. Fourth, isolating a symptom, such as a virus or bacteria, and attempting to suppress or destroy it is counterproductive.

Now let's look at the newer thinking about the nature and function of the immune system itself and the implications this has for the direction of future research as well as the treatment and prevention of disease.

TOWARD A NEW IMMUNOLOGY

A new view of the immune system is emerging. Rather than thinking of the immune system as a security system, a fortress whose function is to defend and attack, Dr. Francisco Varela, professor at the Institut de Neurosciences at the University of Paris and the Ecole Polytechnique, suggests that the immune system is more accurately thought of as a cognitive network analogous to the brain and nervous system. (A primary difference, of course, is that there are no spatially located sensory organs in the immune system.) Rather than a heteronomous (outer-directed) system that responds automatically to something coming in from the outside, the immune system is an autonomous (self-directed) network whose primary purpose is the establishment and maintenance of molecular identity. This means that the immune system is a self-asserting distributive network rather than a defensive device built to address external events. This latter view is the "original sin" of immunology because it was born of the medicine of infectious diseases. It, therefore, had vaccination as its central paradigm—"a heteronomous view par excellence."[20]

This network view "naturally leads to the notion of an autonomous 'cognitive' self at the molecular level as the proper view of immune events." This self, as we know, can recognize, learn, and remember as well as "respond to antigens it has never seen including those which are manmade and hence not even explainable by some form of evolutionary adaptation."[21] In this ongoing network, the antigen is not a determinant but a small perturbation. "This means that, with any perturbation in a rich network, the effects of an incoming antigen will be varied and dependent on the entire context of the network, as is now known to be the case."[22] This means that there is no one-to-one correspondence between antigen and antibody; the doctrine of "one antibody, one antigen" is incorrect, Varela points out.[23]

This, of course, contradicts immunological theories that support mass vaccinations. But it doesn't contradict what many doctors, particularly homeopaths, have said all along. One homeopath, Dr. Stuart Close, puts it this way:

Considered as a technical process, such a method [vaccination] is highly objectionable because it involves so many uncertainties. The living organism is an infinitely complex thing, when we consider the almost innumerable mechanical, chemical and vital processes going on within its constantly changing fluids and solids. There are no means of accurately registering and measuring all these activities; no means of determining exactly what these changes are; nor how they are modified by the introduction of the foreign morbid substance used.[24]

It is precisely this rich configuration of ambiguities that makes the vaccination procedure so potentially destructive.

Seeing the body as a flowing system of interconnected, reciprocal networks continually interacting in molecular biodance is part of the newer contextual thinking. "The mutual dance between immune system and body . . . allows the body to have a changing and plastic identity throughout its life and its multiple encounters."[25]

If we are willing to follow the central importance of the autonomy of process in both neural and biological networks, it "can teach us how we think with our entire body," Varela says.[26]

We not only think with our body, but, according to Dr. Deepak Chopra, we have a thinking body. Mind or intelligence is in every cell of the body.[27] Mind is the enlivening energy that enables cells and body parts to talk to each other, Candace Pert told Bill Moyers on the PBS series *Healing and the Mind*. This communication takes place via messenger molecules—neuropeptides—which are the biochemicals of emotion, so emotion must be the connecting link between mind and body, and mind and matter, she said. Dr. Pert described cellular communication as a highly dynamic system, with cell receptors constantly vibrating and changing shape as they talk to each other.[28]

Thoughts not only create chemicals; they create molecules, Dr. Chopra points out. In other words, thoughts have a physical substrate.

Varela's idea that the immune system and the nervous system are, in many ways, analogs, both being cognitive networks, is restated by Chopra who tells us that the immune system is really a circulating nervous system. The immune cell is a thinking cell, "a conscious little being," he says, adding that the immune cell is just like a neuron; in fact, there is no difference between an immune cell and a neuron. These immune cells are constantly eavesdropping on our internal dialogue. Nothing we are saying to ourselves, even in sleep, escapes the attention of the immune cells.[29]

What are some of the implications of these ideas for the "new immunology"?

First, they point to the physiological correlates of psychosomatic medicine—the power of the mind to create health and disease states in the body. The new science of psychoneuroimmunology—literally meaning from psyche (mind or soul) to nervous system to immune system—studies this linkage between states of mind and states of immunity (see Chapter 8).

Second, these ideas strongly suggest the futility—nay, harmfulness—of attempting to force a treatment on an unwilling person, that is, a person who doesn't believe in its validity or thinks it is harmful. If, as Joseph Chilton Pearce says, the emotional cognitive structure of the brain controls the immune system, as well as learning and memory,[30] then we have again the physiological correlate of an idea expressed by Dr. Mendelsohn. He said that in the absence of parental freedom of choice to accept or reject immunizations for their children, immunization is both improper and *impossible*.[31]

So the new immunology would focus on the totality—physical, mental, emotional, spiritual—of the suffering or susceptible person, rather than merely attempting to isolate and control the mechanisms (symptoms) of disease.

On a physiological level, according to Varela, the new immunology will be organism centered (autonomy) rather than antigen centered (input-output). It will be network centered with emphasis on coordination, rather than event centered with emphasis on specificity. To mobilize the system, the new immunology will attempt to mimic natural events (e.g., spacing antigenic challenges as they occur in nature and entering them into the system through food or drink) rather than using artificial situations. And underscoring all of these ideas, the military model of the immune system will be outgrown. Territorial concepts with emphasis on defense against foreign invaders and internal mutant cells will be replaced with "integrative, adaptive concepts, with emphasis on the stability of internal signals."[32]

"Disease is part of the adaptive process of the whole organism," writes Viera Scheibner in her book *Vaccination: The Medical Assault on the Immune System*.[33] After studying some 30,000 pages of medical papers dealing with vaccination, she came to the following conclusions: First, genuine immunity to disease is developed only when "there is the full expression of the generalized inflammatory process."[34] Second, the normal portals of entry for infectious agents—mouth and nose—are instrumental in producing this generalized inflammatory response, which is part of the natural immunological process. Third, childhood diseases are the priming and challenging mechanisms of the maturation process leading to competence of the immune system. Fourth, these infectious diseases of childhood are, therefore, beneficial "when contracted at a suitable age and allowed to run their course."[35] Fifth, childhood diseases "function to even out differences in rates of development in different body systems and so perform a sort of balancing act in a fast-growing organism." They, therefore, represent important milestones in the development of children.[36]

The new immunology will therefore not seek to eradicate or even avoid childhood diseases but will support the child's natural immune process with home-opathic medicines along with suitable diet, rest, and so on. The attempt by orthodox medicine to eradicate childhood diseases is a sign of ignorance and naivity, Dr. Scheibner contends. The moving forces behind the ritual of vacci-nation are ignorance, irrational fear of illness, and greed.[37]

A group of Swiss doctors seem to concur with Dr. Scheibner's recommen-dations: "We have lost the common sense and the wisdom that used to prevail in the approach to childhood diseases. Too often, instead of reinforcing the organism's defences, fever and symptoms are relentlessly suppressed. This is not always without consequences."[38]

Perhaps the most startling conclusion Dr. Scheibner came to is this: "An extensive study of medical literature reveals that there is no evidence whatsoever of the ability of vaccines to prevent any diseases. To the contrary, there is a great wealth of evidence (direct and indirect) that they cause serious side ef-fects."[39]

Dr. Scheibner later makes a still stronger statement as a result not only of her research into medical literature on vaccinations but her personal research into the breathing patterns of infants before, during, and after stress. Using a micro-processor-based breathing monitor developed by biomedical electronics engineer Leif Karlsson, she and Karlsson discovered that when babies were under stress—whether due to "insult" (vaccinations), cutting teeth, or incubating ill-ness—their breathing changed to episodes of stress-induced or low-volume breathing that occurred in clusters at critical hours while asleep. They found that following DPT vaccinations babies' breathing patterns showed a lot of stress, which continued over a period of at least 45 to 60 days following the injections. This stress-induced breathing pattern was reflected in flare-ups, some-times major, occurring on certain days after the injections. Even though the amplitude of the flare-ups differed, there was a remarkable uniformity with re-spect to the days on which they occurred.

At the time she and Karlsson were doing this research, Dr. Scheibner was not aware of the controversy surrounding vaccination; but after learning from par-ents, who had their babies monitored, that a previous baby had died of SIDS (called "cot death" in Australia) after DPT injection, they realized that a great number of SIDS deaths followed DPT injections. Thus began her "search for the truth" through thousands of pages of scientific journals and other publications on the effectiveness and dangers of vaccines. She concluded:

Immunisations, including those practised on babies, not only did not prevent any infec-tious diseases, they caused more suffering and more deaths than has any other human activity in the entire history of medical intervention. It will be decades before the mop-ping-up after the disasters caused by childhood vaccination will be completed. All vac-cinations should cease forthwith and all victims of their side-effects should be appropriately compensated.[40]

TABLE 3. OLD VERSUS NEW IMMUNOLOGY

OLD IMMUNOLOGY	NEW IMMUNOLOGY
1. Immune system is a security system, a fortress built to attack and defend.	1. Immune system is a cognitive network, a circulating nervous system.
2. Immune system is heteronomous (outer-directed), a defensive device built to address external events.	2. Immune system is autonomous (self-directed), an assertive, distributive network whose purpose is to establish and maintain molecular identity.
3. Immune process is event centered with emphasis on specificity. Antigen is the determinant.	3. Immune process is network centered, with emphasis on coordination. Adaptive and integrative responses of the organism are the determinants.
4. Immunity is antigen-centered (input-output), with a one-to-one correspondence between antigen and antibody.	4. Immunity is organism-centered (autonomy), with the antigen but a small perturbation in a rich and ongoing network.
5. Effects of antigen are generally predictable— antibody production.	5. Effects of antigen are varied and dependent upon context of network.
6. High antibody count indicative of immunity.	6. High antibody count may indicate immune failure. Full expression of generalized inflammatory response necessary for the development of immunity.
7. Focuses on isolating and controlling mechanisms of disease.	7. Focuses on totality of the person and the larger context of his/her life.

TABLE 3. (Continued)

OLD IMMUNOLOGY	NEW IMMUNOLOGY
8. Uses artificial situations to stimulate a single response—antibody production. Massive amounts of concentrated antigens are injected directly into the bloodstream, or, as in the case of oral vaccines, are designed for rapid penetration from the intestines into the bloodstream.	8. Uses—or may mimic—natural events which mobilize the entire system. Spaces antigenic challenges as they occur in nature and enters them into the system by way of food or drink.
9. Disease is threatening, something to be avoided at all costs.	9. Disease is part of the adaptive process of the whole organism.
10. Childhood diseases can be dangerous and must be prevented by the use of vaccines.	10. Childhood diseases lead to immune competence when contracted at a suitable age and immune system is given nutritional and homeopathic support.
11. Aims for disease-specific immunity.	11. Aims for "broad-spectrum" immunity.
12. Views certain microorganisms as pathogenic (disease causing), which must be destroyed.	12. Views microorganisms as "indicators," aspects of a fundamental "life particle" which cannot be destroyed, only changed.
13. Disease is many, each disease being a separate and distinct entity.	13. Disease is one, all diseases having a common functional-dysfunctional principle
14. Atomistic and adversarial.	14. Holistic and unifying.

NOTES

1. Christopher Bird, *The Galileo of the Microscope* (*The Life and Trials of Gaston Naessens*) (St. Lambert, Quebec: Les Presses de l'Universite de la Personne, 1990), p. 42.

2. Ibid., p. 43.

3. Ibid., p. 30.

4. Ibid., pp. 33–34.

5. Ibid., pp. 35–36.

6. Christopher Bird, *The Persecution and Trial of Gaston Naessens* (Tiburon, CA: H. J. Kramer, 1991). This is the American edition of the book referred to in note 1. There are four additional chapters describing later sociopolitical developments.

7. Bird, *The Galileo of the Microscope*, p. 141.

8. Ibid., p. 36.

9. Peter Tocci, "From Bechamp's Microzyma to the Somatid Theory," *Health Consciousness*, October 1991, p. 34.

10. Bird, *The Galileo of the Microscope*, p. 38.

11. Gaston Naessens, *Somatidian Orthobiology*, prod. Tele-université du Québec, Université du Québec, video.

12. Bird, *The Galileo of the Microscope*, p. 35.

13. Tocci, "From Bechamp's Microzyma," p. 35.

14. Michael Sheehan, "What Your Doctor Doesn't Know Can Kill You," *New Frontier*, July–August 1992, p. 10.

15. Harvey Bigelsen, "To Do More Good Than Harm . . . ," *Health Freedom News*, June 1993, p. 15; also see Sheehan, "What Your Doctor Doesn't Know," p. 10.

16. Sheehan, "What Your Doctor Doesn't Know," pp. 11, 12.

17. Barry Lynes, *The Cancer Cure That Worked!* (Queensville, Ontario: Marcus Books, 1987), p. 134.

18. Sheehan, "What Your Doctor Doesn't Know," p. 11.

19. Bigelsen, "To Do More Good Than Harm," p. 17.

20. Francisco J. Varela and Mark Anspach, "Immu-knowledge, the Process of Somatic Individuation," in *Gaia 2, Emergence, The New Science of Becoming*, ed. William Irwin Thompson (Hudson, NY: Lindisfarne Press, 1991), pp. 70–83.

21. Ibid., pp. 71, 70.

22. Ibid., p. 78.

23. Ibid., p. 76.

24. Stuart Close, *The Genius of Homoeopathy*, (Calcutta: Haren & Brother, 1967); quoted by Mary Coddington, *In Search of the Healing Energy* (New York: Warner/Destiny Books, 1978), p. 88.

25. Varela and Anspach, "Immu-knowledge," p. 79.

26. Ibid., p. 83.

27. Deepak Chopra, "Quantum Healing" (talk given at Conference for "Visions of the Future," May 19, 1991, Seattle, WA).

28. Bill Moyers, *Healing and the Mind*, PBS, WHRO-TV, February 22, 1993.

29. Chopra, "Quantum Healing."

30. Joseph Chilton Pearce, "Evolution, Intelligence and the Future," *New Dimensions* Radio, WHRV-FM, September 24, 1993.

31. Letter from Dr. Mendelsohn sent to help parents who objected to having their child vaccinated but were being pressured by "authorities" to have it done.

32. Francisco J. Varela, *Principles of Biological Autonomy* (New York: Elsevier/North-Holland, 1979), pp. 228–237.

33. Viera Scheibner, *Vaccination: The Medical Assault on the Immune System* (Maryborough, Victoria, Australia: Australian Print Group, 1993), p. 240.

34. Ibid., p. 241.
35. Ibid., back cover; also discussion on p. 259.
36. Ibid., p. 259.
37. Ibid.
38. Ibid., p. 89.
39. Ibid., p. 137.
40. Ibid., p. xv.

8 Holism, Epidemics, and Preventive "Medicine"

> We are completely, firmly, absolutely connected with all of existence,
> and . . . the next evolutionary step will involve, at the least, our realizing
> that connection.
>
> —George Leonard,
> *The Silent Pulse*

HOLISM

Is the universe a machine, a battlefield, a thought, or an organism? The metaphor we choose will organize and direct our thinking about ourselves and our relationship to the world around us. The metaphor of the universe as a thought or an organism is, of course, most compatible with the newer holistic models of reality. "Many levelled mind" (Fritjof Capra) and "a great thought" (Sir James Jeans) are some of the terms physicists have used to describe the universe. Physician Lewis Thomas sees our world as a cell. Chemist and inventor James Lovelock sees our planet as a living being whose biosphere and atmosphere constitute a single living system. (He terms this the "Gaia Hypothesis.")

The universe is not only alive and intelligent, but it is a web of interconnections: "Quantum interconnectedness" (John Bell) and "unbroken wholeness" (David Bohm) are again some of the terms physicists have used to describe it. In the world of microorganisms "every creature is, in some sense, connected to and dependent upon the rest," Lewis Thomas points out.[1] Nothing can be understood in isolation; everything is a part of an interrelated, interacting system according to General Systems Theory; and I would add ecology and holistic healing, our concerns here.

I include ecology with holistic healing because, in a sense, holistic healing is the ecological approach to understanding and working with the body. It means seeing any part only in relation to a larger whole, for example, an organ or a function in relation to other organs and functions of the body, and the body in relation to an environment and a lifestyle. Holism is essentially contextuality.

The contextuality of holistic healing has come to mean studying and working with the patient as a whole—her spirit, mind, and emotions as well as her body. I avoid using the term *treating* and use instead the term *working with* because this latter implies conscious participation in the healing process that is one of the distinguishing features of holistic healing, because the primary focus of a holistic doctor is the consciousness of his patient rather than the symptoms of her disease.

The implication here is that mind is the central factor in any healing process. There is abundant evidence that belief in a therapeutic modality is a primary component of the effectiveness of that modality. Medical and anthropological literature is replete with stories of people who have been healed—and "killed"—by the pronouncements of witch doctors in whom they believed. "Now we know that the brain and immune system are 'hard wired' together. Not only are there direct central nervous system links which modulate the expression of immunocompetence, but immune reactions alter brain activity as well.[2] The new science of psychoneuroimmunology—the study of how the central nervous system affects the immune system—shows that the state of one's mind is reflected by the state of one's immune system.[3] It's no longer news that stress impairs the functioning of the immune system and that emotional distress is implicated as one of the causes of disease, infectious as well as degenerative.

Can a physician regard himself as holistic who insists upon giving a patient a treatment he doesn't want? The question seems absurd on the face of it, yet there are doctors who call themselves holistic who think it not inconsistent to disregard a patient's wishes with respect to a treatment. For example, I talked with a woman from Wisconsin who told me she phoned a well-known medical doctor in this area (Virginia Beach) who was listed in several health care publications as a holistic doctor, having had a position of leadership in two holistic health organizations. She and her family were living in Wisconsin and were considering moving to Virginia when she phoned the doctor. She asked him if they chose him for their family doctor, would he exempt the children from the state vaccination requirement? She made it clear that she had studied the matter and did not want her children vaccinated. He told her he would insist that they have at least the polio and tetanus shots!

Why are holism and coercion contradictory? Because coercion excises the patient's mind and spirit from the health or healing process. Coercion is the ultimate assertion of the ego—of hubris and separation—because it treats "the other" as an object. The one who coerces says in effect, "It is okay for me to manipulate you for an end that my superior knowledge, position, or power deems 'right.' ' '

The root of the word *holism* means "holy." According to Marcus Bach, it comes from the Greek word *hololes*, meaning holy, sacred, complete, and implies regarding the other as a holy being, a spiritual entity.[4]

Holism is not new. It is actually a rebirth and a reintegration of the paradigm of holism that reigned prior to the Middle Ages. The functions of teacher, physician, and priest were considered as one, and a healer functioned in all three capacities because he worked with the whole person—the spirit (priest), the mind (teacher), the body (physician). These functions became separated during the Middle Ages with the advent of specialization, and the totality of the individual was lost.[5] Now these functions are beginning to converge, and we see the holistic healer becoming a caring teacher-partner who regards his patients as "holy beings." This perception of "the other" as a holy being who is spiritually inseparable from ourselves is the bedrock upon which we experience "reverence for all life."

If the universe is indeed more like an organism—or a thought—than a collage of disparate objects, then what is implied when a sizable number of people manifest a similar set of symptoms within a specific space–time frame? Let's take a second look at that frightening and puzzling phenomenon known as an epidemic.

EPIDEMICS AND PREVENTIVE "MEDICINE"

"When I use a word, it means just what I choose it to mean—neither more nor less," Humpty Dumpty told Alice.

—Lewis Carroll,
Alice in Wonderland

What is an epidemic? If we lived in Europe in the fourteenth century (around 1350) and we heard of an epidemic of plague, we would know that as many as 75 percent of the people in a given community could be affected. If we lived in the United States in the middle of the twentieth century (around 1950) and we heard of an epidemic of polio, it could mean that as few as .02 percent (1 out of every 5,000) could be affected. Here we will define an epidemic as a set of similar symptoms affecting a noticeable proportion of the population in a given community or communities.

Let's look at some of the more dramatic epidemics, both historical and current, remembering the inevitable distortions that inhere within the act of reporting itself. By looking at these reports, some instructive inferences can be drawn.

That Bug Going Around

The influenza epidemic of 1918 is one of the more dramatic and puzzling epidemics of history. According to an article in the *Los Angeles Times*, it spread to every country of the world, killing an estimated 21 million people and sparing only the Island of St. Helena and Mauritius Island in the Indian Ocean. "Coast Guard searching parties discovered Eskimo villages in remote, inaccessible Alaskan regions that were wiped out to the last adult and child. A British army officer who traveled through northern Persia in 1919 brought a report that in village after village there were no survivors."[6]

"New York City counted 851 deaths in a single day. Chicago did not have enough hearses, and bodies stacked up in the morgues." Dr. Ralph Chester Williams, a former assistant U.S. surgeon general, recalls those fearful days of the 1918 influenza epidemic: "We were swamped with soldiers, sailors, marines and coast guardsmen. They would just collapse in streets downtown and were brought out to us. . . . There was a Marine sergeant. He was brought in unconscious and in three hours that man was dead. Just like that. It was common knowledge that between 400 and 500 people were dying in Chicago each day. More people were dying than could be buried."[7]

The cause—or causes—of this tragedy has been speculated upon but never, to my knowledge, fully resolved. A discussion of this epidemic in the *Journal of the American Medical Association* (September 11, 1920) points out that "those under 35 died in appalling numbers; those over 55 seemed to be relatively safe."[8] This is a reversal of the age incidence of previous influenza epidemics in which the age group most affected was over 55.

What would cause this age incidence reversal? What circumstance was common to people under 35 that was not common to people over 55? Vaccination comes immediately to mind, especially vaccination against typhoid, which was introduced in 1909. People under 35, servicemen, and young women working in munitions factories died in large numbers from influenza; they would be more inclined to be vaccinated than older segments of the population. However, throughout history, plagues have nearly always followed in the wake of war, varying in intensity to the degree that the sanitary and hygienic conditions of the population were healthy or unhealthy.[9] The far-reaching ravages of the influenza epidemic may possibly be explained by the distribution of military campaigns in widely diversified areas. (The number of deaths attributed to this epidemic varies considerably according to reportage.)[10] Water pollution and bacterial modification of typhoid to influenza are possible causes suggested by some researchers.[11]

Whatever the cause, a relatively simple treatment proved to be remarkably effective in curing it. This treatment involves no drugs or medication of any kind, and although simple, it is time-consuming. Probably for these reasons, it was not used by medical doctors.

Dr. R. Lincoln Graham, a naturopathic physician of that period and a recognized authority on hydrotherapy, discusses in his book on that subject how he treated over 400 cases of the flu without a single loss of life. He also tells how during the great diphtheria epidemic in Berlin in 1900 he treated 28 cases of diphtheria without a single fatality. He treated these cases in a clinic operated by a Dr. Guenther who, seeing the remarkable results of this treatment, tried to get the Charities Hospital to adopt this simple yet effective therapy. Dr. Guenther was unsuccessful, and thousands throughout the city died.

Dr. Graham's treatment for flu consists of four basic steps: (1) No food until the disease is over, (2) a glass of water every hour, preferably spring water, (3) an enema or high-colonic irrigation every day, (4) a cold, wet pack around the chest in case of symptoms of pneumonia.

"When I first read this remarkable book," Dr. Wright, another naturopathic physician, said in reference to Dr. Graham's book, "I could scarcely believe the astounding results reported, but since I have been putting his methods into practice the results have never once been disappointing; they are almost routine." He then tells of the first time he tried Dr. Graham's method:

I was called to the home where a six-year old child lay dying of pneumonia. The attending physician told me, 'This child will die before morning.' However, I began the hydrotherapy treatment and within the hour the most remarkable change took place. She had been extremely constipated, was too weak to cough up the mucous that was half choking her, and constantly moaned in pain.

Soon the moans stopped; her bowels moved three times normally and the strangling mucous poured out of her. Her temperature gradually dropped from 104.5° to 97°, and the next morning this dying child was well—completely well! It taught me a great lesson and reinforced my belief in Dr. Graham's methods, which I have continued to use.[12]

How does this treatment relate to the ideas of holistic healing discussed earlier? Holism or contextuality can be applied to micro- as well as macroorganismic life. Lewis Thomas tells us that microbes "live together in dense, interdependent communities, feeding and supporting the environment for each other ... " and that "we can no more isolate one from the rest, and rear it alone, than we can keep a single bee from drying up like a desquamated cell when removed from the hive."[13] Not only are bacteria "groupies," so to speak, they are also, in a sense, chameleons, reflecting an environment from which they are inseparable. Each type of bacteria "has been studied as a pure culture only by isolating it upon a specific nutrient called media," Christopher Bird tells us. "While outside a host or body, bacteria are hard to raise, or culture."[14] It's pertinent to note that to culture bacteria, dead or decaying food must be used.[15]

What does this tell us about rhetoric that refers to "that bug going around" and germs that "attack" people? Isn't it more holistic to think of a substance—which includes microorganisms—that enters the ecological system of either a single body or a community of bodies? If the substance is in a state of decay, the microorganisms will be pathogenic. To the degree that the life-support system of either an individual or a community is unbalanced and toxic, to that degree will the intrusion of foreign substances accelerate pathological change. To the degree that the ecology of the body or community is balanced and "clean," that is, free of accumulated waste material, to that degree will pathogenic bacterial processes be reversed or nullified. The hydrotherapy treatments of Drs. Graham and Wright illustrate that when the body is internally cleansed, pathogenic bacteria have nothing more to feed upon and the disease process reverses itself.

The relationship between imbalance and toxicity is perhaps best illustrated by nutrition. The current emphasis on whole, natural, unadulterated food is part of the contextual thinking that characterizes holism. When food is fragmented, it is no longer balanced and can produce toxic metabolic residues in the body. For instance, refined white sugar and flour produce toxic metabolites such as pyruvic acid and abnormal sugars containing five carbon atoms that interfere with cell respiration and eventually the functioning of a part of the body. This begins the degenerative disease process.[16]

Since any kind of adulteration produces imbalances in our bodies, we can think of purification and rebalancing as correctives that will reverse life-threatening disease processes. To rebalance is, in a sense, to purify, and vice versa. In the next two illustrations we will see how it is possible to create imbalances in the ecosystem by introducing poisons into the system and how it is possible to compensate, to a certain extent, for the adulteration of one part of the life-support system by rebalancing another part of that system.

What's Going Around?

Let's look at symptoms for a moment. Can you guess what disease entities are characterized by these symptoms?

1. Begins with high fever and aching bones. Many cases, after about four days, develop pneumonia. The lungs of victims fill with fluid, causing death.[17]

2. Headache, nausea, vomiting, general malaise, and dizziness.[18]

3. Sharp, recurrent pains in the muscles of the neck, thorax, and shoulders; severe headache; and disturbance in coordination with some motor and sensory disturbances.[19]

4. Unexplained headaches, great thirst, nausea, vomiting, abdominal cramps, diarrhea, seizures that are not epileptic.[20]

The first group of symptoms were the symptoms of the 1918 flu epidemic. The second and third groups of symptoms are the symptoms of pesticide poisoning—the second being the early symptoms of dieldrin poisoning, the third being typical of mysterious "diseases" that occur in heavily sprayed areas, according to chemist and agricultural expert Leonard Wickenden. The fourth group of symptoms are some of the symptoms of early fluoride poisoning, which can occur even at the recommended concentration of 1 part per million for municipal drinking water.

In a recent Hearing, before a Pesticide Committee, a noted medical doctor (Granville Knight), stated under oath that Monitor–4 is of the same chemical family as the defoliants used in Vietnam; the waves of so-called "Virus-X" and similar diseases . . . are caused by exposure to such agricultural chemicals; that it is impossible for doctors to diagnose the difference between London Flu, Virus Conditions, and Pesticide Poisonings![21]

As recently as July 15, 1985, *U.S. News and World Report* came out with an article entitled "Is the Food You Eat Dangerous to Your Health?", which said that American farmers use 1 billion pounds of insecticides every year—nearly four and a half pounds for every man, woman, and child in the United States.[22] That same month, I heard on the news (July 6, 1985) that 300 people had been stricken with flulike symptoms from pesticide-poisoned watermelon grown in California.

Interpreting symptoms of pesticide poisoning as "that bug going around" has been going on for well over 40 years. Dr. F. L. Mickle wrote in the *Connecticut Health Bulletin* (January 1952):

Virus diseases which appear to be increasing are coming to the foreground. They are of much greater importance in the State than formerly. For instance, almost every person you meet on the street or in the homes of your friends speaks at one time or another of having had the "virus that's going around." . . . These viruses cause distressing and incapacitating *upper respiratory symptoms* often accompanied by *diarrhea* and *vomiting*.[23]

The above are some of the symptoms of DDT and related pesticide poisoning. So-called infectious hepatitis has been linked to chlordane poisoning,[24] and as I pointed out in Chapter 4, epidemics of poliomyelitis have been linked to DDT poisoning. Although I am tempted to say that viruses appear sometimes to be the all-purpose dodge, "it should be pointed out that not only may a toxic agent which damages a particular organ simulate infectious disease, but the damaged organ is more susceptible to transmissible agents, if exposure occurs."[25]

How can injury be repaired? What therapy supports the health and vitality of the whole person? What remedial measures can be taken to support the health of the soil and the environment after they have been damaged by toxic agricultural chemicals? The first step, of course, is to eliminate further exposure to the toxin. In the case of injured people, a number of doctors have found the "administration of intensive, complete and persistent nutritional therapy is essential" to repair liver damage. This includes vitamins, liver supplements, lipotropic (fat-utilizing) factors, and a high-protein diet.[26] To heal the soil, organic composting and mulching can be applied.

Are there any preventive measures we can take before exposure to toxic substances? "Medical literature is filled with reports on studies which show that vitamin C can neutralize and destroy toxins in the body and increase the body's resistance to virtually any bacterial toxins as well as drug insults," Dr. Paavo Airola informs us.[27] As with other poisons, immunizations destroy vitamin C in the body. Along with high doses of vitamin C, Dr. Airola recommends garlic, vitamins A and the B complex, the minerals zinc and calcium, as well as certain herbs for several weeks *prior to* and *after* immunizations of infants or children. He recommends this to parents who, after examining the evidence, *choose* to have their children immunized.[28]

In his fascinating and highly readable book *Every Second Child*, Dr. Archie Kalokerinos describes how he found that by giving infants vitamin C *before* they were immunized, SIDS could be eliminated. The book title refers to the fact that as many as 50 percent of the infants in some aboriginal communities in Australia died, usually of SIDS.[29]

"Have you taken an antioxidant today?" pharmacist and nutritionist Earl Mindell asks. He points out that vitamins are our first line of defense against toxic substances. The antioxidants—vitamins A, C, and E and the mineral selenium—are particularly effective.[30]

"The Last Epidemic"

Currently the "epidemic" near the top of our list of concerns is one that has been called "The Last Epidemic." This, of course, is the poisoning from radioactive fallout following a nuclear war or nuclear power plant accident. As with most projections into the future, the assumption is that everyone will be equally or indiscriminately affected. In the case of radioactive poisoning, the only variable would be distance from the blast or protection by some physical shielding agent.

The radiation sickness and disfiguration that affected the survivers of Hiroshima and Nagasaki are legend, but what is not so well known is the fact that not everyone who was exposed to the radiation suffered radiation poisoning. Some who were only a mile from the center of the blast suffered no ill effects.

At St. Francis Hospital in Nagasaki, which was only a mile from the center of the blast, the entire staff suffered no ill effects. The day after the blast, members of the staff went around the city of Nagasaki to visit and care for the sick in their homes—and in the very part of the city that the Americans had declared would be uninhabitable for the next 20 years! How did they escape? For some time prior to the blast, Dr. Tatsuichiro Akizuki, one of the directors of the hospital, had prepared himself and his coworkers by confining their diet to "yang" foods, in this case, miso soup, brown rice, wakame (seaweed), and Hokkaido pumpkin. The strict macrobiotic diet they had lived on apparently protected them. According to macrobiotic theory, nuclear radiation is extremely "yin"; therefore, an extremely "yang" diet is needed to counterbalance it.

Stories of people who recovered from radiation sickness by adopting the macrobiotic diet are sometimes dramatic. A 50-year-old woman in Hiroshima who was near the center of the blast and whose body was burned and penetrated by about 50 glass fragments, recovered by following a strict macrobiotic diet. For one year after the blast, she had a continuous discharge of very black blood from her uterus. Gradually new blood formed, and all the pieces of glass, which were deeply embedded in her body, came to the surface and were removed one by one. At the time her story was written (1979), she was in excellent health.[31]

Later researchers have found other nutritional aids helpful in assisting the body to neutralize the harmful effects of radiation. Some of these are as follows: natural iodine, particularly that found in seaweeds such as kelp; algin, also found in kelp; calcium; vitamin B_6; the B complex as found in Brewer's yeast and liver; vitamin C, including the bioflavinoids and rutin; protein; pectin as found in sunflower seeds; and pure, nonfluoridated water.[32] Vitamin E has been effective in protecting people from X-ray burns and scarring when taken internally and applied to the surface *before* exposure.[33] In fact, all remedies discussed are most effective taken before exposure and could be called preventive medicine. Also, with this kind of preventive medicine, we could say that what will prevent will also cure.

The Endemic

In an old church in Amsterdam, a "hiding church" that was once used by religious liberals escaping persecution, a historic meeting took place. "Only this time it was quite a different group of free thinkers who met, not to discuss religious freedom, but to question and to denounce the 'authorized version' of the disease called the greatest public health threat of the century: AIDS," writes Bob Owen in the August 1992 issue of *Health Consciousness*. Among the attendees were "three dozen renowned scientists, doctors, practitioners, patients, and journalists—along with nearly 400 vitally interested spectators."

Titled "AIDS: A Different View," the article goes on to say, "the May 14–16 Symposium's announced purpose was to define and discuss the syndrome's multiple causes and co-factors." Some of the highlights of the presentations were (1) the refutation of the HIV-AIDS hypothesis by molecular biology, by epidemiology, and by Koch's first hypothesis (for a specific organism to cause a specific disease, "the microorganism must be observed in all cases of the disease"); (2) mounting evidence implicating syphillis as the predisposing factor or cofactor in the immune suppression found in AIDS; (3) the importance of nutrition in affecting immune function; and (4) the implication of drugs, both recreational and prescription, including drugs used to treat the disease, as the real cause of AIDS. This latter view was expressed by Peter Duesberg, professor of molecular biology at the University of California and one of the world's foremost microbiologists, who is one of the most outspoken of the anti-HIV campaigners:

"The cause of AIDS is not sexual activity or associated with viral and microbial infections, all of which we have learned to live with in the last three billion years of life," Duesberg said. "Natural and synthetic psychoactive drugs are the only new pathogens around since the 1970's, and the only disease syndrome around is AIDS, and both are found in exactly the same populations." "Long term drug use," he told conferees, "is at the heart of immune-system dysfunction."

Duesberg and others at the conference who challenged the HIV-AIDS hypothesis are joined by a number of other researchers throughout the world who have observed that many perfectly healthy people test HIV positive, and many full-blown AIDS cases test HIV negative.[34] (The AIDS test doesn't test for the HIV virus but for its antibodies.)

Like the influenza virus that was said to be the cause of the 1918 Spanish flu epidemic, the HIV virus is a normal inhabitant of our blood.[35] But the medical (or allopathic) model demands single-mode causes. Rather than asking the obvious, which is, What cofactors or host-induced predisposition causes these viruses to become harmful? the medical model looks for a microscopic enemy to attack. The name AIDS, itself, which means acquired immunodeficiency syndrome, answers the question. The host-induced predisposition that causes these viruses to mutate into a harmful form is a weakened or damaged immune system.

What causes the immune system to become weakened to the point where an opportunistic infection (*opportunistic* means takes advantage of a poorly functioning immune system) like AIDS can begin to destroy it? Or we might rephrase this to ask, What immunosuppressive factors in our lifestyle and/or environment predispose us to developing AIDS?

Before attempting to answer these questions, we need to get clear about what AIDS is and isn't. The official view is that AIDS is a single disease entity like cancer or polio, but in the view of other researchers, it is a collection of symptoms and/or diseases that have been with us for a very long time. In a 1988 interview in *Spin* magazine, Peter Duesberg affirms this latter view,[36] as does Gary Null, who said that AIDS is really 29 different disease states.[37] Many of the symptoms that have been labeled AIDS are the same symptoms as poisoning from drugs and agricultural and industrial chemicals as are a number of old diseases such as certain forms of cancer, pneumonia, syphillis, and various parasittic and fungal infections that have also come under the AIDS umbrella.[38]

Researcher Dr. Alan Cantwell points to AIDS as simply a form of cancer because both are "caused" by similar-appearing acid-fast bacteria that are found in the affected tissues of both diseases. However, these same bacteria, which Cantwell calls the "cancer microbe," are found within the blood and tissues of all human beings, both healthy and sick, as well as in animals. This microbe— call it HIV or the cancer microbe—is highly pleomorphic, so much so that making a vaccine would be next to impossible. (Dr. Robert Strecker says there are millions of AIDS viruses.)[39] Cantwell quotes several researchers who think that some viruses may be part of the life cycle of a bacterium or a deficient form of it. Some of these researchers describe a "specific life cycle" of the cancer organism very much like the work of Rife and Naessens discussed earlier.[40]

The AIDS virus is chameleonlike. It changes as it reacts with our tissues.[41] So what changes in our tissues cause this harmless virus to mutate into a pathologic form? We're back to our original questions of what factors in our lifestyle and/or environment compromise the immune system.

1. *The drug connection.* Drugs, both licit (prescription and over-the-counter) and illicit (recreational or street) have been most consistently indicted, not only by Duesberg but others as well. Cantwell points to antibiotic therapy, chemotherapy, and radiation (this latter is not a drug, of course, but operates on the same principle—search and destroy).[42] Besides antibiotics, other researchers have pointed to corticosteroids, birth control pills, and synthetic hormones.[43] (Long-term antibiotic treatment unbalances the internal ecology of the body, allowing harmful bacteria to proliferate in the gastrointestinal tract, which, in turn, depresses immune function. But nearly all drugs, including even aspirin, are, in varying degrees, immunosuppressive.)

What about the cytotoxic, immune-destroying drug AZT (azidothymidine) and other experimental drugs used to treat AIDS?

Item: John Kuivenhoven was misdiagnosed as having AIDS. He stopped working, and for six years he lived in a nether world of experimental drugs and their painful side effects, waiting to die. When he finally discovered he never had AIDS, his health was shattered and his livelihood lost.[44]

"If the truth were known there are probably more people dying of the treatment than the disease," writer and researcher Michael Culbert says.[45] The effect of toxic, immunosuppressive drugs like AZT coupled with the immunosuppressive but "politically correct" negative prognosis could easily add up to death-from-treatment although recorded as death-from-AIDS. For how many other diseases is this also true?

Recreational drugs such as marijuana, cocaine, and heroin are known immune suppressors, as are the amphetamines,[46] but some of the most potent immune depleters are "poppers," nitrite inhalants such as amyl nitrite and isobutyl nitrite, used by many homosexual men as an orgasm enhancer and muscle relaxant. This has been suggested as one possible explanation for the apparently higher incidence of AIDS among gay men in the United States.[47] Others would say it is the primary, if not the real, reason for the higher incidence of AIDS among gay men.

2. *The vaccine connection.* As we learned in Chapter 2, mass vaccination programs, particularly those involving live virus vaccines, have been clearly implicated in the increase in immunological and neurological disorders during the past 40 or 50 years. We also learned that because of the phenomenon of transcession these vaccines work immunosuppressively. The toxic chemicals used as preservatives and foreign proteins from the animal tissues in which the viruses are cultured would also add to the immunosuppressive effect.

At this time there are three vaccines specifically linked to the AIDS outbreak:

the polio vaccine, the smallpox vaccine, and the hepatitis B vaccine. Let's begin with the polio vaccine.

"AIDS: Immunization Related Syndrome" was the title of a cover story appearing in the July 1987 issue of *Health Freedom News*.[48] Its author Dr. Eva Lee Snead, described her breakthrough research linking contaminated batches of polio vaccines with AIDS. What were the vaccines contaminated with? A virus, Simian Virus–40 or SV–40, which is found in the tissues of African green monkeys. Remember, the polio virus was cultured on monkey kidney tissue. This virus, which is similar to HIV, is a powerful immunosuppressor, Dr. Snead says, and activator of HIV. It causes a clinical syndrome indistinguishable from AIDS as well as birth defects, leukemia, and other malignancies.

Over 30 years ago I remember reading "horror" stories of the slaughter of thousands—50,000 as I recall—of monkeys to make Salk vaccine, and now I was reading of "a recently discovered virus, unwittingly put into hundreds of thousands, if not millions, of doses of early Salk vaccine." This unknown virus is, of course, SV–40 and the publication is *Science Digest*, 1963.[49] Arthur J. Snider, the author of "Near Disaster with the Salk vaccine," downplays the seriousness of the situation, but I couldn't help thinking as I read Dr. Snead's article, "If AIDS isn't Falwell's revenge for our sexual sins, could it be the monkey's revenge for our cruelty?"

Before leaving Dr. Snead and going on to another substantiating event, some quotations from various professional journals cited in her article are worth noting: "Scientific data have been reviewed which show that the problem of the oncogenic [tumor causing] potential of live virus vaccines should be regarded as an urgent one." "It appears from what has been said that infectious disease and malnutrition are so inextricably interwoven with each other that any attempt to deal with them separately . . . is as futile as trying to separate the effects of heredity and environment." And finally an article from *Public Health Reports* (77, no. 2 [February 1962]) titled "Survey of Childhood Malignancies" points out that "children between the ages 2 and 4 years of age have been more affected by the unfavorable trend of leukemia mortality than any other age group under 70 years." Particularly ironic was the statement that "the recent increase in leukemia deaths happened sooner in technically advanced countries" and that the determining factor was not affluence but "the availability of medical services."[50]

"Smallpox Vaccine 'Triggered Aids Virus' " was the title of a front-page article in *The Times* of London, May 11, 1987. An adviser to the World Health Organization (WHO), the organization that masterminded the 13-year vaccination campaign that ended in 1980, told *The Times*: "I thought it was just a coincidence until we studied the latest findings about the reactions which can be caused by Vaccinia [smallpox vaccine]. Now I believe the smallpox vaccine theory is the explanation to the explosion of Aids."[51]

The smallpox vaccine theory accounts for a number of phenomena: First, the seven central African states most affected are the same states where the most intensive immunization programs were carried out. Second, Brazil, the only South American country covered in the immunization campaign, had the highest incidence of AIDS in that region. Third, there is less sign of infection among 5- to 11-year-olds in Central Africa. Fourth, AIDS is associated with homosexuality in the West, whereas in Africa it is spread more evenly among males and females. Explanation: About 14,000 Haitians who were with the United Nations armed services in Africa were covered in the immunization program. They returned home when Haiti had become a popular playground for San Francisco homosexuals. Fifth, the AIDS organism previously regarded by scientists as "weak, slow and vulnerable" began to behave with the strength capable of creating a plague. Explanation: The use of live virus vaccines, like that used for smallpox, can activate dormant virus infections such as the human immunodeficiency virus (HIV) associated with AIDS.

Because this theory would be devastating not only to the WHO but to other public health campaigns for immunizations as well as the continued use of smallpox vaccine in AIDS research, many experts are reluctant to support it. *The Times* mollifies its readers by pointing out that the 13-year smallpox eradication campaign saved 2 million lives a year and 15 million infections with a global saving of $1,000 million a year. As we learned earlier (Chapter 3), where these figures come from is anyone's guess.

Item: 1985: Two thirds of the physicians eligible for the hepatitis vaccine refused to take it.[52]

Item: August 1, 1988, 8 A.M. News, WTAR-AM: Doctors are hesitant to treat patients with hepatitis virus vaccine because seven years later they could come down with AIDS.

Item: 1988, Dr. Robert Strecker: Epidemiology of AIDS in the United States corresponds with hepatitis B vaccinations.[53]

Item: December 20, 1991, 8 A.M. News, WHRV-FM: The health department is urging parents to get their children vaccinated with a new vaccine, hepatitis B. (This was in response to an "epidemic" of food poisoning traced to a couple of Mexican restaurants in the area.)

Item: 1993: Hepatitis B vaccine "mandated" for newborn infants. (See Chapter 9.)

Because the hepatitis B vaccine is made from human blood, it can carry pathogens from the donors. The concern has been that because the vaccine is frequently made from the blood of male homosexuals, it can carry the AIDS virus. According to Michael Culbert, HIV was first recognized in the United States about 1979, right after the introduction of the first hepatitis B vaccine for male homosexuals, which was derived exclusively from homosexual carriers of the hepatitis virus. The purpose of the vaccine was to protect male homosexuals from hepatitis infection which is "a very real part of modern medical sequelae of homosexual behavior," he says. The hepatitis B vaccine given to these homosexuals in 1978–1980 in New York City and later elsewhere matched the presumed early AIDS cases.[54]

The connection of these three vaccines—polio, smallpox, and hepatitis B— with AIDS has given rise to conspiracy theories.

3. *The conspiracy connection (?)* Is the AIDS virus a "designer bug" given to selected populations as part of the germ warfare program of "enemy agents"? Were the three vaccines—polio, smallpox, and hepatitis B—intentionally contaminated? Is the AIDS virus taken from an animal reservoir of cattle (bovine leukemia virus) and sheep (visna virus) against which our immune system has no defense? Will this genetically engineered virus destroy our immune systems and "wipe out" whole populations?

A yes answer to these questions will give you roughly the AIDS conspiracy scenario.[55] Like all conspiracy theories—at least the ones I'm familiar with— there must be an enemy and the enemy is "out there." In this case, there are two enemies—a microscopic one (the virus) and the human one (enemy agents).

These ideas are inconsistent with the facts and principles discussed in this book. On the level of "fact" (facts are subject to perceptual interpretation, as are ideas), we know that (1) the immune system can respond to antigens it has never seen, even man-made ones (Chapter 7, Varela); (2) the focus on "bad" viruses is misguided; the form and function of a virus are determined by "conditions," now called "associative" or "cofactors" (Chapters 5 and 7); (3) HIV, officially the AIDS virus, is a normal and harmless inhabitant of the blood (Chapter 8); and (4) AIDS is not the threat we have been told it is, and AIDS patients are being cured by natural methods (discussed shortly).

On the level of principle, we know from physics and ecology that the world is a web of living interconnections and that "bad guys" are continually interacting with "good guys" in a mutually supportive "biodance" (Chapters 5, 6, 7). We also know that on an atomic and subatomic level the line between inner and outer is blurry because the observer continually interacts with what he observes (Heisenberg Uncertainty Principle). In other words, there is no vacuum between subject and object; they are interactive. From psychology, we learn that the "out there" is largely a projection of the "in here" (Chapter 9) and that attention and participation are selective and ultimately subject to choice.

This is the real problem with conspiracy theories. Their worldview tends to be atomizing and Newtonian, which can move us into "adrenal consciousness," the consciousness of separation and enemy making. The world becomes a less friendly place where survival is largely a matter of defense and attack—very much like the vaccination paradigm. This worldview is fear inducing, and fear itself is a powerful immune suppressor.

On the other hand, no one can be active in a field such as alternative health care which promotes ideas that certain powerful vested interests perceive as threatening without becoming aware of organized efforts to suppress and misrepresent those ideas. This can include attacking and prosecuting persons engaged in disseminating and/or using these ideas professionally (Chapters 4, 7, 10, 11, 12). Value, worth, and attested benefit to others are almost never a consideration. So conspiracy theories are not without their truth.

And yes, "the AIDS virus," while having much in common with other viruses, is, according to Michael Culbert, "in its totality a unique structure without precedent in the world."[56] But we might also add that drug and vaccine usage, environmental pollution, and unnatural living habits are also without precedent.

Also, it is a matter of record that the military has conducted experiments—or are they attacks?—on unsuspecting civilian populations, as has organized medicine.[57] We actively support these institutions—their programs, their "research," their requests for money. The enemy is real, but it is us. (More about this in Chapter 14.)

4. *Other immunosuppressive connections.* The *toxic effects of agricultural and industrial chemicals on humans*, discussed earlier in this chapter, has been widely discussed and written about. The term *immunotoxicology*, coined during the late 1970s, studies and describes the effects of these chemicals on various components of the immune system. One of the most toxic and insidious is fluoride, a waste product of the aluminum and chemical fertilizer industries, conveniently disposed of in our water supply for the ostensible purpose of preventing tooth decay. Biochemist John Yiamouyiannis points out that fluoride damages various components of the immune system as well as other components and functions of the body, for example, enzyme production, collagen synthesis (forms connective tissue), and bone formation.[58] As his book *Fluoride: The Aging Factor* was being published, he began tracking data on AIDS. He discovered there were three or four times the number of AIDS cases in cities where the water supply was fluoridated than in cities where it was not.[59]

The *overcrowding, lack of sanitation, and malnutrition associated with poverty* are well-documented immune suppressants (see Chapter 4). Less well known, perhaps, is the malnutrition of the affluent caused by the high intake of refined, chemicalized, overcooked food. These processes not only damage the food so that it doesn't deliver the nutrients needed by the body but leave toxic metabolic residues in the body (discussed earlier in this chapter). Did you know that sugar consumption depresses immune function with remarkable rapidity? As little as 100 grams of sugar (less than .004 of an ounce) reduces immune function by 50 percent within the hour.[60] Another research report shows that this same amount of sugar reduces the efficiency of neutrophils (a component of the immune system) in their phagocytic (cell-eating) function for over five hours after ingestion. The effects of sugar consumption begin within a half an hour and at the peak—about two hours after consumption—there is a loss of phagocytic activity of 50 percent.[61]

And yet the average consumption of sugar in the United States is 130 to 150 pounds per person per year.[62] This is over a half a cup a day! (Most of this is in the form of packaged foods, soda pop being the largest single source.)[63]

Once again, the enemy is us.

5. *The disinformation connection.* "African Aids Plague 'a Myth,' " a front-page article in *The Times* of London (October 3, 1993), describes the dramatic testimony of two medically trained charity workers, Philippe and Evelyne Kry-

nen, who were based at the "epicenter" of the AIDS in Africa. "After five years in charge of 230 staff helping 'Aids orphans' in the Kagera province of northwestern Tanzania, Phillipe and Evelyne Krynen have concluded that stories of Africa being in the grip of a new sexually-transmitted disease are a lie." The article continues with the Krynens' discoveries that the HIV test has nothing to do with AIDS. In fact, there is no connection between HIV positivity and risk of illness. Aids is not a sexually transmitted disease. (This is consistent with a number of other researchers, for example, Robert Strecker, Peter Duesberg.) The so-called orphaned children were orphaned not because their parents had died of AIDS but because they were offspring of polygamous marriages or prostitutes whose parents had abandoned them. The AIDS industry is massive, global, and the major source of fear and disinformation. Statistics are kept inflated by (1) listing people who have symptoms of malnutrition, poisoning, and infections, as AIDS victims and (2) people, including children, saying their parents died of AIDS because by doing so they get food, shelter, care, and support. If they say their father died in an automobile accident, there are no privileges. One must play AIDS victim to have access to care.

Studies elsewhere in Africa showing a close correlation between HIV positivity and risk of illness may be the consequence of health workers and patients giving up hope in the face of an HIV "death sentence," the Krynens think. As pointed out earlier in this chapter—and later in the last section—suggestibility is a powerful factor in any human condition.

Philippe now declares: "There is no Aids. It is something that has been invented. There are no epidemiological grounds for it." And yet this is what the AIDS industry is telling us:

A global catastrophe of unimaginable proportions is happening right under our noses. . . . Aids is the biggest human health problem this planet has ever had to face. (Dr. Patrick Dixon, medical director, AIDS Care Education and Training [ACET])

Up to 5.5 million children under 15 in 10 countries of east and central Africa will be orphaned by the year 2000 if present HIV infection trends continue. (UNICEF)

After pointing to millions it believes have been infected with HIV, Dr. Michael Merson, executive director of WHO global program on AIDS, said, "As this decade progresses, the rising number of Aids cases will bring about increasingly severe social and economic consequences."

But Dr. Timothy Stamps, minister of health and child welfare in Zimbabwe, counters: "The HIV industry, which is multi-million-dollar nationwide, is now in my view one of the biggest threats to health." He goes on to point out that this industry is fostering a damaging epidemic of "HIV-itis" in Africa and that it is diverting money, attention, and personnel from real problems such as malaria, tuberculosis, sexually transmitted diseases, and safe motherhood.

And so the lie goes on, begun and propelled by what Philippe calls "fashion,"[64] and "health" organizations continue their lucrative diseasescare business.

Late flash! On the *Gary Null Show* (June 12, 1994, WNIS-AM), Dr. Robert Wilner, author of the book *The Deadly Deception*, was interviewed. Dr. Wilner said that we have known what causes AIDS in humans for over 70 years. It's in the medical texts. The first edition of the *Merck Manual* published in 1954 lists four primary causes of AIDS: (1) starvation and malnutrition, (2) drugs, (3) radiation, and (4) chemotherapy. It lists a few other very minor causes of AIDS as well.

Citing major research and the work of many distinguished scientists, Dr. Wilner made some startling statements that are contrary to everything we have been told: First, HIV does not cause AIDS. It is a virus that has never been proven to do anything and is found in less than 50 percent of all AIDS patients. Second, AIDS is not contagious. You cannot give it to anyone, and you cannot get it from anyone. Third, AZT is the number-one cause of AIDS in the world. It is 1,000 times more toxic than reported by Burroughs-Wellcome, the company that has made multiple billions of dollars selling it. (AZT destroys the immune system by interfering with the replicating ability of the immune cells.) Fourth, drugs—both doctor-prescribed, which includes AZT, and street drugs—are the number-one cause of AIDS. Fifth, AIDS is not an epidemic. It's an endemic. From 1985 to 1992, 12,000 people (government figures) died each year of AIDS in the United States. In a population of 255 to 270 million people, this is not an epidemic. (Compare this to the well over 1 million people in the United States who get cancer every year.) Sixth, the AIDS scam is the real cause of AIDS. There are well over 500 doctors in the United States who are aware of this, and their number is growing.

Dr. Wilner told shocking stories of news blackouts, hidden agendas, dishonest scientists in Washington, incredibly flawed research, and an irresponsible, criminal FDA. Did you know that Peter Duesberg, the most honored virologist in the world, has had his research grants taken away, and recently the University of California at Berkeley has taken away his laboratory? Why? He was too outspoken. He had the "nerve" to tell what he saw: AIDS in the United States is caused by drugs; in Africa, it is caused by starvation.

So universities must "discipline" their "errant" scientists for not conforming to the line of the Commercial Party.

6. *The healing connection.* Dr. Roger Cochran was dying of AIDS. He had lost 65 pounds and could hardly walk. Although a heavy user of recreational drugs, a habit he became hooked on during his service in Vietnam, he recovered his health by the simplest of natural methods. His story is compellingly told by Bob Owen in *Roger's Recovery from AIDS.*[65]

The story has other unusual features. Instead of taking medically prescribed drugs and going to the hospital where the fatality rate for AIDS patients was virtually 100 percent, Dr. Cochran went to his old friend, Dr. Bob Smith, who had graduated with him from UCLA Medical Center and had served as a physician with him in Vietnam. Dr. Smith was a general practitioner who knew almost nothing about AIDS, but his friend's pleading caused him to undertake a thorough study of the subject. He banished all preconceived notions from his mind in this search for information on AIDS.

On the political side, Dr. Smith found that the publicity given to AIDS was all out of proportion to its incidence, while other deadly diseases were practically ignored. Dr. Smith also discovered that AIDS is not a disease epidemic; it does not destroy the immune system; and the combination of symptoms called AIDS is the result of a ravaged immune system. Opportunistic infections or diseases like AIDS are the body's way of getting rid of toxins a normal immune system would have disposed of.

Among the books Dr. Smith turned to was the classic *Toxemia Explained*, written in 1926 by John H. Tilden. Dr. Tilden made the case that the single cause of disease was a chain of pathology beginning with body saturation of toxic material, which usually consists of dammed-up body wastes and other poisons taken into but uneliminated from the system. What is called disease is essentially the body's effort to free itself from these encumbrances.

Dr. Tilden's recommendations included fasting, bed rest, and giving up enervating habits, mental as well as physical. This would allow nature the chance to eliminate the accumulated toxins. Then, if enervating habits are relinquished and a health-promoting lifestyle is adopted, health will return. This principle applies to any "so-called disease."

So Roger went to Dr. Smith's home for total bed rest in a sunny room with lots of fresh air. He began fasting, alternating between water only and fresh fruit juice. For 35 days he did nothing but drink, urinate, and sleep. His bodily energies were almost totally available for detoxification and restoration.

At the end of 35 days, Dr. Cochran's blood pressure and white cell count were normal. He was pain free and symptom free, and his self-esteem had returned.

Now both Drs. Cochran and Smith are aiding those who have symptoms diagnosed as AIDS. This brings us to one more important discovery Dr. Smith made in his search for an AIDS "cure."

To help an AIDS sufferer, there are three hurdles he must surmount.

1. The patient must recognize that he is responsible for both the condition and the recovery.

2. All contributing causes of the syndrome must be determined and removed.

3. A course of action must be chosen that will enable the body to recuperate its vitality and restore immune function.

This way of thinking and treating disease is known as *natural hygiene*. Its practice, in its purest form, includes a vegan (no meat or animal products) diet of fresh, uncooked, unrefined, organically grown food and periodic short fasts on pure water. In practice, few hygienists can afford to be this strict. Harvey

Diamond and Marilyn Diamond, for instance, recommend short raw food and juice fasts and some cooked food.[66] Moderate exercise and positive thinking are, of course, part of this lifestyle.

Other natural healing systems would say, in effect, that because we live in such an unnatural, polluted world and live such unnatural, sedentary lives that our bodies, including our immune systems, have become weakened and need extra support. Dr. Laurence E. Badgley, author of *Healing AIDS Naturally*, has been successful in treating AIDS patients using nutritional supplementation, homeopathic remedies, herbal therapies, acupuncture, and dietary changes, along with meditation and positive thinking. Also important is teaching patients how to avoid negative cofactors such as nutritional deficiencies, drugs, and *vaccinations*. In common with the hygienists, uncooked "live" food, much of it in the form of freshly squeezed vegetable and fruit juices, is stressed, as is exercise, and the patient's sense of being "in charge" of his or her situation. Mind and spirit are so intimately involved in the healing process, Dr. Badgley feels, that doctors who give their patients death sentences are inhibiting immune function.[67]

"Research is showing that it is impossible for a deviate or unhealthy cell to attach itself to a healthy one. That is why it is so important to maintain a healthy body," Janet Zand says. Dr. Zand, who has treated many viral patients in her practice, uses herbal remedies, diet, and homeopathy. Because extreme fatigue and digestive problems—specifically chronic bowel syndrome—are common with most viral patients, she prescribes acidophilus, for stabilizing the digestive tract, and suma, a South American herb, for building up the patient's strength. Other herbs Zand has used successfully in normalizing elevated lymphocyte levels common in immune-weakened patients are a combination of echinacea, goldenseal, red clover, and burdock.

As for diet: "Sugars and fried foods are lethal for the viral patient," Zand says. She also points to the importance of mental strength as well as physical. "A patient who is surrounded by loving, caring, and positive people will do much better."[68]

These are just a few of the doctors using natural methods who have been successful in treating AIDS. Remember the Koch, Naessens, and Enderlein therapies? The Koch treatment has been resurrected, *in principle*, in the form of hyperoxidation therapies, both oral and intravenous, which have shown impressive results.[69] Again, a common denominator of these therapies is that they work from the inside out, rather than from outside in, as do "adversarial" or drug therapies. In other words, the focus is on building from the inside, strengthening the natural healing energies of the mind-body, rather than fighting something originating outside.

The Mind Connection

No discussion of the relationship between holism and epidemics would be complete without underscoring the pivotal role of the mind. A number of scientists have said that what we call "reality" is perceptual agreement, that is, consensual reality. The world of our interpretation of sensory data is just that—consensual perception. One of the more bizarre epidemics of history illustrates this point, which is, to paraphrase Rupert Sheldrake, that much of what we consider truth or "laws of nature" may be only habits of perception. Our "knowledge" is part of our culture; we see and look for what we "know."

A strange malady occurred during the Middle Ages in the southeastern part of Italy known as Apulia.

People, asleep or awake, would suddenly jump up, feeling an acute pain like the sting of a bee. Some saw the spider, others did not, but they knew that it must be the tarantula. They ran out of the house into the street, to the market place dancing in great excitement. Soon they were joined by others who like them had just been bitten, or by people who had been stung in previous years, for the disease was never quite cured. The poison remained in the body and was reactivated every year by the heat of summer. People were known to have relapsed every summer for thirty years.[70]

"Music and dancing were the only effective remedies, and people were known to have died within an hour or in a few days because music was not available. A member of Dr. Ferdinandus' own family, his cousin, Francesco Franco, died thus within twenty-four hours because no musician could be found after he had been stung."[71] "After having thus danced for a number of days, the people were exhausted—and cured, at least for the time being. But they knew that the poison was in them and that every summer the tunes of the tarantella would revive their frenzy."[72]

Though the malady reportedly continued for several centuries, it wasn't until the seventeenth century that the disease was studied and recorded. The physicians of the day accepted the popular theory that the disease was due to the bite of the tarantula; however, when these same tarantulas were shipped to other parts of the country, they seemed to lose their venom. The spider was venomous in Apulia only. According to one report, a wasp, a rooster, and even the tarantula herself danced whenever she heard the music. However, this phenomenon occurred only in Apulia.

According to another report, a skeptical physician in Naples had himself bitten in the left arm by two Apulian tarantulae in August 1693 before six witnesses and a public notary. The arm became somewhat swollen, but otherwise he felt no ill effects. People rationalized that it was the scorching heat of Apulia that activated the virus and gave it its specific effect; but again, in other countries just as hot as Apulia where the same tarantula occurred, there was no such thing as tarantism (the name given the malady).

The doctors tried the usual treatments of the day: scarifying the wound with a lancet or cauterizing it with a red-hot iron; however, the great majority of the patients had no wound. Internally the doctors gave antidotes such as treacle or brandy. Finally, the doctors had to admit there was no cure except music, not any music, but only the tunes played in Apulia for centuries as the treatment for tarantism. They theorized that the dances created by the music caused the patients to perspire, thereby driving out the poison and curing them—at least for the season. Sometime during the middle of the eighteenth century, the disease died out.[73]

What could have caused this strange malady? Historian Epiphanius Ferdinandus gives us a clue. "He said that according to some people tarantism was not a disease at all, a view that he refuted immediately with the argument that if tarantism was a mere fiction, there would not be so many poor people, and particularly women, spending nearly all their money on the music."[74] Henry Sigerist, medical doctor and historian, apparently unravels the mystery when he suggests that tarantism was a nervous disorder, a kind of neurosis brought about by the conflict between the beliefs and customs of the Greek tradition, which had been strong in Apulia, with the new Christianity that inundated the old culture. The old dieties such as Dionysus, Cybele, and Demeter and the orgiastic rites that were part of their worship were buried; but the primitive instincts and the need to express the emotions associated with them did not disappear. Instead, they became legitimatized in the form of dancing as victims of tarantism. (The similarity of these rites to the symptoms of tarantism is striking.)

The power of the mind and emotions to create and correct disease states has been widely discussed. "Every thought you have creates changes in the body," according to Dr. Norman Shealy.[75] He says that joy increases the strength of the immune system, and sadness or depression decreases the strength of the immune system.[76] Shealy illustrates his point by telling stories of people who, by following a meditation-visualization program, recovered from often serious and incapacitating illnesses. (Counseling, autogenic training, and good nutrition were also part of his program.)

"We use hypnosis like a surgeon uses his scalpel. We cut into a person's psyche to find the root cause of his physical disease. Then we remove it . . . curing the disease," Dr. Pavel Bul, therapist at Leningrad's Pavlov Medical Institute, revealed. He said his studies show conclusively that almost all cases of asthma, allergy, and hypertension have strong emotional roots.[77]

If mind and not matter is primary and if we are all connected in some transpersonal sense, then transfer of mental and emotional states, sometimes called *psychic contagion*, can occur.

In March 1982, I heard on the news that in the previous year Norfolk Catholic High School in Virginia had experienced an epidemic. At first it was called the flu, then doctors suspected carbon monoxide poisoning, and finally an epidemiologist in the area said the disease was psychosocial. People "caught" the disease by seeing their friends get it.

If the thought patterns in our mind affect the thought patterns of all other minds, could consensual reality be thought of as a contagion or confluence of mental images? Quantum theory reveals that we live in an ocean of force fields, that fields generate objects, and that an object is simply a highly concentrated aspect of a field—thought (the field) structures matter (the body). The mind and the images of reality it holds are the pivot upon which the destiny of the body turns; the images of many minds can be the pivot upon which the destiny of a group or even the world turns.

The power of the mind—or is it, more accurately, belief?—to create our reality is nowhere better illustrated than with the AIDS endemic. In the interview with Dr. Wilner, referred to earlier, he pointed to the two major causes of death from AIDS: (1) If a person is told he is HIV positive, he is probably about 50 percent dead just from being told that; it's a death sentence; (2) this is usually followed by taking the doctor's advice and getting on AZT; in this scenario, AIDS is largely an iatrogenic disease caused by the blind belief of both doctor and patient.

Robert Ingersoll once remarked that had he been God he would have made health contagious instead of disease. "When shall we come to recognize that health *is* as contagious as disease," an Indian contemporary responded. Virtue is as contagious as vice, and cheerfulness is as contagious as moroseness, he continued.[78] When the mental images of a community of minds are filled with pictures of health rather than disease, the possibilities for the realization of health become practically limitless. This interconnectedness and blurring of boundaries is beautifully expressed by Dr. Larry Dossey:

Isolated derangements at the level of the atoms simply do not occur. . . . All information is everywhere transmitted. Crisp, causal events that were once thought to characterize each and every human disease fade into endless reverberating chains of happenings. . . . We see the molecular theory of disease causation as an outmoded, picturesque description. Discrete causes never occur in individual bodies for the simple reason that discrete individual bodies do not themselves exist.

Dr. Dossey refers to the "space-time" model of health in which the body is not regarded as an object surrounded by empty space but as a pattern and process whose boundaries are "always fading, reforming, and fading again in the endless round of biodance." Because of the "profound interrelations between consciousness and the physical world," we should strive to maximize rather than minimize the subjective element in the healing process, he points out. Purposeful change can be initiated by patients as well as professional healers. "Each patient has the potential of being his own healer. Healing becomes democratized."[79]

NOTES

1. Lewis Thomas, *The Lives of a Cell* (NY: Bantam Books, 1974), p. 6.

2. From a flier announcing a conference to be given at the New York Academy of Medicine on the subject "Mind and Immunity," April 1982.

3. "Psychoimmunology: For Each State of Mind, a State of Body?" *Brain/Mind Bulletin,* December 10, 1984.

4. Marcus Blach, "Holistic Healing" (lecture at Association for Research and Enlightenment, Virginia Beach, VA, December 29, 1976). Sometimes the word *holism* is

spelled "wholism." The focus here is on the idea of wholeness, the whole person, rather than his consciousness per se or the idea that he is a holy being.

5. Ibid.

6. "Spanish Flu of 1918 Worst Killer of All," Atlanta (UPI), *Los Angeles Times*, January 12, 1969, p. 7.

7. Ibid., p. 7.

8. *Foreign Letters*, "The Great Influenza Epidemic," *Journal of the American Medical Association*, September 11, 1920, p. 755.

9. "It is said that when plagues decimated millions in Europe throughout the Middle Ages, many survived by eating garlic cloves daily. They would disinfect areas by scattering the potent cloves over waste pileups." More recently, Russian doctors cured so many infections with garlic that it has been called "Russian Penicillin." In the 1965 flu epidemic in Russia, a 500-ton emergency shipment of garlic was distributed throughout the danger areas. The government-controlled newspapers urged people to eat more garlic. See Carlson Wade, "Country Kitchen," *Better Nutrition*, March 1982, p. 30.

10. Henry E. Sigerist, *Civilization and Disease* (Ithaca, NY: Cornell University Press, 1943), p. 236. Dr. Sigerist gives us the figure of 10 million lives lost to the influenza epidemic of 1918–1919. Ethyl Hume gives us the figure of 8 million lives lost, excluding China, Japan, South America, and great tracts of Asia and Africa. See Ethyl Douglas Hume, *Bechamp or Pasteur?* (Essex, England: C. W. Daniel Company Limited, 1947), p. 220.

11. Hume, *Bechamp or Pasteur?* pp. 220–226. Also see R. B. Pearson, *Fasting and Man's Correct Diet* (Mokelumne Hill, CA: Health Research, 1921), pp. 136, 37–39.

12. "How One Doctor Cured the 1918 Flu," *Organic Consumer Report*, October 5, 1976.

13. Thomas, *The Lives of a Cell*, pp. 6–7.

14. Christopher Bird, "What Has Become of the Rife Microscope?" *New Age Journal*, January 26, 1976, p. 42.

15. Royal E. S. Hays, "The Germ Theory," *Homeopathic Review*, May 1947; reprinted by Nell Rogers and Guy Rogers, *The Medical Mischief, You Say!* (Pasadena, CA: Health Research, 1953), p. 35.

16. William Dufty quoting William Coda Martin, *Sugar Blues* (NY: Warner Books, 1975), p. 154.

17. "Spanish Flu of 1918."

18. Leonard Wickenden, *Our Daily Poison* (NY: Hillman Books, 1961), p. 57.

19. Ibid.

20. "Are You Getting Too Much Fluoride?" *Better Nutrition*, December 1981, p. 49.

21. From a flyer from Eden Ranch, publishers of *Organic Consumer Report*, n.d. (probably published in the early 1960s).

22. "Is the Food You Eat Dangerous to Your Health?" *U.S. News and World Report*, July 15, 1985.

23. Italics mine. Morton Biskind, "Public Health Aspects of the New Insecticides," *American Journal of Digestive Diseases*, November 1953, p. 333.

24. Ibid., p. 338.

25. Ibid., note.

26. Ibid., p. 338.

27. Paavo Airola, *Everywoman's Book* (Phoenix, AZ: Health Plus, 1979), p. 290. Dr. Airola gives us six scientific references as a sample.

28. Ibid.

29. Archie Kalokerinos, *Every Second Child* (New Canaan, CT: Keats, 1981).

30. Earl Mindell, *Vitamin Bible* (New York: Warner Books, 1979).

31. Leonard Jacobs, "Natural Ways to Survive a Meltdown," *East West Journal*, June 1979, p. 66.

32. Linda Clark, *Stay Young Longer* (NY: Pyramid Books, 1971), p. 117. Also see idem, *Linda Clark's Handbook of Natural Remedies for Common Ailments* (NY: Pocket Books, 1977), p. 176.

33. Adelle Davis, *Let's Get Well* (NY: Harcourt, Brace & World, 1965), p. 381.

34. Michael L. Culbert, *AIDS: Hope, Hoax and Hoopla* (Chula Vista, CA: Bradford Foundation, 1989). Also see Jon Rappoport, *AIDS INC.* (San Bruno, CA: Human Energy Press, 1988): T. C. Fry, *The Great AIDS Hoax* (Austin, TX: Life Institute, 1989); *Gary Null Show*, WNIS-AM, September 26, 1993, and October 31, 1993.

35. *Gary Null Show*, September 26, 1993.

36. Interview with Peter Duesberg in *Spin* magazine 3, no. 8 (1988); reprinted by Fry, *The Great AIDS Hoax*, p. 148. Duesberg said that AIDS is "a bank of old symptoms."

37. *Gary Null Show*, October 31, 1993.

38. Culbert, *AIDS*, chaps. 7, 8, 12.

39. Robert Strecker, *The Strecker Memorandum*, 1988, video.

40. Alan Cantwell, Jr., *AIDS: The Mystery and the Solution* (Los Angeles, CA: Aries Rising Press, 1986).

41. *The Strecker Memorandum*.

42. Cantwell, *AIDS*.

43. Culbert, *AIDS*, chap. 7.

44. "For 6 Years, Man Thought He Had AIDS," *Virginian-Pilot/Ledger-Star*, October 24, 1992.

45. Culbert, *AIDS*, p. iv.

46. Ibid., chap. 7.

47. Ibid., chap. 6; also see Rappoport, *AIDS INC.*, chap. 5.

48. Eva Lee Snead, "AIDS: Immunization Related Syndrome," *Health Freedom News*, July 1987, pp. 14–17, 22, 44–45.

49. Arthur J. Snider, "Near Disaster with Salk Vaccine," *Science Digest*, December 1963, pp. 40–41.

50. Snead, "AIDS," pp. 16, 22, 44.

51. "Smallpox Vaccine 'Triggered Aids Virus,'" *The Times* (London), May 11, 1987, pp. 1, 18.

52. Robert S. Mendelsohn, "The Drive to Immunize Adults Is On," *Herald of Holistic Health*, September–October 1985, p. 2; cited by Neil Z. Miller, *Vaccines: Are They Really Safe and Effective?* (Santa Fe, NM: New Atlantean Press, 1992), p. 44.

53. *The Strecker Memorandum*.

54. Culbert, *AIDS*, pp. 170–171; also see p. 126.

55. A number of medical doctors have promoted these ideas. For instance, Robert Strecker, *The Strecker Memorandum*; William Campbell Douglass "Who Murdered Africa," *Health Freedom News*, September–November 1987; Sean Seale, "Origin of the AIDS Virus, Fact or Fiction?" *Health Freedom News*, January 1989.

56. Culbert, *AIDS*, p.6.

57. Ibid. p. 178; also Rappoport, *AIDS INC.*, chap. 3; Jessica Mitford, *Kind and Usual Punishment* (NY: Alfred A. Knopf, 1974).

58. John Yiamouyiannis, *Fluoride: The Aging Factor* (Delaware, OH: Health Action Press, 1983). Note: Chapter 15 of his book shows that fluoride does not prevent tooth decay.

59. Culbert, *AIDS*, p. 157.

60. Marian Tompson, "Another View," in Robert S. Mendelsohn, *The Risks of Immunizations and How to Avoid Them* (Evanston, IL: The People's Doctor, Inc., 1988), p. 96.

61. Leon Chaitow, *Vaccination and Immunization: Dangers, Delusions and Alternatives* (Essex, England: C. W. Daniel Company Limited, 1987), p. 135.

62. *Gary Null Show* WINIS-AM, August 8, 1993. Gary Null puts the figure at about 150 pounds per person. *Heritage Newsletter*, September 1989, puts the figure at 120 pounds average.

63. *Heritage Newsletter*, September 1989.

64. Neville Hodgkinson, Dar es Salaam, Africa, "African Aids Plague 'a Myth,' " *The Times* (London), October 3, 1993. Note: The term *diseasescare* is mine.

65. Bob Owen, *Roger's Recovery from AIDS* (Malibu, CA: Davar). The information for the discussion of this book is taken from a book review by Fry, *The Great AIDS Hoax*, pp. 267–269.

66. Harvey Diamond and Marilyn Diamond, *Living Health* (New York: Warner Books, 1987) p. 320. Also idem, *Fit for Life* (New York: Warner Books, 1987) (paperback edition), pp. 248–249. Recipe section in both books includes both raw and cooked foods.

67. Laurence E. Badgley, "A Study on the Immune System," *Health World*, November–December 1988, pp. 40–41.

68. "Natural Healing and AIDS," *Heritage Newsletter*, March 1988.

69. John P. Dobbins, "AIDS Cured by Hyper-oxidation," *Health Freedom News*, February 1992, pp. 27, 46; Bill Thomson, "The AIDS-Ozone Connection," *East West Journal*, September 1989, pp. 73–74, 112; see also interview with Robert Atkins, M.D., on the *Gary Null Show*, WNIS-AM, July 4, 1993. Dr. Atkins said he's had 500 patients go from HIV positive to HIV negative using ozone therapy. Articles discussing orally administered oxygen therapies are Bill Thomson, "Do Oxygen Therapies Work?" *East West Journal*, September 1989, pp. 70–75, 110–111; literature from the International Association for Oxygen Therapy, Priest River, ID.

70. Sigerist, *Civilization and Disease*, p. 218.

71. Ibid., p. 219.

72. Ibid., p. 221.

73. Ibid., pp. 222–224.

74. Ibid., p. 224.

75. Norman Shealy, "Autogenic Training," Association for Research and Enlightenment, Virginia Beach, VA, August 30, 1977.

76. Negative emotions trigger the release of norepinephrine, an immune suppressor. See "Psychoimmunology: For Each State of Mind, at State of Body?" *Brain/Mind Bulletin*, December 10, 1984, p. 3. Also, Dr. Larry Dossey points out that "thought and emotion affect the immune system at cellular and subcellular levels." See *Brain/Mind Bulletin*, July 29, 1985, p. 2, insert.

77. "Organic Seeds for Thought," *Organic Consumer Report*, September 28, 1982.

78. Huston Smith, *The Religions of Man* (New York: Harper & Row, 1965), p. 117.

79. Larry Dossey, "Space, Time, and Medicine," *ReVision*, fall 1982, pp. 54–55.

9   "Beautiful" and "Ugly" Solutions

Anything which is forced or misunderstood can never be beautiful.
                                                    —Xenophon

THE "BEAUTIFUL" SOLUTION

The Aesthetic Criterion

"Beauty is truth, truth beauty," wrote the poet John Keats over 150 years ago in his "Ode to a Grecian Urn." Now, twentieth-century scientists are telling us that beauty is a means of discovering truth as well as a standard by which it is recognized. In science you can recognize truth by its beauty and simplicity, physicist Richard Feynman points out. "Werner Heisenberg declared that beauty 'in exact science, no less than in the arts, is the most important source of illumination and clarity.' "[1] As a standard in physics, beauty even takes primacy over experiment.

The three elements of beauty specified by physicists are simplicity, harmony, and brilliance. Contained within the principle of simplicity are completeness and economy; contained within the principle of harmony is symmetry; and contained within the principle of brilliance are clarity and resonance or the ability to shed light on other phenomena.[2]

"A beautiful solution or proof is one that is simple, direct, that goes to the very nature and essence of the problem. An ugly one, though perfectly correct and usable, somehow misses this essence."[3] John Holt refers here to mathematics, paraphrasing a point made by Wertheimer in his book *Productive Think-*

ing. Can we apply this standard, as well as the standard of beauty specified by physicists, to the more humanistic fields, specifically the field of health care?

Let's begin by asking the obvious: Does the practice of vaccinating people— or searching for a vaccine—for every identifiable disease go "to the very nature and essence of the problem?" Is this solution the simple and direct one? Is it conducive to a sense of harmony within oneself and with the natural world? Is it economical, not only in terms of money but in terms of time and energy expenditure?

Since vaccination programs are central to the raison d'etre (justification for existence) of the public health departments, the practice of pediatrics, and much public-funded research, we might ask these questions of our entire healthcare system. Let's apply to the healthcare system our three criteria of beauty: simplicity, harmony, and brilliance.

Simplicity. A beautiful healthcare system would be based on theories that are simple without being simplistic. The fundamental ideas could be understood and applied by most people. The theories would be economical; that is, they would explain a wide range of phenomena in the simplest, easiest, most direct way possible. The theories would be complete in that they would be logical and consistent. In practice, the program would be economical, not only in terms of money but in terms of time and energy expenditure.

Harmony. A beautiful theory of health would promote a sense of harmony with the natural world. It would perceive other life forms as intelligent, responsive, and life supporting; our relations with them would be dependent upon our own actions and perceptions. We now know, for instance, that even microorganisms show signs of intelligence as well as responsiveness to human thought and emotion.[4]

The principle of harmony is implied in the idea of holism. If we think of a disease process as part of a larger process or whole, we know that a part cannot be altered without altering the whole. This suggests that any action directed to a part must be harmonized with the welfare of the whole. For instance, a holistic doctor would know that a treatment either to prevent or correct a disease would change the body-mind, not only in relation to the disease being treated but in relation to other diseases as well. Therefore, his treatments would be directed toward enhancing the life of the body as a whole as well as the life of the person as a whole.

The elegance of balanced proportions is suggested by the principle of symmetry. It is suggested not only anatomically—for example, duality and complementarity of right and left sides of our bodies—but in the idea of balancing our lives. As we discussed earlier, lifestyle and "thinkstyle" are primary determinants of health or its lack.

Brilliance. Implied in the above discussion.

An elegantly simple and harmonious healthcare system would be conducive to personal growth and empowerment. Therefore, its theories and practices would be directed toward personal autonomy, creative and egalitarian interaction with others including healthcare professionals, and the promotion of a sense of harmony and relatedness to one's own body-mind as well as the natural world. It would focus on the characteristics of health rather than on the characteristics of disease, promoting the former rather than fighting or avoiding the latter. It would be oriented toward correcting causes rather than treating symptoms; therefore, it would encourage long-term rather than short-term or "quick-fix" solutions; for, like great works of art, beautiful solutions stand the test of time.

Are there any healthcare systems or schools of healing that have most of the above characteristics? Generally speaking, any of the "natural"[5] schools of healing will promote personal autonomy and independence, nonauthoritarian ways of relating to healthcare professionals, and a sense of harmony and relatedness to one's own body-mind as well as the natural world. These schools of healing are called natural, not so much because they generally make minimal use of technological intervention, but because they work directly with the natural healing energies of the body and the natural world.

Natural therapies generally assume a life or mind principle—variously referred to as the "vital force," the "innate," "mana"—that sustains and heals the body-mind. Central to the philosophy of natural healing is the idea that the body is self-healing and that the purpose of a therapeutic modality should be to arouse and support this healing energy.

Energy and Natural Healing

"I sing the body electric," said the poet, Walt Whitman (*Leaves of Grass*). "The body is electrical in nature," Dr. William McGarey told his audience. "The medicine of the future will be electrical in nature."[6]

Understanding and treating the body as energy rather than as mass is an idea as old as civilization. Forty-five centuries ago, a Chinese physician named Koai Yu Chu identified the unity of matter and energy and described a "primordial energy that gives birth to all the elements and is integrated into them." This energy, which the Chinese later called *Ch'i*, is the life force of the universe as well as the healing and sustaining energy of the body.[7] When this energy is blocked, illness results. The purpose of the healer is to release the blockage so the energy can flow freely. This is the theory behind acupuncture and acupressure, of course. If we think of healing as balancing as well as restoring the energy within the body, we can include such healthcare systems as macrobiotics, chiropractic, homeopathy, naturopathy, and herbology.

In general, natural schools of healing, such as these, avoid the use of toxic substances such as drugs and vaccines, because they interfere in subtle ways with the free flow of this energy, or vital force. Any toxic substance, whether exogenous (originating outside the body) or endogenous (originating inside the body) is part of the problem, not the solution. Also, natural schools of healing generally interpret disease symptoms as part of a healing process, not as an enemy to be fought, so a toxic system of weaponry would have no place.

A number of writers have mistakenly identified the principle of vaccination with the principle of the law of similars in homeopathy. The law of similars asserts, "Like will be cured by like—a like remedy in minimum dose." In other words, that substance that produces the same symptoms in a healthy person as the symptoms in the sick person, if given in sufficiently small doses, will cure the illness. (This makes sense only when we abandon the adversarial view of disease and see its symptoms as part of a larger healing process.) The differences between the application of this principle and the principle behind vaccination are major:

1. The homeopathic dose is much smaller than that used in vaccines; in fact, the homeopathic medicine is diluted to the point where there is no trace of the original substance—only an energy pattern. (This is achieved by a process known as "potentization" in which the dynamic energy latent in a substance is liberated by a succession of dilutions and mechanical agitation.) So the homeopathic dose is essentially an energy therapy designed to arouse and strengthen the natural healing energy or vital force of the body. It is not directed at microorganisms or their destruction but to the patient and the strengthening of his vital forces.

2. The homeopathic remedy is holistic; it addresses the uniqueness of the patient as well as his wholeness. The patient as a mental and spiritual being is studied and treated as well as the patient as a physical organism. [Herd treatment and prescriptions, such as those prescribed by compulsory immunization laws, would be contrary to the homeopathic philosophy and ideals.]

3. Homeopaths generally do not use injections. It is contrary to the homeopathic philosophy "to violate the integrity of the body by forcibly introducing medicinal agents by other than the natural orifices and channels."[8]

Homeopaths can use oral immunizing agents, however. Certain of these highly attenuated, harmless preparations can be used as immunizing agents for most transmittable diseases as well as to counteract the undesirable side effects of conventional immunization antigens.

A sense of harmony, relatedness, and personal empowerment is promoted by the philosophy of homeopathy. It assumes a Life or Mind entity that creates and sustains the physical organism. The working principle of this Life or Mind is the Law of Reciprocal Action, otherwise known as the law of balance. It is variously called the law of compensation, rhythm, polarity, vibration, or just action-reaction, and it is operative in the mental and spiritual realms as well as in the physical realm. The expression of Life or Mind is the Law of Love, which is always beneficent, creative, and harmonizing. "Hence, the consistent practitioner of homeopathy never uses, and has no need to use, any irritating, weakening, depressing, infecting, intoxicating or injurious agent of any kind in the treatment of the sick.''[9]

Perhaps the baseline of all schools of natural healing is naturopathy, or Nature Cure, as it is known in England. Its "medicines" are such things as sunshine, fresh air, pure water, natural foods, and regular periods of internal cleansing through juice or water fasts and colonics. Manipulative therapies such as chiropractic and reflexology, nontoxic herbal and homeopathic medicines, and hydrotherapy (the therapeutic uses of water) are also part of the naturopathic "tool kit." Recently, iridology, the science of reading the degree of tissue activity of the various organs of the body by the markings in the iris, has been used by many naturopaths.

Iridology bears out one of the basic premises of naturopathy, namely, that disease develops through an orderly progression of increasing toxic encumbrance in the body. All forms of disease are caused by an accumulation of toxins in the system, according to naturopathy, and the purpose of any therapeutic program is to assist the body to rid itself of these poisons.

Through iridology we can trace the progression of disease from acute to degenerative, the acute stage being the active discharge stage and the degenerative stage being the stage of tissue destruction. The model works something like this: First we have a cold or some acute mucous elimination. We take a cold remedy to stop the discharge of mucus. The cold disappears, but later—sometimes many years later—bronchitis, flu, boils, cysts, or a running ear develops. Again we take suppressant drugs, and the symptoms disappear. Later—again, sometimes many years later—we develop hayfever or pneumonia. Years later, after dosing with more shots and drugs, we develop asthma or rheumatism. Finally, after further physiological insult with drugs and shots, we develop degenerative diseases such as cancer, arthritis, and gangrene. We have progressed from an acute illness to a subacute one and from there to a chronic, then subchronic, and finally degenerative disease.

To "cure" a disease we have to cleanse the body so the body can replace degenerative tissue with new. We must retrace the disease process and arrive at the acute stage again wherein the body regains the vitality necessary to throw off what doesn't belong to it. When we take drugs to stop the discharge—a symptom of elimination—we push not only the toxic material but the drugs as well back into the tissues and create "toxic settlements."

One of the pioneers in researching and teaching people the principles of health is distinguished nutritionist, iridologist, naturopath, and chiropractor Dr. Bernard Jensen. In his book *The Science and Practice of Iridology*, he presents case histories illustrating the retracing process. Dr. Jensen told one woman, for instance, whose iris showed a great deal of sulfur settlement in the brain area, that she would probably have a sulfur elimination during the course of her therapy. Her gray hair turned completely yellow as the sulfur was eliminated through her scalp. During this elimination crisis, she developed diarrhea and remembered when, as a child, her grandmother had given her sulfur and molasses as a spring tonic. In a couple of months after the elimination process, her hair returned to its natural black color.

Another case describes a very thin young man with a stomach ulcer who wanted to know how to gain weight. During the healing crisis, he developed a high fever and delirium, a painful headache, and extreme pains in the head around the ears. He then remembered having this same condition one time on a trip to Alaska. Nothing was done for the condition while on the trip except that drugs were administered. During the eliminative process, he tasted the same drugs he had taken years before. After the crisis, he gained 15 pounds and felt wonderful.

Even mental disturbance can be corrected by a process of cleansing and rebalancing the body. One woman, after trying a number of different schools of healing including medicine and chiropractic, was healed of compulsive and intermittent crying by fasting, living on natural foods, and exercising regularly. During her healing crisis, she developed a fever, her crying returned, and her head became infested with lice! In questioning this patient, Dr. Jensen found that when she was a child, she had head lice and kerosene had been used to destroy them. This had suppressed the condition, and the lice lay dormant beneath the scalp. The healing crisis caused the crying spells and lice to resurface as part of the retracing process.[10]

Could we say that sickness is something trying to come out? Seen in this light sickness is a complement to health. It is the body-mind's attempt to (1) cleanse itself, (2) heal itself, (3) rebalance itself, and (4) teach us. From Hippocrites, who saw the primary function of disease as the body's attempt to reestablish harmony within itself, to Freud, who saw the healing of the psyche as resulting primarily from the discharge of negative emotions that were locked into painful experiences in the past, the theme of purgation and rebalancing—both physical and mental—in healing is perennial. We might call this the Healing Archetype.[11]

What about "childhood disease," and why do children seem to be more "susceptible" to colds and runny noses than adults? The conventional explanation of this susceptibility is that their immune systems are immature and they haven't built sufficient "resistence" to the "bugs going around." Quite the contrary, Dr. Jensen maintains. Precisely because children usually have more runny noses and colds than the adults with whom they live indicates their bodies are vital enough to throw off toxic material; whereas adults, whose bodies are generally less vital and more encumbered, tend to store toxic materials. The capacity for acute illness, either initially or in a healing crisis, indicates a comparatively high level of energy and physical vitality. Childhood diseases are really a subacute form of disease, the initial cold or runny nose being the acute form that was suppressed by drugs or other unnatural substances.

It has been said, usually pejoratively, that naturopaths don't believe in germs or vaccinations. Certainly vaccinations would be contrary to the naturopathic philosophy. Dr. Jensen, for instance, devotes over two pages of his book *You*

Can Master Disease to the destructive effects of vaccinations. He quotes a number of eminent medical doctors and studies that point to a link between childhood immunizations and the later appearance of polio, meningitis, and cancer. "Artificial immunizations and drugs injure the nerves, the cerebral cortex, the heart, the kidneys, and the glands, and chronic disease is the result," Dr. Jensen states.[12]

Classical naturopathy doesn't agree with the medical interpretation of germs. It maintains that bacteria (germs) are created by dead and decaying tissue. Their function is a cleanup one—to feed upon toxic material until it is gone, hence, the naturopathic emphasis on keeping the body clean. Dr. John Christopher, an outstanding herbalist and naturopathic doctor, would encourage a fever in his patients so the germs could do their work better![13]

Recent Research

Recent research bears out many of the premises of natural healing. The idea, for instance, that disease results from energy blockage has been corroborated by the researches of Dr. Otto Warburg, two-time Nobel Prize winner in cellular physiology and medicine, and Dr. William Frederick Koch, whom I discussed in Chapter 4. Energy production on the cellular level, they have found, is the key to health or disease. This energy production is the same as the cell respiration referred to in Chapter 4 as the oxidation process. The blocking of this process is "the most important cause of malignant, viral, bacterial and allergic diseases," they point out. "Effective prevention and treatment of these diseases depends upon the restoration and maintenance of the normal oxidation process." Dr. Koch also proved that "blocked oxidation in microorganisms causes them to be pathogenic and parasitic, and that when this condition was corrected these organisms become non-pathogenic, non-parasitic and non-virulent."[14] What blocks the oxidation process in the body? Oxygen deficiency and the presence of certain toxic substances. To restore health, the following modalities are used: (1) an oxidation catalyst in conjunction with colonics; (2) organically grown food—food grown without toxic fertilizers and pesticides—eaten mostly raw; and (3) chelated minerals.[15]

A simple illustration of the pleomorphic nature of microorganisms can be found in the bacteria of the human intestine. Healthy intestinal bacteria manufacture many nutrients, including vitamins B and K, and "strongly influence the internal balance of cholesterol and the biliary compounds (digestive juices) made from it." Dr. Miles Robinson goes on to say that "it is important that the intestinal bacteria be properly fed (and not overfed) because a new generation occurs about every four hours, and it is characteristic of all bacteria to develop unsuitable and even virulent strains depending on how they are fed."[16] When the diet contains too much sugar and too little fiber, the intestinal bacteria develop abnormal strains. This can lead to various diseases such as diverticulitis, colon infections, digestive and circulatory problems, diabetes, obesity, appendicitis, and gall bladder infections.[17]

The pertussis vaccine, which has been implicated in so many cases of vaccine injury, is particularly difficult to produce precisely because the pertussis organism—*Bordetella pertussis*—is so mutable! It has the ability to mutate unexpectedly and change its character. Even carefully selected strains perform differently when grown in different media, John Cameron of the University of Quebec tells us.[18]

Can the human mind induce mutations in bacteria? At St. Joseph's University in Philadelphia, 52 human volunteers, not known to be psychically gifted, promoted the mutation of bacteria from one strain to another simply by "wishing." Conversely, they were able to inhibit the reverse mutation by the same mental intention.[19]

If thought, which is energy, can influence matter, then light, which is another form of energy, can also influence matter. All matter—atoms, molecules, microorganisms—gives off radiant energy, which, under certain conditions, can be made visible. Royal Raymond Rife discovered that microorganisms give off a monochromatic wavelength of invisible ultraviolet light and that by subjecting a particular type of microorganism to a specific short-wave frequency the microorganism disintegrated. Other frequencies would cause the microorganism to illuminate or give off visible light, implying that these frequencies were vitalizing to the microorganism. Dr. Rife found he could save the lives of test animals that had been given lethal doses of pathogenic organisms by subjecting their bodies to the proper wavelength of electrical energy, in this case, the oscillatory rate that would destroy the particular pathogen.[20] Are we moving toward the time when health care programs will include periodic exposure to specific life-enhancing radiation frequencies? We know that certain sounds and certain kinds of music have a therapeutic effect, while other sounds and other kinds of music have a disabling or debilitating effect.[21] And, of course, color therapy is an ancient art from which many have benefited.

"There is a surfeit of clinical information suggesting that we have literally become malnourished and sickened by the habitual diet of an outmoded view of the world, the classical Cartesian-Newtonian [The world seen in terms of discrete objects and subject/object dualism] description of the universe," writes Dr. Larry Dossey. He goes on to say that "this fragmented and alienated world view has directly contributed to fragmented and alienated life styles—with corresponding disease-ridden results."[22] The remedy, he says, is to incorporate a truer, more health-inducing picture of the world.

We know, for instance, that matter originates from and disappears into energy or force fields. "The world at bottom is a quantum energy world," physicist John Wheeler points out.[23] Yet we still think and act as though biochemical analysis were the final revelation. Most medical doctors and chemists, for example, have insisted that synthetic (man-made) food supplements are the same as "natural" food supplements (derived from food sources and processed in such a way as to retain enzymes and other nutrients) because their chemical formulas are the same. Now we know that not only do the atoms in the molecules of the synthetic product rotate differently from the atoms of the natural one,[24] but the natural product has a more dynamic energy pattern than the synthetic.

Two researchers, Drs. Justa Smith and Ehrenfried Pfeiffer, have demonstrated with a series of chromatograms—photographs that reproduce the energy patterns of an object (somewhat like Kirlian photography)—that natural substances have an energy pattern characterized "by radial lines and fluted edges, while the pattern of the synthetic product is almost entirely concentric and relatively dull looking."[25] Looking at these chromatograms, one begins to feel that natural is indeed beautiful.

The characteristic pattern of the natural substance, for example, orange juice or grape juice, is destroyed by pasteurization and some preservatives. The living pattern is diminished or weakened by freezing and by other preservatives. In other words, as a method of food preservation, freezing is less destructive than heat, and some preservatives are more destructive than others. Even food grown in soil in which the compost had been sterilized showed fewer "live" elements than food grown in compost that was not heat treated. "There is a delicate and admirable balance of components in all the kingdoms of nature, Dr. Smith points out. And this balance is disturbed not only by refining out nutrients but by adding preservatives like BHA and BHT."[26]

What are the "live" elements that give the natural product its characteristic pattern and look of "aliveness"? They are enzymes and, as we learned earlier, they are destroyed by heat above 122^0 Fahrenheit.

Over a hundred years ago, Bechamp discovered the difference between natural and synthetic substances. He found that chalk buried in limestone brought about fermentation, whereas chemically "pure" chalk (calcium carbonate) made in his laboratory would not. What was that "something" in the natural chalk, buried for thousands of years in the ground, that did not exist in the chemically pure chalk? It was the microzymas, of course; their secretions—products of metabolism—are the enzymes that cause fermentation.

Fish or sea vegetation cannot live in synthetic "sea water," although it is chemically identical with the real thing; however, when just 1 ounce of real sea water is added to 20 gallons of the synthetic substitute, that "something" the chemists were unable to isolate or analyze changes the water so that fish and sea plants can live in it.[27] Is this living "something" the microzymas (somatids, protits, or bions of later researchers)?

It's tempting to ask, At what point does matter become energy? Royal Raymond Rife discovered when he looked into his Universal Microscope that cells "are actually composed of smaller cells, themselves made up of even smaller cells, this process continuing with higher and higher magnification in a sixteen-step, stage-by-stage journey into the micro-beyond."[28] Bechamp stressed the almost invisible size as well as the "immeasurableness" of microzymas. Are they the elemental living principle?[29]

Generally, doctors using natural methods of healing have long advocated the use of natural substances in preference to their synthetic counterparts, saying, in effect, that because these substances are biologically active, they are more effectively utilized by the body. Medical literature contains numerous reports confirming this idea. One report, for instance, states that cases of scurvy failed to respond to synthetic vitamin C and that a cure was effected only when the patients were given a natural food substance containing vitamin C.[30]

Part of the "aliveness" of natural foods and food supplements is that they are holistic; that is, they contain associated nutritional elements such as enzymes, coenzymes, and trace minerals, as well as vitamins and minerals that assist in the process of assimilation. Many of these food elements have yet to be discovered.

A beautiful healthcare system would be holistic on many levels, focusing on parts only as they relate to and the harmonize with a larger whole. It would see the body-mind as a purposive, dynamic energy field to be responded to, not a machine or an inert mass to be manipulated. A beautiful healthcare system would focus on the patient and his uniqueness, not on disease and herd "remedies" such as mass inoculations. And above all, it would be open-ended, aware that truth has many dwelling places and that our senses and our intellect apprehend only a fraction of the living universe.

THE "UGLY" SOLUTION

> Whoever has the mind to fight has broken his connection with the universe.
>
> —Terry Dobson quoting his Aikido teacher,
> "A Soft Answer"

Disease Wars

We speak of "delivering a knockout punch to leukemia," "fighting multiple sclerosis," "battling muscular dystrophy," and "waging a war against cancer." In fact, we not only "fight" disease; we fight litter, poverty, pornography, crime, mediocrity, and, yes, even fat. If we are confronted with a challenge—usually called a problem—we must fight it.

At the Center for Attitudinal Healing in California, children with "life-threatening" diseases draw pictures of "getting well." One picture shows "bad cells" lining up on one side and "good cells" lining up on the other. All cells are carrying guns. Another drawing shows two "bad cells" being attacked by a fighter plane driven by "good cells." In the bottom right-hand corner is a tank labeled "good cells" that are also attacking the "bad cells." In another drawing, a circle with the label "angel" is sending lightning darts to a figure labeled "devil."[31]

For over a century, we have used metaphors of *fight, attack,* and *defend* to describe our relationship with disease. The military mentality that creates these metaphors is also the mentality that designs weapons. A "good" weapon is supposed to destroy the "enemy" without harming the soldier who uses it. The problem is, it doesn't quite work that way. Aside from the more subtle levels of psychic and quantum energies in which the universe reveals itself as a tissue of interconnections and reciprocal relationships, there is the gross, sensate level of reality in which the entrance of destructive energies at one level of an eco-system reverberates on many levels of that system and even other systems as well. Simply stated, any remedy powerful enough to destroy "the other" de-stroys the host as well. The destruction of the host may be slower, the debili-tating effects more subtle and long range, but the weapons approach to a challenge—whether on a microscopic scale involving cellular particles or on a macroscopic scale involving international relations—signifies the old conscious-ness of separation, materiality, and inanimacy.

"If there should be life on the moon, we must begin by fearing it. We must guard against it, lest we catch something," Lewis Thomas tells us after describ-ing the elaborate, antiseptic ceremony through which the astronauts must pass on their return to earth in order to become members once again of the human community. "It is remarkable that we have all accepted this, without hooting, as though it simply conformed to a law of nature. It says something about our century, our attitude toward life, our obsession with disease and death, our hu-man chauvinism." Further on, he points out that "most of the associations between the living things we know about are essentially cooperative ones, sym-biotic in one degree or another." In discussing bacteria, he says that "they should provide nice models for the study of interactions between forms of life at all levels. They live by collaboration, accommodation, exchange, and bar-ter."[32]

Back in 1903, Russian biologist Peter Kropotkin wrote a book called *Mutual Aid: A Factor of Evolution* in which he amassed almost as much evidence that animals cooperate as Darwin did that each is engaged in a selfish struggle for existence.[33] Are we reaping the final fruits of our predisposition to interpret events in combative, competitive terms in an armaments race that threatens to extinguish life on this planet?

"War is an old habit of thought, an old frame of mind, an old political technique, that must now pass as human sacrifice and human slavery have passed," writes Herman Wouk in his preface to *War and Remembrance.*[34] Will we outgrow this habit, this old frame of mind before it is too late? As Buck-minster Fuller has reminded us, "We are in our final exams."[35]

It is probably no accident that one of the major drug cartels, I. G. Farben (Germany), is also a major munitions manufacturer and a former designer and operator of the concentration camps used in Nazi Germany.[36] The weapons mentality wages wars on many levels.

The war game is, as many have observed, exceedingly profitable for the munitions industry, in this case, the pharmaceutical-medical industry. In 1981, for instance, vaccine distribution of eight major vaccines in the United States generated over $300 million for the drug industry.[37] The figure is several times this amount now, of course.

Propaganda to keep enlistments up and money rolling in is part of the war machinery. The appeal to fear and the necessity for technological intervention and management of disease is illustrated in much of the literature distributed by state departments of health. "The hidden menace" and "killer and crippler" are some of the terms used to describe certain childhood infectious diseases from which children must be "protected" by immunizations. "Danger," "warning," "allowed to strike" are some of the scare terms used to intimidate parents into getting their children vaccinated. The more serious consequences as well as the frequency of the diseases for which children are vaccinated are maximized, if not grossly exaggerated, while the frequency of serious complications resulting from vaccinations is ignored or greatly minimized.

Superstitions, like old soldiers, never die. They simply change clothes and sit in the seats of respectability. Medical historian Henry E. Sigerist points out:

Primitive man found himself in a magical world, surrounded by a hostile nature whose every manifestation was invested with mysterious forces. In order to live unharmed, he had to use constant vigilance and had to observe a complicated system of rules and rites that protected him from the evil forces which emanated from nature and his fellow men.[38]

Let's look at a folder distributed by the Virginia State Department of Health in 1982. In the middle section is a schedule that reads as follows:

2 months: DPT, TOPV (trivalent oral polio vaccine)

4 months: DPT, TOPV

6 months: DPT

15 months: Measles, Rubella, Mumps

18 months: DPT, TOPV

4 to 6 years: DPT, TOPV

14 to 16 years: Td (tetanus and diphtheria)

Does this look a bit like a reappearance of the "complicated system of rules and rites" primitive man lived by in order to protect himself from the evil forces that surrounded him? Have the "miracle" cures primitive man sought in the spells and potions of the witch doctor become the miracle cures of drugs and vaccines?

The 1993 schedule has been expanded to look like this:

RECOMMENDED SCHEDULE OF VACCINATIONS FOR CHILDREN UNDER 2

- One vaccination against measles, mumps, and rubella (MMR)
- Four vaccinations against diphtheria, pertussis, and tetanus (DPT)
- Three vaccinations against polio (OPV—oral polio vaccine)
- Three vaccinations against hepatitis B
- Three or four vaccinations against *Haemophilus influenzae B* (Hib) (causes meningitis)[39]

All of these immunological assaults when the child's nervous and immune systems are most vulnerable and immature! In fact, it takes 10 or 12 years for the immune system to become "strong and resistant," which it does by running "a gauntlet of infectious challenges."[40]

What about an infant whose immune system is relatively undeveloped and is dependent for about the first six months on the immune factors it receives from its mother?[41] The recommended schedule for these infants is two doses of oral polio vaccine; three doses of DPT; three doses of Hib; and two, perhaps three, doses of hepatitis B, one dose of this latter to be given at birth![42]

Did you know that the hepatitis vaccine attacks the newborn liver, which may become dysfunctional for 14 days or more after the injection?[43]

Did you know that groups at high risk for contracting hepatitis B are prostitutes, sexually active homosexual men, intravenous drug users, institutionalized children and adults, some health workers, the military, and people on hemodialysis?[44] Hardly newborn infants! But then babies are "accessible"![45]

Did you know that "all studies of efficacy of Hib vaccines admit that the vaccine is ineffective in children younger than 18 months"?[46]

Did you know that when Japan raised the minimum vaccination age to 2 years, SIDS and infantile convulsions disappeared in that country and "Japan zoomed to the lowest incidence of infant mortality in the world"?[47]

Did you know that the United States has one of the highest infant mortality rates in the world[48] and that vaccination commences earlier in the United States than in any other country?[49]

There are more shots, of course: OPV, DPT, and MMR before the child starts school (4 to 6 years) as well as Td every 10 years (called adult booster).[50]

It wasn't many years ago that Hib vaccine was recommended. Now it is mandated in at least 44 states.[51] It's a short step from recommending to mandating, as anyone familiar with the history of vaccination can attest. Will chickenpox vaccine be next? Will children be routinely administered MMRV (*V* for varicella zoster virus)? What will be next? A cancer vaccine? Did you know that, excluding accidents and their effects, cancer is the number-one cause of death for children ages 1 to 14[52] and that there has been a 20 percent increase in childhood cancers?[53]

But is any of this surprising? Once the paradigm is bought into—the idea that we need internal "weapons" to combat the evil forces that surround us—

the possibilities for additions and multiplications of protections needed are almost endless, as is the potential for long-term damage.

Did you know that vaccination did not begin with Edward Jenner but had its origin centuries earlier, the Druid priests of ancient Britain and Germany being among its earliest practitioners? The priests used "isopathic diluted exudate from smallpox victims, in trying to instill protection."[54] This practice was continued through the Middle Ages and was taught by the physician Paracelsus. One historian describes an old Circassian woman who "would cut a cross in the flesh of the applicant and then use smallpox exudate on the wound, announcing that this was an unfailing preventative of the disease."[55]

Now we have a technology that makes this practice far more destructive on both a personal and a cultural level, this latter because it enables misinformation and coercion to penetrate more completely throughout a society. And like the habit of war and other forms of violence, will we outgrow this mentality before it is too late?

At this point it is redundant to ask, Does the pharmaceutical-medical approach go to the very core and essence of the problem? So let's ask, Why are these unnatural approaches to health—vaccines and drugs—not beautiful compared with the more natural approaches we discussed earlier? Not only do unnatural (meaning dependent on synthetic drugs and a complex technology) treatments ultimately complicate the disease process, but they escalate cost, dependency, and concentration of power outside of oneself. Perhaps, even more important, they promote a sense of alienation from one's own body and the natural world that sustains it. The body is seen not as an extension of one's consciousness and part of a larger continuum that includes all life but as an isolated object that must fight for survival and defend itself against a hostile environment.

The "ugly" solution is fragmented, superficial, and short-ranged. It looks for the immediate, the obvious, the "quick fix." (See Table 4 for a comparison of the two approaches.) Because it focuses on the management of symptoms rather than the correction of causes, it lacks a unifying principle. Like the old pantheon of deities and devils, the ugly solution externalizes causality and promotes feelings of victimization and dependence on the "expert." Geared to profits for the professional, it eschews the promotion of self-responsibility and independence.

As we move from a mass to an energy consciousness, from the model of the body as a machine composed of discrete parts set on automatic to a model of the body as an energy ecosystem directed by a consciousness, a monolithic, adversarial healthcare system will be increasingly hard to justify. How can we begin to transform a limited vision and ugly solutions into a larger vision suggesting more beautiful solutions?

"Nature is a part of us, as we are part of it. We can recognize ourselves in the description we give to it,"[56] physical chemist and Nobel laureate Ilya Prigogine points out. We need to recognize the combativeness within ourselves when we see the world as a mosaic of adversarial relationships. As author and educator Noel McInnis said, "Complete emancipation of our latent powers is

TABLE 4. TWO APPROACHES TO HEALTH CARE

THE "UGLY" SOLUTION	THE "BEAUTIFUL" SOLUTION
1. Atomized, fragmented.	1. Holistic—parts integrated and understood in relation to larger wholes.
2. Focuses on data and effects.	2. Focuses on principles and underlying causes.
3. Adversarial—promotes feelings of alienation.	3. Harmonious—promotes feelings of connection and relatedness.
4. Focuses on negative—engenders fear.	4. Focuses on positive—inspires.
5. Circuitous—skirts around the real problem.	5. Direct—goes to the core of the problem.
6. Obfuscating, complicating.	6. Clarifying.
7. Externalizes causality.	7. Internalizes causality.
8. Capricious, arbitrary.	8. Orderly, logical.
9. Superficial and simplistic.	9. Elegantly simple and multidimensional.
10. Addictive—creates dependency.	10. Empowering—supports autonomy and self-responsibility.
11. Wasteful—cost escalating.	11. Economical—cost-effective.
12. Closed shop—authoritarian.	12. Open-ended—egalitarian.
13. Short range.	13. Long range.
14. Side effects.*	14. Side benefits.

*A friend of mine, Dr. E. Dana Congdon, told a group of us that since he switched from using drugs in his practice to using herbs, he no longer worried about side effects in his patients but could look forward to seeing side benefits.

not possible as long as we are enthralled by the mentality of attack."[57] When we transform an adversarial consciousness—the consciousness of attack and defend—into a consciousness of connectedness, cooperation, and compassion, the beautiful solution will reveal itself.

NOTES

1. "Beauty, Simplicity, Harmony Keys to Physics, Neuroscience, Art and Music," *Brain/Mind Bulletin*, December 10, 1984, p. 2.

2. Ibid.

3. John Holt, *Instead of Education* (New York: E. P. Dutton, 1976), p. 91. Holt is discussing a point made by Wertheimer in his book *Productive Thinking*.

4. Paul Pietsch, "The Mind of a Microbe," *Science Digest*, October 1983, pp. 69–71, 103; also " 'Wishing' Spurs Genetic Mutation in Bacteria," *Brain/Mind Bulletin*, September 10, 1984, p. 1.

5. *Natural* in this context means using no toxic substances such as drugs and vaccines and no invasive procedures such as surgery.

6. William McGarey, "The Temple Beautiful" (talk given at the Association for Research and Enlightenment, Virginia Beach, VA, July 6, 1981).

7. Mary Coddington, *In Search of the Healing Energy* (New York: Warner/Destiny Books, 1978), p. 14.

8. Ibid., pp. 80–100. Quotes are on p. 98.

9. Ibid., p. 98.

10. Bernard Jensen, *The Science and Practice of Iridology*, (Escondido, CA: Bernard Jensen Products Publishing Division, 1952), pp. 31–32.

11. This idea was perverted by the medical profession into practices of bloodletting, violent purging, and leeches and cupping.

12. Bernard Jensen, *You Can Master Disease* (Solana Beach, CA: Bernard Jensen Publishing Division, 1952), p. 208.

13. An interesting experiment with lizards demonstrates the importance of the cleansing function of fevers. Lizards were injected with potentially fatal doses of bacteria. When the lizards crawled under a heat lamp, which raised their body temperature 3°, 75 percent of them survived. When no heat was available, the lizards couldn't raise their body temperature, and 75 percent of them died. See Ronald Kotulak, "Desert Lizards Led Researcher to Theory That Fever May Help Body Fight Disease," *Miami Herald*; reprinted by *Health Science*, April–May 1981.

14. Robert C. Olney, "Blocked Oxidation," *Cancer News Journal* 8, no. 5 (1973), reprint article on inside front cover.

15. Ibid.

16. Miles Robinson, "On Sugar and White Flour . . . the Dangerous Twins!" *Executive Health* 11, no. 6; referred to and quoted from in the article "Don't Eat Sugar!" *Better Nutrition*, April 1980, pp. 19, 38.

17. Ibid., p. 38. Dr. Robinson tells of a year-long experiment in which five groups of baboons were fed different kinds of carbohydrates. The first four groups were fed refined carbohydrates—either glucose, fructose, sucrose (table sugar), or starch. The fifth group was fed natural foods such as bananas, yams, oranges, carrots, and bread. Only the

animals in the first four groups showed demonstrable damage to the heart artery and a 35 percent rise in cholesterol.

18. Harris L. Coulter and Barbara Loe Fisher, *DPT: A Shot in the Dark* (New York: Harcourt Brace Jovanovich, 1985), p. 27.

19. " 'Wishing' Spurs Genetic Mutation in Bacteria," *Brain/Mind Bulletin*, September 10, 1984, p. 1.

20. Royal Lee, "The Rife Microscope or 'Facts and Their Fate' " (Reprint no. 47, Lee Foundation for Nutritional Research, Milwaukee, WI); also Christopher Bird, "What Has Become of the Rife Microscope?" *New Age Journal*, March 1976, pp. 41–47.

21. Steven Halpern and Louis Savary, *Sound Health: The Music and Sounds That Make Us Whole* (San Francisco: Harper & Row, 1985).

22. Larry Dossey, "Space, Time, and Medicine," *ReVision*, fall 1982, p. 57.

23. Ibid., p. 56.

24. "The plane of a beam of polarized light is rotated by all natural substances either to the left (*l*-form) or to the right (*d*-form). Substances not occurring in nature may not cause rotation of the plane of polarization and these substances are said to be optically inactive (*dl*-form)." See Beatrice Trum Hunter, "Synthetic Vitamins," *Consumers' Research Magazine*, March 1974, p. 19.

25. Jane Kinderlehrer, " 'Natural' Is Beautiful—and Better!" *Prevention*, January 1974, p. 97.

26. Ibid., p. 99.

27. "Natural vs. Synthetic: What Is the Real Answer?" *Organic Consumer Report*, February 27, 1962.

28. Bird, "What Has Become," p. 41.

29. Thomas Edison apparently had an understanding of this principle when he wrote, "Take our own bodies. I believe they are composed of myriads and myriads of infinitesmally small individuals, each in itself a unit of life, and that these units work in squads—or swarms as I prefer to call them—and that these infinitesmally small units live forever. When we die these swarms of units, like a swarm of bees, so to speak, betake themselves elsewhere, and go on functioning in some other form or environment." See Thomas Alva Edison, *The Diary and Sundry Observations of Thomas Alva Edison*, ed. Dagobert D. Runes (Westport, CT: Greenwood Press, 1968, reprint), pp. 235–236.

30. Hunter, "Synthetic Vitamins," p. 18.

31. Center for Attitudinal Healing, *There Is a Rainbow Behind Every Dark Cloud* (Millbrae, CA: Celestial Arts Publishers, 1979).

32. Lewis Thomas, *The Lives of a Cell* (New York: Bantam Books, 1974), pp. 6–7.

33. Tom Bethell, "Burning Darwin to Save Marx," *Harpers*, December 1978, p. 38.

34. Herman Wouk, *War and Remembrance* (Boston, MA: Little, Brown and Co., 1978).

35. Buckminster Fuller, "Bringing the Universe Home," Interview with Buckminster Fuller, *The Graduate Review*, December 1976.

36. Peter Barry Chowka, "Pushers in White: The Organized Drugging of America," *East West Journal*, March 1979, p. 32.

37. Coulter and Fisher, *DPT*, p. 406.

38. Henry E. Sigerist, *Civilization and Disease* (Ithaca, NY: Cornell University Press, 1943), p. 131.

39. Schedule from the National Immunization Campaign. See Diane Tennant, "Fearing Reactions, She Says No to Shots," See *Virginian-Pilot/Ledger-Star*, April 30, 1993.

40. Harold E. Buttram, M.D., foreword, *Vaccines: Are They Really Safe and Effective?* by Neil Z. Miller (Santa Fe, NM: New Atlantean Press, 1992), p. 10.

41. Ibid.

42. "Give Your Child a Shot . . . at Good Health," Bureau of Immunization, Virginia Department of Health, 1992, p. 6.

43. Viera Scheibner, *Vaccination: The Medical Assault on the Immune System* (Maryborough, Victoria, Australia: Australian Print Group, 1993), p. 1.

44. Ibid., p. 2.

45. Ibid., p. 7.

46. Ibid., p. 128.

47. Ibid., pp. 263, xix.

48. WHRV-FM, October 11, 1991. According to this report, only Greece and Portugal had a higher infant death rate. On March 3, 1989, *CBS News* reported that we had the world's highest infant mortality rate, with 40,000 babies dying before age 1. Some doctors and researchers have blamed this high mortality rate on teenage pregnancies and drug abuse, but others, as we have shown, have linked it to vaccinations.

49. Coulter and Fisher, *DPT*, p. 32.

50. "Give Your Child a Shot."

51. "Updates: Vaccine Use Extended to Infants," *FDA Consumer*, January-February 1991, p. 2. Reported by Miller, *Vaccines*, p. 43.

52. *Monthly Vital Statistics Report for the Centers for Disease Control*, 1991, per phone call to the American Cancer Society, November 23, 1993.

53. National Cancer Institute Report, 1992, reported by Gary Null, *Gary Null Show*, WNIS-AM, November 7, 1993. The National Cancer Institute reported—per phone call September 28, 1994—that the incidence of cancer rates among children has increased less than 1 percent per year from 1970 to 1990 (*Book Seer Statistical Review* from 1970 to 1990). Another source (*Cancer Statistics Review*) said the same thing except the years were from 1973 to 1990.

54. Leon Chaitow, *Vaccination and Immunization: Dangers, Delusions and Alternatives* (Essex, England: C. W. Daniel Company Limited, 1987), p. 4.

55. Ibid.

56. Quoted by Larry Dossey, in *Space, Time and Medicine* (Boulder, CO: Shambhala, 1982), p. 82.

57. Noel McInnis, "Living Without Attack," *Green Light News*, May 1984, p. 6.

PART III Free to Choose

A free society, if it is to remain free, cannot permit itself to be dominated by one strain of thought.

—William J. Baroody, Sr.

10   Appointment with Tyranny

The condition of freedom in any state is always a widespread and
consistent skepticism of the canons upon which power rests.
                                                —Harold J. Laski

"IT'S THE LAW"

On August 19, 1981, a social worker rang the doorbell at our residence in
Virginia and informed us that a member of our family, a young person in excellent health, was required by law to submit to a medical procedure that not
only was fraught with risk but was not even guaranteed to be effective! The
medical procedure was immunization, and the young person was my two-and-
a-half-year-old grandson Isaac, who was living with us at the time. Tanya,
Isaac's mother and my daughter, was also living with us. (She was separated
from her husband.)

Since Tanya was at work, the social worker left a letter in a sealed envelope
for her. The letter told her to call and make an appointment to see the social
worker, Deborah Balak, within the next two days.

"The social worker was certainly pleasant and agreeable," I told Tanya. "But
she did say it was against the law not to have your child vaccinated. I told her
it was not against the law because I had a copy of the Virginia law, and it
allowed two exemptions—medical and religious. I also told her there was an
impressive body of medical opinion and empirical evidence indicating that this
practice was harmful. I told her we had never had our children vaccinated. She
said she didn't want to harass us but was merely doing her duty."

"So this is what happens when you tell the truth. I probably should never have taken him to the hospital!'' Tanya replied. She was referring to the emergency hospital where she had taken Isaac a few days earlier (August 14) to see if he needed stitches. (He had fallen from the couch and had cut his head on the edge of the coffee table.) During the course of the examination, the nurse asked if he were "caught up with his shots." Tanya, being "oriented" on this issue, replied, "Ohhhhhhhh no!''

"This shouldn't take long, Tanya. Just give her a copy of the exemption form we used in California, stating that immunizations are contrary to your beliefs,'' I told her.

On August 21, Tanya went to see the social worker and presented her with the signed vaccination exemption form I had used in California. Naively, I had assumed this was a national provision. Deborah told Tanya her stand was contrary to law and she would have to report it to the judge. She gave Tanya a copy of the law, and Tanya said in parting, "This better not take much of my time!''

A few days later, Tanya received a summons to appear in court with Isaac on September 8, 1981.

When we read the summons, we were shocked. It stated that the parents or guardian of William Isaac Turner "observe reasonable conditions of behavior pending final determination of custody to wit: to refrain from acts of commission or omission which tend to endanger the child's life, health or normal development.'' When Tanya read this, she had nightmares of someone taking her beautiful, adored Isaac away from her. I must confess that I shared some of this nightmare myself, particularly when I remembered the Chad Green case.[1]

WE GO TO COURT

September 8: Tanya, Isaac, and I sat for two and a half hours on the hard benches of Room 201, District Courts Building, waiting for the name "Turner" to be called. I went along to help take care of Isaac and to give my daughter moral support. As it turned out, however, I did everything I had counseled my daughter not to do: I lost my cool.

We had brought along a folder full of medical statements indicating both the harmfulness and ineffectiveness (ineffective in terms of doing what it is supposed to do) of the practice of vaccination. Most of these statements were taken from material that appeared in Chapter 2 of this book. We also had a letter from our local medical doctor, Paul Monroe (not his real name). The letter stated that the child did not need routine vaccinations because of "possible dangers to his health'' based on "national medical statements indicating the dangers of vaccinations.'' We also had another exemption form signed by Tanya which stated that vaccinations were contrary to her religious beliefs. We thought we were covered. We would present the letter and the evidence to the judge and that would be the end of it. How naive we were!

At 1:30 the name "Turner'' was called, and we went to another courtroom.

Tanya sat on one side, Deborah Balak and a gentleman whose function we did not know sat on the other side, and Isaac and I sat in the audience section facing the judge. After the charges were read, Tanya opened her folder and presented the letter from Dr. Monroe to the judge. The judge waved it in the air and said, "Who is this Dr. Monroe? What does 'F.A.C.S.' mean? This is no exemption letter." Approximately the next 5 or 10 minutes went something like this:

Judge: We need a statement from a pediatrician. Where is the child's pediatrician?

Me: We don't have one. This is an invasion of privacy.

Tanya: There is a great deal of evidence that vaccinations are harmful.

Me: Yes, Rutgers; U.C., California; Dr. Mendelsohn.

Judge: Well, we'll see. I've had all my children vaccinated.

Me: There is a religious exemption.

Judge: (*Waving his arms*) Ohhhh no!

A few exchanges with the social worker and Tanya, which I have forgotten, and then the judge said, "Well, you'll need to get a lawyer."

Me: This better not cost anything. We're not paying a cent!

At this point the judge reprimanded me for being disorderly and ordered me to leave the court. Tanya told me to take Isaac with me, which I did. In his reprimand the judge said that this case was between the Commonwealth of Virginia and Mrs. Turner, not me. As I was walking out into the parking lot with Isaac, I thought, "This case is not between the state of Virginia and Tanya; it is between freedom and tyranny."

After the court hearing was adjourned, Tanya talked in the hall with Deborah Balak and the gentleman who was with her in the courtroom. Later we discovered he was Michael Soberick, the prosecuting attorney. When Tanya came to the parking lot, she told me, "That man with Deborah wanted to see the letter from Dr. Monroe. He told me to get him to rewrite the letter to read more like the law, and he would be satisfied and drop the case. But I don't want to bother Dr. Monroe anymore. I told them I could take the religious exemption. The man asked me what my religion was, and I told him, 'My own private religion.' He sort of snickered when I said that." Tanya also told me that he seemed to want to get the whole thing over with and that it was Deborah who was pressing the issue.

Tanya also told me the judge appointed a lawyer for Isaac and asked her how much she made so he could suggest a lawyer for her. She declined to divulge her salary because she felt it was none of the court's business. (She was working as a computer programmer.) The judge, therefore, did not suggest a lawyer.

When Tanya told me this, I was outraged. So this was going to cost money as well as more time and energy! We had broken no law that I knew of and yet Tanya was being charged with the expense not only for a defense attorney for herself but very possibly for the state-appointed attorney for her child. (The summons stated on the reverse side that the parents could be charged with the cost of the legal services for their child.)

Perhaps the real irony of the whole affair was that it would be hard to find a child more loved and carefully reared than Isaac. Tanya stayed home from work for over two years to nurse him, and he was fed only fresh, whole, "natural" foods and food supplements.

That night I had insomnia. The specter of possible large legal fees and more time and energy down the drain kept me awake. (Our financial resources could best be described as modest.) My daughter told me the next morning that she also slept poorly. To people uninitiated in the ways of the mindless machinery of the state legal system, the experience of confronting its police powers can be frightening. (When I use the term *mindless* I mean mind plugged into automatic and thereby disconnected from its perceptive and reflective powers.)

FIRST AID ARRIVES

The next day I called the National Health Federation in Monrovia, California. This is an organization whose purpose is to promote freedom of choice in health matters. When I explained our problem, the secretary connected me to Clinton Miller, the federation's legislative advocate. We discussed both the medical and religious exemptions that were allowed in the state of Virginia, and it became apparent that taking the religious exemption was by far the easier and less expensive way to go. Clinton had a letter written to Deborah and a statement for us to sign that said that "the administration of immunizing agents conflicts with their religious tenets and practices." He would have sent a letter to the judge, had we known his name.

Talking with Clinton was very therapeutic. The tension of being alone and not knowing drained out of me. Tanya had much the same experience when I relayed the information to her that evening.

Three days later Clinton's letter arrived. We—both parents and maternal grandparents—signed the statement. Monday morning, September 14, Tanya delivered to the social worker the envelope containing the letter, the signed statement, and the religious exemption form that she had not had a chance to present to the judge the week before.

On September 21 Deborah called Tanya at work to make an appointment to discuss the letter Tanya had given her. Two days later Tanya and Alan (her husband) visited Deborah in her office. She said she felt the letter misrepresented her because Tanya had merely said that vaccination was against her beliefs, not religious beliefs. She inquired about Tanya's religious beliefs. Tanya said that the specific religious tenet that the practice of vaccination violated was her belief that the body was the temple of God and the use of immunizing agents polluted the body. In other words, her religious practices included not using immunizing agents. Deborah was not sufficiently impressed to call the whole thing off and said to Alan, "You know, of course, it's important to have the child protected." Tanya told me she seemed genuinely concerned about the welfare of the child.

Lawyers and Churches

On September 25 Tanya called Clinton Miller to tell him that the letter did not deter Ms. Balak from pursuing legal action against her and to ask him what course of action he would now recommend. He recommended we engage Gerald Norton (not his real name) as our attorney. Tanya then asked if there were any possibility of our losing the case. Clinton implied it was not inconceivable because we were up against a tyranny. Tanya replied she would leave the state before she would have Isaac vaccinated. Clinton mentioned the possibility of raising funds for the defense.

Tanya went to see Gerald Norton about taking the case. He said he couldn't because he was going to Europe, and besides, he would charge too much. (He said this after questioning her as to her financial status.) He recommended that she consult Joseph Connelly (not his real name), another lawyer, saying that the case was interesting and could easily go to the Supreme Court.

When Tanya went to see Joe Connelly, he read my account of the proceedings thus far and looked over the pertinent documents. Then he asked Tanya about her financial resources. When he found that these were inadequate, he recommended that she join the Christian Science Church "to take care of the immediate situation" (translate: "get the law off your back"). When Tanya remonstrated that she would like to fight this very unjust law—which violates the very essence and spirit of democracy—and "open a few eyes," Joe said that the most feasible way for her in her financial position to go about doing this would be to write legislators and contact key people after the trial.

Earlier, Joe Connelly had contacted the city attorney who was sitting with Deborah Balak at the initial hearing. The attorney said that being a member of the Christian Science Church would satisfy the law. He also said that getting the doctor to write a letter stating that the child had some specific physical condition for which inoculations were contraindicated would satisfy the law. Obviously, we couldn't ask a doctor to lie because Isaac is a healthy child.

The disappointing aspect of this experience for Tanya was that no one seemed really interested in her case, not even the principle of the thing, which is our real bone of contention. (The principle being, of course, the right of freedom of choice in personal health care matters.) The lawyers were only interested in somehow satisfying the letter of the law and obtaining money for their services. She finally learned that hiring lawyers and going to court—especially for the purpose of defending a principle—is a rich man's game.

She told us she planned to go to the Christian Science Church and get an application for membership.

That Sunday, October 4, Tanya came home early from an out-of-town trip in order to go to the Christian Science Church. She had been to the Christian Science Reading Room earlier in the week and had gotten some literature and read it. The ideas, for the most part, were congenial, and so she went to the church. She came home happy with what she found, saying the people were warm and friendly. She got an application for membership.

The next day I called the American Civil Liberties Union in Richmond, Virginia, to see if they would take a case like ours. The girl answering the phone told me that they were so far behind in litigation that they could take no new cases; and before they could take our case, it would have to be reviewed by a board. She gave me the impression that it was not beyond the realm of possibility for them to take a case such as ours, the only criterion being whether a civil liberty was being violated.

On Wednesday, October 7, Clinton Miller called. In essence, he said that he felt it was wrong for anyone to join a church under coercion and that the advice the lawyer gave Tanya is referred to in legal parlance as "expeditious" advice. In other words, if you don't have the money to afford a lawyer, just do something to get yourself off the hook. I gave him Joe Connelly's phone number, and he said he was going to write some letters and make some phone calls. He told us to call him at his home on Saturday if we hadn't heard from him. We decided, however, that we would simply go to court, and Tanya would say in effect, "I can't afford a lawyer. These are my religious tenets and practices, and this right is protected by the Constitution. Religion is a very private and personal thing, not to be defined or limited by the state." Also, Clinton said that it was not beyond the realm of possibility that the Christian Science Church would not accept her—and then where would she be? Certainly, his own church would turn down an application if the person applying appeared motivated by any other reason than deeply felt commitment to the tenets of the church.

When Tanya got home she called Clinton and told him of her "conversion" to the Christian Science Church. She said that the ideas of the church were congenial for the most part and that joining this church might solve other problems for her such as providing a Sunday school for Isaac. Clinton questioned the sincerity of her convictions, but when he realized that she seemed content with this solution, he said he would drop the case. He told her to call Michael Soberick, the prosecuting attorney, and maybe they would drop the hearing.

Tanya called Michael Soberick the next day and told him she had applied for membership in the Christian Science Church to satisfy the law. He said that in that event the case would be continued for six months, at which time it would be reviewed to be sure she was still a member of the church in good standing. He asked for the name of a person from the church who knew her and knew of her intentions to join. He also said they would require verification of her attendance.

Tanya then called me and was indignant. She said, "Well, I'm back to square one." The realization that she was going to be monitored and her sincerity checked shattered her former enthusiasm; she recognized she had been motivated by expediency. I told her to call Clinton Miller and get his advice. She did, and he laughed at her sudden "unconversion." They discussed writing a press release and getting publicity. He also mentioned Kirpatrick Dilling, the National Health Federation's (NHF) lawyer in Chicago, and implied that the case would not be at all difficult for him to win. However, the concern was more with raising the level of public awareness than just winning the case. He told Tanya to have me write a press release and to call back later that evening with the article. He gave her the first sentence.

The next day Clinton called, and we worked over the press release. I also talked with Jo Ludwig about starting an NHF chapter here. They said they would send a packet of materials I would need to start a chapter.

Two days before the second court hearing (October 11), I awoke at 2 A.M. I went downstairs, took a pencil and several pieces of scratch paper, and wrote Tanya's defense speech. Later that morning I typed it up; Paul, my husband and Tanya's father, edited it, and Tanya made a few changes. She practiced the speech in front of us. We made a few suggestions.

IN COURT AGAIN

October 13: Second hearing. Tanya, Alan, Isaac, Paul, and Ingri (Tanya's younger sister) attended the hearing. I didn't go into the courtroom because I was too angry, embarrassed, and frustrated. Angry, because to me this whole business was such an obvious violation of civil liberties, and these people couldn't see it. Embarrassed, because I had misbehaved in a court of law. Frustrated, because I felt like an anthropologist who had stumbled into a tribe of primitives and found herself forced to pay homage to their taboos and fetishes. Yes, my prejudices were surfacing.

We were better prepared for this hearing than we were for the first one. Not only did Tanya bring the speech we had prepared, but she brought additional medical evidence as well. We also knew the name of the judge (Frederick Aucamp) and the identity of the prosecuting attorney, Michael Soberick.

After the hearing, Tanya, Alan, Paul, and Ingri told me what happened in the courtroom. Like the Japanese film *Roshomon*, each had a different version of the drama. Alan thought Tanya's inability to handle the rebuttal and cross-examination disastrous; Paul thought everything worked out beautifully; and Ingri, although critical of Tanya's delivery, was generally pleased at the way things went. Tanya herself told a reporter, "I was really happy with the judge. He listened to all my arguments." This is part of the speech she read to the court:

Your Honor, Judge Aucamp, Assistant City Attorney, Mr. Soberick, and Ms. Balak from the Virginia Beach Department of Social Services. If it pleases Your Honor, I would like approximately seven minutes of your time to state my case.

I, Tanya Turner, am appearing *pro se* (prō-sāy) before this court today. I am appearing in my own defense because I cannot afford the services of a lawyer. The state has appointed an attorney, Mr. Alan Rosenblatt, for my son Isaac. Because I cannot afford his services either, I do not accept the services of Mr. Rosenblatt.

I am appearing in this court today because I am charged with failure to have my two-year-old son Isaac vaccinated. I believe this charge comes under the category of medical neglect. Since I deliberately *chose* not to have my son vaccinated, this is not a case of neglect but of educated choice. I *chose* not to have my son vaccinated for both medical and religious reasons. The state law of Virginia allows both these exemptions. I tried to satisfy the medical exemption by presenting to you, at the first hearing on September 8, 1981, a letter from our doctor, Paul Monroe, a general surgeon. You would not accept this letter. I would have attempted to satisfy the religious exemption at that time but was prevented from doing so.

. . . As an American citizen whose right to worship according to the dictates of his own conscience is protected by the Constitution of the United States, I object to the surveillance procedures Mr. Soberick has suggested. I refuse to be coerced into a particular form of worship.

Virginia State law says *nothing* about *organized* religion in the "religious tenets or practices" allowed in the first exemption. The notion that this exemption applies only to members of an organized religion is only an interpretation of some lawyers. This *interpretation* violates the First Amendment of the Constitution of the United States, which I will read in part.

"Congress shall make no law respecting an establishment of religion, or prohibiting the free exercise thereof . . . "

The state may not define what a religion is and is not. A religious tenet or practice is not limited to a tenet or practice of an *organized* religion. Religion is a personal and private matter and includes any sincerely held belief.

While I will continue to investigate the Christian Science Church, I will base my defense at this time on my *own personal* religious tenets and practices. I believe that the body is the temple of God. This is a religious tenet, found in the Bible, First Corinthians, Chapter 6, Verse 19.

I, myself, have never been vaccinated. I do not believe in the injection of foreign and, therefore, toxic substances into the human body. My religious practices, therefore, include not using immunizing agents.

I have another religious tenet that is the very bedrock upon which this country was founded. I believe in freedom of choice. I believe the right of the individual to decide for himself how he will conduct the affairs of his life is sacred and inalienable as long as he injures no one else. If a person does not have the right to choose what shall be done to his own body and how he shall rear his own children, what right does he have?

Thank you, Your Honor.

The judge listened courteously and asked for any witnesses. Ingri described how sick she became and how her hair fell out after a smallpox and cholera vaccination in India. After consulting *Black's Legal Dictionary* for the definition of *religion*, Judge Aucamp said that Tanya's objection to vaccination was really philosophical rather than religious and therefore didn't come under the protection of the First Amendment. He said in effect, "At the next hearing, then, you'll have to present medical evidence that vaccinations are harmful, or I'll have no other choice but to order shots for the child unless you appeal." He instructed Tanya to take the necessary medical evidence to the prosecuting attorney two weeks before the third hearing.

PUBLICITY AND NEW CONTACTS

On October 14, Tanya and Isaac's picture appeared in the *Virginian-Pilot* with an accompanying article entitled "Woman Challenges Required Vaccinations."[2] "I refuse to be coerced into a particular kind of worship," she told the reporter after telling him how the city attorney's office had advised her that her membership in the Christian Science Church would be monitored over a period of months.

A number of people called expressing concern and sympathy. Several of them—including a local nurse and a chiropractor—gave us some valuable information that we included in our exhibit. We were also urged by several people to get a lawyer.

I wrote to Thomas Finn, head of the Freedom of Choice Law Center in Georgia, in reference to his article in the *Vegetarian Times*, "How to Avoid Compulsory Immunizations."[3] I asked a question that the article raised and enclosed a newspaper article about our case.

A few days later Tom Finn called and offered to represent us without charge if we would pay his travel expenses to and from Virginia Beach and his lodgings. He pointed out several possible pitfalls with the way we were proceeding and seemed very concerned that we not jeopardize the freedom of choice health movement by losing our case. I assured him we would not lose and would call him back after discussing this matter with the rest of the family and Clinton Miller.

After consulting with the family and Clinton, we agreed to have Tom Finn represent us. This choice also required a Virginia lawyer because Tom is not licensed in the state of Virginia. Tanya was relieved because she had been uneasy about appearing *pro se* in court again.

On October 30, about two and a half weeks before the court hearing, Paul and I delivered to Michael Soberick's office almost 90 pages of scientific evidence and medical opinions attesting to the harmful effects of vaccination. After I sent Tom Finn the pertinent papers and my account of the case as well as a copy of the exhibit we sent to the prosecuting attorney, Tom phoned the prosecuting attorney and told him to give the exhibit to the judge.

On November 17, Isaac's birthday and the evening before the court hearing, we picked Tom up at the airport. Because we didn't know what he looked like, Isaac carried a sign reading "Welcome Tom Finn." Between Tom's briefcase and our sign, recognition was easy. Tom was friendly and congenial, and we enjoyed our visit with him.

COURT AND VERDICT

At 1 P.M. on November 18 we were in court. Outside the courthouse, Tanya was interviewed by TV reporters; inside the courthouse, she was interviewed by newspaper reporters. After about 15 or 20 minutes we all filed into the courtroom, newspaper and TV reporters filling the second row and family and friends the third row. A sandy-haired, bespectacled man, whom I later found out was an official of the health department, sat in the second row.

Judge Aucamp immediately asked for the doctor's letter. Tom gave it to him, and the judge suggested we try to get it reworded to comply with the law. Tom said he would call Dr. Monroe to get him to reword the letter. Because Wednesday is Dr. Monroe's day off, Tom called him at his home. When Dr. Monroe said he would rewrite the letter, the health officer took the phone and read him the "riot act." He told Dr. Monroe that people would now get the idea that all they had to do was go to him and they wouldn't have to be vaccinated. The prosecuting attorney made the same objection when Tom told the court we were getting the letter from the doctor rewritten as requested. Dr. Monroe told the health officer that shots would be detrimental in this case because the family was so opposed to them. (I wasn't present at this scene since it took place "offstage." Tom told us this later, saying that Dr. Monroe was really a "strong man.")

Judge Aucamp made a motion to adjourn the court and reconvene when we could present the letter from the doctor. After several suggestions, we finally agreed to meet the next day. Tom asked if it were necessary for him to be there, and the judge said no. All that was necessary was for the letter to be reworded and turned in.

A couple of unusual elements in this scenario are worth comment. The first was that the letter did not have to state a negative physical condition for which vaccinations would be contraindicated. Tom pointed out that the law did not specify that the condition had to be negative. (Our exhibit presented evidence that vaccinations could be harmful to *any* child.)

The second was that after setting a date for readjournment and before dismissing the court, the judge made the statement that he didn't want to get into the medical aspects of this case because that would be "opening a can of worms." I couldn't help but translate this rather revealing statement as, "I have seen the evidence and found that it does exist—vaccinations are harmful—but I'm stuck with a law I have to uphold and constituents I don't want to antagonize, so let's all get off the hook as gracefully as possible."

November 19: The Day of the Chestnuts. Second part of the third hearing. Michael Soberick turned in a spirited performance. Once again he objected to the "hearsay evidence" of the letter that the judge had said the day before was precisely what the law called for. He wanted to cross-examine the doctor. He objected to the "contradiction" of the two letters (really the second was simply more specific than the first). And finally, he repeated again the old chestnut,

"Society has rights." He put Tanya on the witness stand and quibbled about the difference between "status" and "condition" and objected again that there was no health problem with the child for which shots would be contraindicated. Tanya replied that the condition that the law referred to could be positive or negative—the law didn't specify.

Before the final ruling, more chestnuts fell:

Michael: Society has rights.

Judge: The individual has rights, too.

Michael: The child should be protected.

Judge: That's the responsibility of the parents.

When Michael made the statement that failure to vaccinate Isaac threatened public health, I wondered if he had read any of the material we turned in to him. When the judge finally ruled in our favor, he turned to Mike and said, "Well, Mike, I know you feel like you've been railroaded." The judge also said that the responsibility to prevent similar exemptions rests with the legislature, not him. "Hmmmmmmmm," I thought, "so the name of this game is *Win, Don't Rock the Boat,* and *Pass the Buck.*"

After the hearing, I went up to the judge and thanked him for his decision and apologized for my behavior at the first hearing.

FALLOUT

The next morning when we tuned in to the 8 A.M. news broadcast, the first news we heard was:

Three-year-old Isaac Turner won a victory in the Virginia Beach courts yesterday. The mother maintained that the risks involved with vaccination do not warrant vaccinating a healthy child.

When we opened the front page of the local news section of the *Virginian-Pilot*, we read the headline: "Judge Exempts Child from Inoculations."[4] In the article Judge Aucamp was quoted as saying, "The risks of the shots outweigh the benefits." The article went on to say that a spokeswoman for the health department said that studies by the Federal Center for Disease Control show there are greater risks in failing to vaccinate children. She said that one half of 1 percent of the children eligible for vaccinations are granted exemptions on medical or religious grounds each year and that about 65,000 children were vaccinated in Virginia last year.

When I read these figures, I couldn't help being appalled. How can a nation of sheep be a free people? Apparently no one questions the wisdom of a theory that says in effect that the best way to build health—and disease prevention subsumes under health—is to poison the body. (Vaccines are poisons by definition.) And even worse, apparently no one questions the studies and pronouncements of a monolith, particularly a monolith with such an obvious vested interest in perpetrating a particular point of view. I was reminded of what Alvin Toffler said: "We need to begin thinking like the same revolutionaries who made the American form of government in the first place."[5]

The afternoon paper, the *Ledger-Star*, printed an article with the suggestive title "Doctor's Note Saves Boy from Vaccination."[6]

Three days later (November 23), the *Virginian-Pilot* published a letter to the editor written by Dr. Thomas Rubio, professor of pediatrics, Eastern Virginia Medical School, entitled "Children Haven't a 'Right' to Disease."[7] The letter echoed the same ideas as the editorial, saying that the judge's ruling "disregarded the rights of the child to be protected against serious illnesses." He took exception to the judge's statement that "the risk of the shots outweigh the benefits" by referring to "the extensive experience with vaccinations in this country" and the "well documented" studies of the U.S. Public Health Service and the "recommendations of the American Academy of Pediatrics." He also warned of dire consequences of failure to comply with the required immunization program.

On November 27 an editorial appeared in the *Virginian-Pilot* called "Immunize Immunizations," which objected to both the decision of the judge and the letter of the doctor that exempted Isaac from vaccination.[8] The arguments were typical: the recitation of statistics that show a decline in the number of infectious diseases and the attribution of this decline primarily to the practice of vaccination. The editor warned of epidemics to come if the practice of compulsory mass immunizations is not strictly adhered to: "Whenever an epidemic of childhood disease occurs, the outbreak is nearly always traceable to a falloff in inoculations." The editorial concluded by saying, "If the General Assembly values the health gains from mass immunizations, it will inoculate the system against subversion by a physician's say-so."

On December 6 the *Virginian-Pilot* published my rebuttal under the title "Vaccination Is a Political Disease."[9] Even though my letter was considerably shortened, the editor managed to extract the salient points, which were: (1) The decline in infectious diseases was not due to vaccination; (2) the harmful effects of vaccination are not negligible, nor do they affect just a minuscule percentage of the population; and (3) advocates of compulsory immunization are, in fact, "advocating taking away one of our basic freedoms—the freedom of choice referred to in the Declaration of Independence as the right to 'life, liberty and the pursuit of happiness.' " My letter continued, "you advocate imposing your medical beliefs—and they are beliefs—on others in violation of the Constitution."

On December 10 Tanya received a letter from her Virginia lawyer, Hank Sadler. He informed her that Michael Soberick, the prosecuting attorney, was appealing the ruling of the judge. When Tanya first showed me the letter, my reaction was visceral: "How could he," I thought. "Did he read any of the material we gave him? . . . Maybe he's under pressure from the health department . . . or is it pressure from the ego?'' The real point of the exhibit, as I saw it, was not so much to show how harmful vaccinations are but to show what a wide latitude of disagreement there is among doctors—the ''experts''—themselves. Some refuse to give this shot or that shot, and some give only one shot at one time and not at another, and some, in agreement with us, say ''no thanks'' to the whole business. Gray areas like this are hardly places where the police powers of the state belong.

Shortly after we received this letter, I wrote to Clinton Miller, telling him we had already spent over $800 on this case and simply couldn't afford to spend any more. The National Health Federation sent out a letter to raise funds for Tanya's legal expenses. Included in the letter was a reproduction of the newspaper article with Tanya and Isaac's picture, a press release written by Clinton Miller and me, and an eloquent letter written by Dr. Mendelsohn.

A few weeks after the letter went out, we began receiving calls from sympathetic and interested people from all parts of the country. Some of them sent valuable literature, which I have included in the second chapter of this book. One woman from Michigan told me we should be working with our legislators to get the law changed. Some wanted to send money, and I told them to send it to the NHF Legal Fund for Tanya.

Among the many letters and phone calls that came in during the next few months, a particularly heart-rending letter told of ''a dear friend'' whose beautiful, healthy 6-year-old son, who had never been ill, ''died a hideous death'' after vaccination. Subsequent letters described the mother as being adamantly opposed to vaccinations. She had let herself be pressured into submitting to the vaccination because otherwise her son would not have been admitted to school in New York. Shortly after the vaccination the child went to sleep and slept all afternoon. Each day thereafter he ''became more and more listless until excruciating pains and high fever forced his admittance to the local hospital. After numerous operations and unbelievable suffering for seven months, the child died a hideous death.'' The writer of the letter went on to say that the mother ''did not sue the doctor as he was, by New York State law, required to vaccinate the child before he would be permitted to enter school.''

For the first time in my life, I could fully identify with people all over the world who are struggling for freedom and with the founders of our country who dedicated their lives to create a constitution that would guarantee liberty for its citizens. Somehow I realized on a deeper level that the central theme of human history was indeed freedom, as Lord Acton[10] had said, and that life without it wasn't worth living.

NOTES

1. See Peter Barry Chowka, ''A Matter of Life, Death, and Freedom,'' *New Age*, January–February 1980.

2. "Woman Challenges Required Vaccinations," *Virginian-Pilot*, October 14, 1981, p. C3.

3. Thomas Finn, "How to Avoid Compulsory Immunizations," *Vegetarian Times/Well-Being*, no. 48, 1981.

4. "Judge Exempts Child from Inoculations," *Virginian-Pilot*, November 19, 1981, pp. C1. C4.

5. From a talk by Alvin Toffler reported in the University of Utah *Review*, November 1975.

6. "Doctor's Note Saves Boy from Vaccination," *Ledger-Star*, November 20, 1981, p. C3.

7. "Children Haven't a 'Right' to Disease," *Virginian-Pilot*, November 23, 1981, p. A14.

8. "Immunize Immunizations," *Virginian-Pilot*, November 27, 1981, p. A14.

9. "Vaccination is a Political Disease," *Virginian-Pilot*, December 6, 1981, p. C4.

10. Lord Acton was an eminent Cambridge historian who began in 1880 a series of books in which he planned to expound human freedom as history's central theme. He is the author of the famous saying: "Power corrupts and absolute power corrupts absolutely."

11 "Let My People Go"

When Israel was in Egypt land,
Let my people go.
Oppressed so hard, they could not stand,
Let my people go.

—"Go Down, Moses,"
Negro spiritual.

"Let my people go." I could still hear our high school glee club singing those lines. "Go down, Moses . . . Tell old pharoah/To let my people go." Yes, freedom is the central theme of human history.

THE MEDICAL PHARAOH

What happened to the participants in our drama? Dr. Monroe almost lost his license. The Virginia Beach Medical Society cited him for unethical conduct for the exemption letter he wrote for us. "Personal choice means absolutely nothing to these people," he told me. "They want complete control over you."

To Dr. Monroe it was unethical to force a medical treatment—and particularly a risky medical treatment—upon an unwilling patient. To the Virginia Beach doctors it was unethical to break rank—go outside one's specialty and go against the party line.

Tanya and Isaac fared better than Dr. Monroe. Through a simple legal maneuver, Tom Finn got Mike Soberick to call off the appeal. We were free . . . for the time being.

Among the many phone calls I received—mostly from people wanting more information about vaccinations and how to avoid them—a particularly interesting and helpful one came from a woman in Wisconsin. She said that she and her family wanted to move to Virginia (her husband had an excellent job offer) but would not consider it if they were going to be hassled about immunizations, as we were. She described the struggle they had in Wisconsin getting the exemption based on personal conviction reinstated. The exemption had been part of the law once—the result of the hard work of many people—and suddenly they discovered it wasn't there anymore. A legislator told her the pressure was from the federal level and I said, "Of course. In 1962 there was a compulsory immunization bill before Congress that would have exempted no one, but it was defeated because of the efforts of such groups as the Christian Scientists, the National Health Federation, the Natural Hygienists and others." "Yes," she said. "The legislator here told me that they are now going about it by getting just a few states at a time."

Later she sent me a tape of a doctor speaking out against immunizations at a Natural Hygiene Convention, part of which I used in Chapters 2 and 3 of this book. She also sent me some literature and a remarkable book entitled *The Hazards of Immunization* (1967) by Sir Graham S. Wilson, published by the University of London, which chronicles complications and fatalities from the use of serums and vaccines.[1] The accounts are relayed simply and dryly, most of the mishaps being attributed to such things as bacterial contamination or faulty preparation. Opening the book at random, we read on page 88: "Olin and Lithander (1948) describe an incident in which three children injected intramuscularly at the same time with convalescent measles serum prepared at a hospital laboratory became ill within 6 to 8 hours. They suffered from high fever, vomiting and diarrhea, followed by somnolence, agitation and cyanosis. Two of them died 14 and 18 hours after the injection." Further down the page we read, "In this incident, which occurred in India in October 1902, 19 persons injected with plague vaccine contracted tetanus 5–6 days later and all died within 7–10 days of their injection." Similar incidences are recounted for 290 pages reinforced by 20 pages of references.

Perhaps the most depressing feature of this book is not so much the bloodless numbers, statistics, and recitations of cripplings and fatalities but the discouraging realization that man learns very slowly; his ability to penetrate the multiple layers of data and phenomena and arrive at a clearing where principles reveal themselves is apparently very limited at this time. Dr. Wilson makes it clear that he is no antivaccinationist, saying that even though "all forms of active and passive immunization are potentially dangerous, [it] is no condemnation of their use" (p. 6).

A NEW BEGINNING

It was now time to contact legislators and formally open an area chapter of the National Health Federation. On January 4, 1982, I mailed letters to the five

House of Delegates and the three state senators of our district, requesting that Section D of Article 3, Chapter 2 of the Code of Virginia (the compulsory immunization law), be amended to include an exemption based on personal beliefs. I cited a number of other states that had this exemption as well as the unconstitutionality of the present law. Three delegates replied, saying they would investigate the matter, and our senator from this area, Joe Canada, said he would send my letter to Legislative Services to have a bill drafted.

On May 13, 1982, the Tidewater Chapter of the National Health Federation had its first meeting. Our first project was getting a petition signed which requested that the compulsory immunization laws of Virginia be amended to provide for an exemption based on personal conviction. The petition mentioned that there were 19 states that already had this exemption. An accompanying sheet listed, with references, some of the diseases and disabilities that have been linked to immunizations and pointed out that there are natural and harmless ways of preventing and treating the so-called dread diseases for which vaccines are given.

By the third meeting, it became apparent that we weren't getting enough signatures, so I handed out samples of a form letter to be sent to state legislators in September. The letter was checked by the group.

A couple of interesting confrontations occurred in connection with our petition-signing activities. Several people told stories of an occasional person who was hostile and indignant when confronted with the petition. One person, who is a member of a church that is health and nutrition conscious, told how her fellow church members shied away from her when she approached them with the petition, saying in effect that their pediatrician knows best.

Another incident occurred with regard to getting publicity for our meetings. The first time I submitted an announcement of our meeting to *The Beacon*, a section of our leading local newspaper, for inclusion in their "Community in Action" section, the editors deleted the phrase "freedom of choice in health matters." The second time I submitted the notice of our meeting, I included the above phrase plus "Speaker and discussion: Compulsory Immunization." This notice never appeared in the paper. When I inquired as to why our notice was not published, I was informed by the girl in charge that it had been omitted at the downtown offices, probably for reasons of space, and besides, *The Beacon* does not guarantee publishing all notices anyway. When I remonstrated that several notices much longer than mine were printed, she replied that it is easier to delete a whole notice than to delete part of a longer one.

The third time I submitted the notice of our meeting, it was printed, but both the phrase "freedom of choice in health matters" (which explains what the Health Federation is all about) and the name and subject of the speaker were omitted. (The speaker was speaking on "Alternate Cancer Therapies." She had been cured of terminal cancer by using a combination of the laetrile and Gerson therapies, and her story had been printed by both the *Virginian-Pilot* and the *Ledger-Star*.)

I decided it was time to write the editor. When we remember that Virginia is a state that is proud of its colonial heritage, of the monuments and relics associated with the founding of our country—which was founded upon the ideals of freedom and brotherhood—the story I am telling seems particularly ironic. *The Beacon* frequently publishes stories featuring the history and current use of these historical relics. In fact, the edition in which our truncated notice appeared featured a story on a historical park here. So after describing our problem with the "Community in Action" section of *The Beacon*, I said to the editor:

Could it be that freedom is a dirty word when used in the "wrong" context? Is it a noble, inspiring and beautiful word when associated with historical names, places and objects; but does it become obscene, irrelevant and cumbersome when applied to current events that threaten the power and prerogative of one of the tribal gods?

The founders of our country established a system of checks and balances to ensure equitable treatment of people and issues. They knew that unless they established checks on power and prerogative these easily become abusive. Where are the checks and balances in the area of the healing arts? Only one school of healing—medicine—is recognized in a court of law and only their particular point of view is endorsed and disseminated by the media. Stories are legion of doctors—medical or otherwise—who either break with that point of view or never bought it in the first place and who are remarkably successful in "curing" people of all manner of maladies, including "incurable" ones. Their reward: ostracism, persecution and, in many cases, confiscation of materials and loss of license. This abuse of power, because it is unchallenged by a system of checks and balances, is precisely what the National Health Federation was organized to counteract. Does *The Beacon* align itself with this abuse of power?

About a week later I received a phone call. No, it was not from the editor but from the girl who takes the notices. "The problem is with 'freedom of choice in health matters,' " she said. "You have freedom of choice. You can choose the doctor and the hospital you want." "But you can't choose the kind of therapy or even the kind of doctor you want," I said. "What if I wanted to go to a naturopath or a homeopath? The former aren't even licensed in this state and the latter aren't even represented in this area, as far as I know. Also, what if I had cancer and decided I wanted laetrile or some other metabolic therapy? At best I would have a very difficult time getting it." I also pointed out that freedom to choose includes the right to treat and prevent illness in different ways, the compulsory immunization law being an obvious violation of this principle. "So it's a right to pursue a different philosophy of health. Your objections are philosophical," she said. "You might put it that way," I replied.

We had no more trouble getting notices of our meetings in *The Beacon*.

POLITICS

We sent form letters to Virginia legislators asking them to introduce legislation to amend the compulsory vaccination law to allow for an exemption based on personal belief. The letter quoted statements from Dr. J. Anthony Morris, former chief vaccine control officer of the FDA, that "there is a great deal of evidence to prove that immunization of children does more harm than good" and that "there is no rationale for forcing immunization."[2] We also included the famous statement on vaccination by Clarence Darrow: "If vaccination does what its advocates claim for it, the person who is vaccinated ought to be safe no matter whether anybody else is vaccinated or not."[3] We pointed out that 19 states already have a personal exemption and concluded by saying "the practice of vaccination is controversial and is hardly an area where the police powers of the state belong."

Most legislators didn't reply. Of the three that did, one said he agreed and would support our position, but he was up for reelection and lost. One said he would study the matter, and another said he "had occasion to pursue this matter in some detail with the State Health Commissioner who presented overwhelming evidence that a voluntary immunization program would not be successful or worthwhile to maintain"; therefore, he could not support our position. When I read that letter, I couldn't help thinking, "What an admission! So the program can't stand on its own merits; it has to be forced."

On November 15, I went to see Joe Canada, one of our state senators, to see about introducing an amendment to the compulsory immunization law to allow for an exemption based on personal belief. He suggested I would be wise to be satisfied with a "study" for the next year or two because if I tried to push the bill through this time, it would very likely be defeated. This bill will be tough to pass, he pointed out, because the law has been in effect for so long. He explained to me some of the convolutions of the legislative process and how even the simplest, most obviously needed legislation takes two and sometimes three years to get enacted.

At our January 1983 Health Federation meeting, I spoke on "The Four Myths of Vaccination," and at our February meeting, we showed the videotape *DPT: Vaccine Roulette*. Ellen Jacobs (not her real name), a teacher of natural childbirth, brought her class to both meetings. She told of two women she knew who lived in this area whose babies had died the very night after receiving their first DPT shot. Another person described a friend's child who died the night after receiving the DPT shot. Ellen also related that a woman, a former student of hers, with a 5-month-old baby girl called her recently to tell her that her baby died one week after receiving the DPT shot. "The baby was breast fed, and the parents were really into nutrition, too," Ellen said. In all these cases, the doctors denied any connection between the shot and the death, insisting the shot had nothing to do with it. "What else could they do?" I pointed out. "If they admit a connection, they not only could be sued, but their license and practice could also be threatened."

During the course of the four years since the last court hearing, I have received many phone calls from parents who were determined not to have their child immunized and wanted to know how to avoid it. Many had an older child who had been immunized and had suffered various side effects, some apparently permanent. For instance, one mother who "knew better" let her son be immunized for admittance to school. He went into anaphylactic shock. She was determined that her younger child would never be immunized even if she had to keep her out of school. Another mother told how her baby girl became paralyzed on the left side after her third DPT shot. The child, who was 7 at the time the mother talked to me, had a stiff left hand and a slight speech defect. Another mother who had a healthy 6-year-old daughter who suddenly came down with rheumatoid arthritis remembered she had let her be immunized for German measles a month earlier. With the exception of the shock case, the doctors, as usual, denied any connection between the shot and the disability.

In many cases of parents with a vaccine-injured child, the parent was opposed to, or at least hesitant about, immunizations but let herself be pressured into consenting. There is a bond between mother and child that is particularly strong during those early years, and any anxiety or resentment the parent feels can be picked up by the child. Surely there is a connection, no matter how subtle, between parental objection to a procedure and the child's subsequent negative reaction to it. After all, we are not decapitated bodies anymore than we are disembodied minds.

When doctors speak of "herd immunity," they use the same terms we use to describe cattle or sheep. They forget that humans are mental and emotional individuals as well an anatomical and biochemical ones.[4] We might say that mass, compulsory immunization programs treat not only fictional, standardized, textbook bodies but headless ones as well.

During these same four years, I was surprised to discover the subterfuges people used to "protect" their children from the vaccination steamroller. I won't describe these because I don't want to jeopardize the only escape route many people know.

When a woman from Pennsylvania called and wanted both more information on immunizations as well as how to avoid them, I looked at my list of exempt states and said, "Oh, you don't have anything to worry about. Pennsylvania is one of the free states." Afterward I thought, "Hmmmmmm . . . *free* and *slave*, terms used to describe states over 100 years ago. We even have an 'underground railroad,' parents—and doctors, I might add—who use subterfuges." When we are unconscious, history is doomed to repeat itself.

POWER AND PRIVILEGE SPEAK

On April 7, 1983, I phoned Joe Canada to inquire about the bill. He said he couldn't get enough support for the bill, that no one was interested, but would try to have hearings on it between now and January 1984. I told him I would give him some literature on the subject. A few days later I dropped off a copy of an early draft of Chapter 2 of this book as well as copies of some articles.

On May 6, 1983, the *Virginian-Pilot* came out with a front-page article entitled "Schools Will Require Students to Show Proof of Shots This Fall."[5]

"Pupils Not Immunized to Be Barred" was the title of an article that appeared in the *Ledger-Star* the previous day.[6] The articles stated that there was a new and tougher immunization law passed by the general assembly in 1982! For instance, private schools and day care centers must comply and students' records checked for the exact dates of immunizations. A vice principal interviewed in a later article said he could get fined $10,000 for admitting a student who hadn't complied with the law. The articles did mention, however, the medical and religious exemptions.

By August, headlines were reading "Thousands of Students Still Need Shots"[7] and "Tidewater Schools Bar 3,700."[8] Various articles told of deluged clinics, vaccine shortages and borrowings from other cities, and harried personnel. I, as president of the local chapter of the National Health Federation, was interviewed and Tanya's case was mentioned. I was also interviewed on television.

I went to the library to get a copy of the new "tough" law. Sure enough, the legislature had amended the section pertaining to the medical exemption, saying that the certification by a licensed physician would have to specify "the specific nature and probable duration of the medical condition or circumstance that contraindicates immunization." Another interesting amendment to the law occurred in the first paragraph of the section on immunization requirements: "Neither this Commonwealth nor any school or admitting official shall be liable in damages to any person for complying with this section." What more is there to say?

UPDATE

Our chapter is no longer active. Two of our most dynamic and effective supporters, the vice president and the publicity chairpersons, moved out of state. The energy that kept the chapter alive gradually dissipated. I, for one, had the growing realization that real change in a society comes about not by legislation but by education. Passing a law when the consciousness of a critical mass of people does not accord with the law would be a holding action at best. The big issue here was not immunization, per se, but freedom of choice. The consciousness that is capable of grasping what this really means is a consciousness that understands that reality is relationships, that man is a spiritual being with the divine right to choose, and that truth is essentially harmonizing and liberating.

A society can change its direction only when a critical mass of people are capable of grasping a larger truth, of having a greater vision. A few lectures on immunization won't do it. The scientific aspects alone are too much for a simple public lecture. No, a book was required.

This was brought home to me even more emphatically when I took a trip to Arizona recently. I gave a public lecture on immunization—"Immunization: Miracle or Myth?"—and met with a group of people who were working with the immunization issue there. Arizona is one of the more recent states to become "free," to exempt students from the vaccination requirement on the basis of personal belief. Yet, I was told, the schools and the media were ignoring the law, telling parents that it was a "no shots, no school" situation. Furthermore, parents told of children who were in school with the vaccine waiver but were forced to stay home and miss many important school activities, including, in some cases, graduation activities. They were excluded because the board of health declared an emergency—an epidemic. Where the evidence was for this epidemic is anybody's guess. As we have learned (Chapter 3), epidemics are not difficult to manufacture.

While I was there, a number of people on different occasions told me what I had heard before: There is constant pressure to get the personal belief exemption in the compulsory vaccination law rescinded. Where does the pressure come from? The health department and, behind them, the federal government. I was reminded of an elderly woman who attended a couple of our Health Federation meetings. Many years ago—I believe it was in the 1960s—she and others had worked very hard to get the personal belief exemption clause inserted into the vaccination law in Virginia, only to have it rescinded shortly afterward. (She, incidentally, was a registered nurse whose healthy baby daughter became cross-eyed shortly after her DPT shot.)

The story I have told here is an old story, one that has been repeated over and over throughout human history and is now being repeated daily, hourly upon this planet. It is the story of coercion, of power using privilege to impose "benefits" upon those who do not want them. It is the story of egotism, greed, and blind belief. Without the last, the imposition of these benefits on a large scale would be impossible. Liberating ourselves from the nursery of nonthink in which blind belief flourishes is to begin the journey, not only to freedom but to maturity.

UPDATE II

October 1993: The Good News and the Bad

The good news is that more people are waking up—or is it growing up? In 1991, a newspaper article in Washington State (Associated Press), read: "Parents Rebelling Against Immunizing Their Children."[9] A comment from the *Boston Herald* on Neil Z. Miller's book (see Appendix G) states: "A growing number of people are refusing to have their children immunized. Mr. Miller believes this issue is about to explode." Unfortunately, too many people have arrived at this position after having experienced the tragedy of a vaccine-damaged child. If we haven't learned to question "authority" figures by the time we are adults, nature can exact rather harsh penalties.

More good news: More people are winning cases in court, not just after the fact of a vaccine-damaged child but before the fact. That is, people are winning the right to say "No thank you." Not to have this right in the first place is so outrageous that I have seriously wondered whether we have lost our capacity for outrage. Or maybe tunnel vision is just too pandemic.

Now the bad news: "On April 1, 1993, White House legislation (S 732, HR 940) was introduced into Congress which would establish federal 'tracking and surveillance' of American families through their children's Social Security numbers to increase vaccination rates among preschoolers."[10] Big Brother? This legislation would remove all exemptions except medical,[11] which opens the door for child abuse charges against parents who consciously choose not to vaccinate their children.[12]

In spite of the objections of many people and groups, this bill unanimously passed the Senate on November 16, 1993. As of this writing, the bill has been stalled in the House for months after an intense information campaign mounted by the National Vaccine Information Center and Dissatisfied Parents Together (NVIC/DPT) and other parent groups; however, the bill may become law as early as the end of 1994. Due to the efforts of these groups, there is a provision for parents to "opt-out" of the tracking system; but again, parents who choose not to vaccinate their children with one or more of the federally recommended and state-mandated vaccines risk eventually being targeted with charges of child neglect.[13]

Those who responsibly represent the "other side" of the vaccination issue are almost totally eclipsed from the media, the schools, and many government hearings. For instance, House and Senate hearings on the above legislation barred healthcare professionals concerned about the safety and efficacy of vaccinations from testifying. Parents were purposely forbidden to speak by those controlling the hearings, although individual parents and parent organizations asked days before the hearing for permission to testify.[14]

Freedom of Speech (First Amendment)?

Who was permitted to testify? Four presidents of companies that produce vaccines, the American Academy of Pediatrics, and public health officials, along with Donna Shalala, secretary of health and human services, and Marian Wright Edelman of the Children's Defense Fund.[15] At least one TV network news channel I saw made much of the "fact" that vested interests such as the AMA weren't permitted to testify at the meetings.

Don't think this vaccination bill was new to or initiated by the Clinton administration. The vaccinators have tried for many years for this kind of control over people. President George Bush, for instance, proposed "increasing immunization funds by 40 million to 258 million and making children's immunization a condition of welfare."[16] Wasn't it Gore Vidal who said this country needs two political parties?

Government (of the People?)

During the 1993 legislative session in Virginia, a bill was introduced that would require home-schooled, excused, or exempted children to submit to the same "health"—translate *vaccination*—requirements as those attending school. Several parents called to inform me about this bill and give me phone numbers of legislators to call. This I did along with registering my reasons for opposing the bill. When I phoned our state senator, Ken Stolle, to register my objection, an office worker informed me that they had received a lot of calls from people opposed to it.

Several weeks later (February 24, 1993), I received a letter from Ken Stolle, saying that he voted for the bill (H.R. 1954), "which passed both the House of Delegates and the Senate unanimously." What happened? Maybe not enough people registered their objection. No. A friend of mine told me that at least 250 people in this area were actively opposed to it and named a couple of organizations involved.

A few days later I phoned Ken Stolle's office to register my disappointment that a bill that was opposed by a considerable number of people was passed so easily. "This sure tells us who's running this country—special interests!" "You got it!" the office worker replied.

Education? (Fall 1990)

A friend of mine was teaching a course in early childhood development at Cuyahoga College in Ohio during the fall of 1990. Since the course was geared for parents and teachers involved with the Head Start program, one of its purposes was to familiarize the students with the laws and regulations governing the program. My friend, therefore, decided to discuss the vaccination laws of the state. At the time, Ohio was listed as one of the "free" states. Even though she read this in my book, she checked with the law library to confirm it. When she informed the class of the state law, a student reported her to the supervisor. A few days later she was called into the supervisor's office and told that the policy of the college is that vaccinations are mandatory and not to tell students otherwise! Any child enrolled in the Head Start program must be vaccinated, the supervisor told her.

A Healing Profession? (Fall 1990)

This same friend took her toddler to the pediatrician because she was having difficulty breathing. When the pediatrician asked if the child had had her shots, my friend replied, "No, I'm waiting until she gets a little older when her immune system is more mature." The doctor excused himself to consult with his colleagues in the office. When he came back, he said, "I'm sorry, but we don't treat children who aren't immunized."

Her experience is not unusual. I've heard of others.

When another friend of mine took her daughter to the hospital for emergency treatment and was met at the admittance desk by the usual "Is she caught up with her shots?" she simply said yes to avoid a hassle. When the child's siblings later came to the hospital to visit their sister, the mother told the truth and said no to the question. Result? The children couldn't visit their sister because they "might spread disease." "Isn't that ridiculous?" the mother said to me. "Ridiculous, yes, but sad," I replied.

Now let's look at a story that ends on a somewhat more hopeful note.

Turnabout (1991–1992)

In the middle of March 1991, the media reported a measles outbreak at a Christian Science school in Pennsylvania where four students died because, as the editorial in the *Virginian-Pilot* put it, "their parents refused medical care on religious grounds." The editorial referred to measles as a "killer disease" easily preventable through vaccination and argued for the deletion of the religious exemption clause from the Virginia vaccination code. The state shouldn't "stand aside as they [parents] impose deadly beliefs on their children," the editorial stated.[17]

November 19, 1991: A call from a woman in Pennsylvania, whom I will call Marti, told me the personal belief exemption clause was currently being threatened. In fact, the subject had already gone into committee, and the senator who was pushing for its deletion would not return her calls. (I told her I had the same experience with our state senator [Joe Canada] after the tougher vaccination requirements went into effect.) She asked for my advice on how to handle this challenge. Among other things, I stressed the importance of organizing and sounding "official" when communicating with legislators, preferably giving yourself a title such as "President, Citizens for Healthcare Democracy." I asked her to let me know how the situation was resolved.

December 12, 1991: Another young mother from Pennsylvania called and asked the same question as Marti. She, like Marti, was a young mother who was determined not to have her children vaccinated. During the course of our conversation, she gave me some interesting information about the widely reported measles outbreak in her state. She said her aunt, who lives close to the school, along with some other people investigated the report. They discovered that two of the deaths were children who had cystic fibrosis and another was a boy who had been badly abused—beaten, starved, dehydrated. The grandmother of this child was one of those pushing for the deletion of both the personal choice and the religious exemption clauses from the Pennsylvania vaccination code. "Instead of addressing the real problem, the maltreatment of the child, she thinks a shot will do it." "No, people don't want to take responsibility," I remarked. "Yes, I think she wants to protect her daughter."

The statistics the caller gave me varied considerably from the ones reported in the newspaper editorial. The editorial said that Philadelphia officials reported "500 cases of measles this year, 134 of them among the 201 students of a private, religious school."[18] The caller said that 10 children in the school got measles, and 5 of them died. She said she didn't know how the other 2 died. (Two years later I was told by a couple of residents in that area that the children who died received no healthcare at all.)

April 1, 1992: I received a letter from Marti thanking me for my support and giving me an update on the vaccination bill (S. 1205) in Pennsylvania. The bill, which was currently in the appropriations committee, was amended to include the following exemptions: (1) medical, (2) religious, (3) homeopathic, and (4) strong moral or ethical objections similar to a religious belief. She said, "We are trying to get a chiropractic exemption added also. . . . The homeopathic society is actively engaged in the battle as is the chiropractic association and various grassroots organizations."

Amazing what people can do when they work together for a common goal! However, in the latest listing of personal exemption states, Pennsylvania was not among them. Apparently, similar blockage to this legislation occurred in Pennsylvania as in Ohio when a more definitive personal exemption clause was sought by concerned citizens. (See Chapter 14.)

NOTES

1. Sir Graham S. Wilson, *The Hazards of Vaccination* (London: University of London, 1967).

2. *Organic Consumer Report*, October 23, 1979, p. 2.

3. Clarence Darrow, from an article in the *American Bureau of Chiropractic News*, "Clarence Darrow on Medical Control," February 9, 1928.

4. For an excellent discussion of this point, see Roger J. Williams, *You Are Extraordinary* (New York: Pyramid Books, 1974).

5. "Schools Will Require Students to Show Proof of Shots This Fall," *Virginian-Pilot*, May 6, 1983, p. 1.

6. "Pupils Not Immunized to Be Barred," *Ledger-Star*, May 5, 1983.

7. "Thousands of Students Still Need Shots," *Virginian-Pilot*, August 9, 1983, p. 1.

8. Code of Virginia 22.1–254.1, 22.1–256 or 22.1–257.

9. "Parents Rebelling Against Immunizing Their Children," New York (AP), CBH (Moses Lake, WA), May 17, 1991.

10. Kristine Severyn, "Parents 'Shut Out' of Congressional Vaccine Hearings," reported by Barbara Mullarkey, "Government Support of Vaccinations Continues to Prick Parents," *Wednesday Journal*, June 9, 1993. (Mullarky also follows the statement quoted with "Big Brother?")

11. Diane Tennant, "Beach Woman Opposing Immunizations," *Virginian-Pilot/Ledger-Star*, April 30, 1993.

12. Diane Tennant, "A Healthy Risk," *Virginian-Pilot/Ledger-Star*, August 14, 1993.

13. "Vaccination Tracking System Back on Track in Congress," NVIC NEWS, August 1994, p. 8. Also, *Florida Chiropractic News* 217 (November-December 1993). Reprinted by *The International Vaccination Newsletter*, March 1994, p. 13.

14. Severyn, "Parents 'Shut Out.' "
15. Ibid.
16. Editorial, "How to Lick Measles (Again)," *Virginian-Pilot*, March 14, 1991.
17. Ibid.
18. Ibid.

12   Waking from the Propaganda Trance

What luck for the rulers that men do not think.
—Adolf Hitler

Ralph, what did you do [in school] today? Think or believe?
—Ralph Nader's father

SNOW JOB PREVENTION

How do we keep from being duped and doped? Is there some way we can become immune to the vast epidemics of mindlessness that perennially sweep through our society? A good place to begin is to take a second look at "what everybody knows." Begin to ask questions: How do I know this? From what source am I getting my information? From what point of view is this idea true? From what point of view is it not true? As Alfred Korzybski, Polish engineer, mathematician, and founder of General Semantics, used to say, "Whatever it is, it also isn't."[1]

If an idea is present as *the* explanation for some event or *the* solution to some problem, say to yourself, "That is one explanation. There are others." Or, "That is one solution. There are others." Try playing with other explanations that will lead to other solutions such as reversing cause-effect relationships. When you read about scientists looking for a virus that causes a disease, say to yourself, "Maybe we should look for the disease that causes the virus." (Or better yet, "Maybe we should look for the condition that causes the virus.")

When you read or hear statements such as "doctors say" or "experts agree," the implication is that *all* doctors say or *all* experts agree. Say to yourself, "Have you interviewed every doctor—or 'expert'—in the world? Likewise, with the expressions "nobody knows" or "no known cure" or "no evidence for," talk back to them. Say to yourself, "Nobody you know knows" or "There is no cure you know of" or "There is no evidence you know about."

We are speaking, of course, of the proverbial "sweeping" or "glittering" generality, familiar to students of advertising and propaganda. General Semantics refers to these expressions as "allness" statements because they imply that someone knows everything about something. Try substituting *someness* for *allness* and say to yourself, "Some doctors agree" or "Some scientists say." Be alert for words like *all, everybody, no one, no, never, always, entirely, totally, completely,* and *absolutely.* They frequently signal an allness statement.

These little exercises are simple but subtle. They open rather than close the mind, which, in turn, can lead to inquiry and discovery. As a number of people have observed, great contributions are made not by people who know the answers but by people who know how to ask questions. The art of asking questions is largely the art of uncovering and challenging the assumptions hidden in our habitual patterns of thinking.

GOING SANE

Are language habits a pivot that can balance or unbalance the mind? Can we become "unsane" (Korzybski's term) by being ignorant of the nature and disciplined use of language? Can understanding the nature of language and using it in a disciplined, conscious way contribute to one's health and maturity?

In 1933, Korzybski published a ground-breaking book, *Science and Sanity,* which, in essence, answered the above questions in the affirmative.[2] This book originated the science of General Semantics, which is the study of symbols—and words are symbols—and how we use and react to them. Man, as a symbol-using creature immersed in a world of symbols, can become unsane when he misuses them or reacts to them inappropriately. While most of the theory and principles of General Semantics are beyond the scope of this discussion, a look at some of the principles should be enough to keep us from being mesmerized by many of the messages the mainstream culture sends to us.

The Non-Allness Principle we just discussed, for example, points to the idea that "no one knows everything about anything" because not only is human cognition and sense perception limited, but language, or any symbol system for that matter, is reductionist. The details of any given event that we choose to perceive and communicate are abstracted from an infinite number of possible details. Hence, interpretations are idiosyncratic—personal and peculiar to the observer-participant.

The allness statement has many faces. Can you recognize the allness statement in these two examples? First: "the most perfect man who has ever entered the Kingdom of Science."[3] This is an example of the unqualified superlative and was spoken by the great British physician Sir William Osler. He was referring to Louis Pasteur. Second: The Salk vaccine has been hailed as "the most dramatic breakthrough of the 20th century."[4] Here, the unqualified superlatives assume that the speaker is familiar with (1) all the scientists who ever lived and/ or (2) all the breakthroughs of the twentieth century. The statements also assume that a purely objective standard of superiority exists. This doesn't mean that we shouldn't use superlatives. Without them, strong feeling would be hard-pressed for expression. It only means we should qualify our superlatives. Instead of saying "the greatest" or "the most," we should preface our statements with qualifiers such as "as far as I know" or "the greatest scientist I ever knew." This simple reminder that our viewpoint is only one of many helps to promote humility, openness, and flexibility.

"Watch when you feel depressed," a friend of mine, psychologist, author, and teacher of General Semantics Gina Cerminara, used to say. "If you'll watch closely you'll find you are thinking in allness terms [e.g., 'I *never* do *anything* right' or '*No one* cares about me']. Allness statements box us in." Applying the Non-Allness Principle will not only contribute to mental health, my friend used to point out, but it will help us to become more tolerant and less precedent bound. We will begin to ask, "Why am I doing this?" Then we will begin to examine some of the assumptions that have shaped our lives and open the door to alternative explanations and solutions.

One of the most pervasive and deeply embedded assumptions in our society—and probably most human societies—is the idea that some people have the right to tell other people what to do. These people have that right because they have greater knowledge or skills of a certain kind than the rest of us. How do they get that knowledge, what does it mean, and why do most people acquiesce to their pronouncements?

THE AUTHORITY MYSTIQUE

Pronouncements by "experts"—frequently representatives of established professional organizations—are another source of propaganda. When we see this appeal to authority, we need to ask, "How do you know? What original research have you done? Are there vested interests behind your position?"

What really is an "expert"? How does one become one? The term itself implies "allness"—someone who knows everything about something. If we look closely, we will discover that an expert is usually a person who has passed through certain academic rituals and has learned to see a segment of reality from a certain perspective. He has also learned to communicate ideas as seen from that perspective in a certain code or form of rhetoric. The limitations of a perspective can be disguised by exotic rhetoric.

What about the perspective of most medical doctors? They are probably the only group of experts whose orders we are enjoined to follow—"doctors's orders"—and whose pronouncements on the cause and treatment of disease are almost sacrosanct. This enormous amount of power and privilege blinds most of them—and most of us—to the obvious fact that their knowledge, like the knowledge of the rest of us, is limited and represents only one way of seeing and interpreting a set of data.

Some limitations of the medical (or allopathic) perspective are these:

1. In medical school the focus of study is a cadaver, a dead body. Hence, the vital processes and energy patterns of a living body are lost, and the student tends to think of the body in static, mechanistic terms.

2. The focus again is on dissection and analysis of tissue; the relationship of the parts to the whole, therefore, tends to be lost. These limitations of perspective—which apply also to number 3 below—are camouflaged by esoteric language, the Greek and Latinate terminology used by the medical profession. This is part of the distancing process that creates the "authority" of the professional. In my more impertinent moments, I have said that a medical education is largely learning some skills and a stance and dressing them in exotic nomenclature.

3. Perhaps the most crucial limitation of the medical perspective is the built-in assumption that disease is an enemy that must be fought with weapons, that is, drugs and vaccines. A number of writers have pointed out that medical schools in the United States are subsidized by the foundations and grants of the multibillion-dollar drug industry and that that same industry spends an average of $6,000 a year on every doctor in the United States to get him or her to prescribe their drugs.[5] With a built-in bias like this, is it any wonder that the medical profession is disease rather than health oriented, and that we spend 30 to 40 percent more on health care than any country in the world?[6] In 1993, the cost will exceed $1 trillion.[7]

Does this enormous expenditure buy better health? A cursory glance at a few statistics will dispel any notion that it does. (These numbers are increasing.)

Forty million Americans suffer from arthritis.[8]

Fifteen million Americans have asthma.[9]

One million people die annually from heart disease.[10]

Over one million new cancer cases are diagnosed annually; at least one half of these cases will be fatal.[11]

In 1987, Americans had 1.12 chronic diseases per person, excluding cancer and osteoporosis, and the number is increasing![12]

The United States leads the world in degenerative disease.[13]

One hundred and thirty thousand persons a year die from doctor-prescribed drugs.[14]

To put some of these figures in perspective, heart ailments in the United States kill more people than died in World Wars I and II and the Korean and Vietnam Wars.[15] Despite the fact that we have spent over $1 trillion on cancer research and treatment since December 1971 when President Richard Nixon declared the War on Cancer,[16] the incidence of cancer has increased 30 to 300 percent, depending on the kind of cancer referred to.[17] The Figure of $1 trillion is more than 58 times enough money to provide adequate food, water, education, health, and housing for everyone in the world.[18]

Is there any profession, other than the medical profession, where the disparity between cost and benefit is so great?

The maintenance of the authority mystique depends to a great extent on limiting access to information and choices that challenge the position of the authority. Isolation is a well-known technique of brainwashing. Because the intellect learns by comparison, when it is presented with only one point of view or other points of view are denigrated, it looses its capacity to discriminate and ultimately its capacity for fully rational thought. We forget to our peril that there are many orders, degrees, levels, and kinds of realities that correspond to the many different minds that perceive and create those realities. When we forget this, we develop tunnel vision. We see only one way of doing or thinking about something. The remedy, of course, is this: Whenever you see only one way of doing or thinking about something, that is the time to look for alternatives.

Anything perfectly obvious should, to some extent, be suspect. Nowhere, perhaps, is this better illustrated than in the myth of the objectivity of science and scientists. Not only is absolute objectivity an impossibility,[19] but scientists, being human, are emotionally and promotionally involved in what they are doing. So called conflict-of-interest stories are by now proverbial. When a group in power has a vested interest in sickness, is it too much to suggest that their approaches to the solution of this problem will be as expensive, circuitous, and complex as possible?

But is medicine a science? Can anything that deals with so many unknown and uncontrollable variables be a science? "[P]hysicians are not scientific in any meaningful sense. They get very technologic," Dr. Thomas Preston reminds us.[20] When the primary subject of a field is as rich and resonant with ambiguities as a human being, we have moved into the realm of art. Isn't this why we refer to the field of healing as the healing arts, not the healing sciences?

HARDENING OF THE CATEGORIES

"A rose is a rose is a rose" goes the famous statement by Gertrude Stein.[21] General Semantics would say, "$Rose_1$ is not $rose_2$ is not $rose_3$." Each is different and unique. We might say that a person who tends to deal with people and objects in terms of their similarities and neglects their differences has "hardening of the categories." A more colloquial expression for this tendency is "lumpism," because the person with this tendency "lumps," certain people or ideas together into neat little categories where they harden into stereotypes. That these stereotypes have little to do with reality can easily be illustrated by the example of a simple object such as a carrot. Carrots differ not only in size, shape, and color but in chemical composition and molecular arrangement. A carrot grown in one kind of soil will have different nutritive values than one grown in another kind of soil. This, of course, is true for other foods as well.

If this is true for roses and carrots, think how much more true it is for complex entities like human beings. Award-winning biochemist and professor emeritus Roger Williams points out in his book, *You Are Extraordinary*, how very different people are, not only anatomically but physiologically and biochemically as well.[22] On page 36, for instance, we see 12 pictures of "normal" livers, each with a distinctively different size and shape. On page 34, we see 11 diagrams of the chemical constituents of the blood of 11 healthy young men. Each diagram is distinctly different, and each contrasts with the "textbook" diagram. In fact, as Dr. Williams points out throughout his book, the textbook standard is a fiction. So are words like *average*, *typical*, or *normal*. Each of us is uniquely individual and different from any other individual.

This uniqueness extends to minds and temperaments. We each have different life needs—for food, recreation, rest, stimulation, and so on. One person might require 20 to 30 times more of a certain nutrient than another; a drug that might make one person drowsy would keep another awake. What is work for one person is play for another. Dr. Williams deplores the tendency to "average" people, to reduce them to a statistic, and warns that "we as individuals cannot be averaged with other people. Inborn individuality is a highly significant factor in all our lives—as inescapable as the fact that we are human."[23] To ignore the uniqueness of a human being is to ignore part of that very essence that makes him human.

What about mass bureaucratically administered programs such as mass vaccination programs? That the uniqueness of the individual tends to get lost in these programs is suggested by an article that appeared in the *International Medical Digest* (July 1969) that states: "There is no sound basis for the assumption that every child or infant must be inoculated with every available vaccine; on the contrary, there may be a valid reason for omitting any or all available antigens. Each patient is an individual, and deserves evaluation on this basis, rather than as an epidemiologic statistic." The article goes on to point out that "the incidence of vaccine-induced morbidity has increased alarmingly" and that the medical profession "must re-evaluate the principles, purposes, and hazards of immunization and reassess current procedures."[24] Assembly line medicine is bad medicine.

That mass vaccination programs create epidemics of nonthink was eloquently expressed by Clinton Miller in his testimony against H.R. 10541 in the House of Representatives (May 17, 1962). After pointing to some of the problems with mass vaccination programs such as (1) serious side effects—for example, encephalitis, coma, and death—suffered by some children, (2) little-known or publicized contraindications for vaccination, and (3) some statistical "hanky-panky," Clinton Miller said:

In mass vaccination programs, it is common practice to omit or ignore such information in presenting the case for vaccination to the public. There is a tendency to let the "experts" make the decisions, after which they summarize the evidence with such press release statements as "absolutely safe," and other statements designed not to educate, but to inspire absolute confidence.

We point out that the tendency of a mass vaccination program is to "herd" people. People are not cattle or sheep. They should *not* be herded. A mass vaccination program carries a built-in temptation to oversimplify the problem, to exaggerate the benefits, to minimize or completely ignore the hazards, to discourage or silence scholarly, thoughtful and cautious opposition, to create an urgency where none exists, to whip up an enthusiasm among citizens that can carry with it the seeds of impatience, if not intolerance, to extend the concept of the police power of the state in quarantine far beyond its proper limitation, to assume simplicity when there is actually great complexity, to continue support of a vaccine long after it has been discredited, to make a choice between two or more equally good vaccines, and promote one at the expense of the other, and to ridicule honest and informed dissent.[25]

Just as people and objects are unique, so are events. And as with objects and people, the shared characteristics of any two events—or situations—are fewer than the differences between them. When a person wants to make a point by comparing these shared characteristics, we call this "reasoning by analogy." Legal arguments that use precedents are using this kind of reasoning. Likewise, people who suggest a particular remedy for a current problem, because a problem similar to it occurred many years ago and was apparently corrected by the recommended course of action, are reasoning by analogy. People use this kind of reasoning when they point to epidemics that occurred many years ago and were apparently corrected by vaccination and warn that these same epidemics could occur now if there is a falloff in vaccinations. The problem with reasoning by analogy is again the problem of ignoring differences, some of which could be crucial. Certainly a past condition and a present condition are dissimilar in many important respects. We learned, for instance, in Chapter 4 that the conditions that created the epidemics of "yesterday" were very different from those that prevail in the civilized world today.

Using faulty analogies to support an argument is common: equating what happens in a test tube with what happens in a human body, for example, or equating humans with animals, such as supporting an argument for certain dietary practices because certain animals have these practices. Not that these observations and experiments don't have value; it's that they should be regarded as suggestive rather than prescriptive.

Post hoc reasoning that assumes a causal relationship between two events is also illustrated by the immunization example just discussed. Since this was discussed in Chapter 3, let's look now at the "black and white syndrome" or "hardening of the polarities."

HARDENING OF THE POLARITIES

To some, the world is divided into two camps—black and white, right and wrong. There is no middle ground, no gray, no alternative(s). This is the world of the person with, what I call, hardening of the polarities. General Semantics refers to this as either/or or two-valued thinking.

Two-valued thinking can be very useful for the propagandist because it creates false dilemmas. I once saw a pediatrician on television say that he explained to parents who were concerned about the dangers of vaccination that the risks of the disease outweighed the risks of vaccination. He was saying in effect that there is only one way of preventing certain diseases, namely, vaccination. He was also inferring that these diseases are irredeemable "bad guys" from which our children must be protected by medical technology. The propagandist creates the impression that there are only two solutions to a disastrous or potentially disastrous situation—his solution and the wrong solution. There are no alternatives.

CARD STACKING

Card stacking is really an extension of the two-valued thinking discussed above. The art of carefully selecting and presenting ideas and data—data that may or may not be true—so that only the best or worst possible case is presented is known as card stacking. There are no ambiguities; other possibilities are either ignored or discredited. The object is to get you, the reader or the viewer, to react strongly for or against an idea, an issue, a person, or an object. The pediatrician just spoken of buttressed his advice to parents by "reminding" the TV audience how vaccination "wiped out"—or nearly did—such "dread" diseases as smallpox and whooping cough. No credit was given to the contribution of such things as improved sanitation, personal hygiene and the increased consumption of fresh fruits and vegetables. The detrimental side effects of vaccinations were barely mentioned.

Professor Gordon Stewart of Glasgow University remonstrates against this card stacking on the part of those who unreservedly recommend vaccinations:

What kind of immunisation is this for which success is being claimed? . . . What kind of epidemiology is this which advocates immunisation by excluding consideration of factors other than immunisation? . . . What kind of editorial policy is this which publishes incomplete data and promotes far reaching claims about the efficacy of immunisations but refuses to publish collateral data questioning this efficacy?[26]

Card stacking can be concealed by misleading use of words. For instance, a free "newspaper" bearing the masthead of one of the two leading newspapers in our community was delivered to our home every Wednesday. Opening the newspaper, we found headlines on such medical topics as "Safe Exercise OK During Pregnancy, Experts Say" (May 22, 1985) and front-page articles on medical topics such as "Nation Marks 30th Year Free from the Specter of Polio" (April 17, 1985) and " 'Remedies' for Arthritis Called Fake" (May 9, 1985). Anywhere from two thirds to three fourths of the articles were about medical "breakthroughs" and related topics such as medical advice and stories of people struggling with some disease or disability that is medically managed. Is this really a newspaper? I would call it medical advertising.

Misleading video pictures and "discussions" where only the spokespersons for a particular group are present are other examples of card stacking. For instance, I saw on television a segment of a news program that had been "advertised" earlier in the day as a "discussion on chiropractic." The discussion turned out to be a medical doctor telling the viewers that orthopedic care of serious back problems was more effective than chiropractic. He conceded that chiropractic was more effective for minor back problems than orthopedic care, but only because the chiropractor, unlike the orthopedist, took time to discuss appropriate exercise and nutrition with his patient. At the beginning of this "news" segment, the viewer was shown a picture of a patient lying face down on a chiropractic table, being adjusted by a woman "chiropractor." The woman wore dark-red lipstick and had long dark-red fingernails. Need I say more?

LOADED WORDS AND PICTURES

Perhaps the easiest way to get people to do what you want them to do—and this is the goal of the advertiser and propagandist—is to "stack the deck" with "loaded" words and pictures, that is, words and pictures with emotionally charged meanings or connotations. Referring to a disease as a "hidden menace" or a "killer and crippler" is an example of loaded language. The picture of the chiropractor just described in an example of a loaded picture.

Whatever the picture of the chiropractor with long red fingernails suggests to you, it hardly suggests a healthcare professional who works primarily with her hands and fingers. To refer to a relatively benign, self-limiting disease of childhood such as rubella or German measles as a "hidden menace" or a "killer and a crippler" is again using language to mislead. (No doubt, the writers were referring to the birth defects associated with rubella if contracted during the first trimester of pregnancy. But, as Dr. Moskowitz points out, vaccines for childhood diseases can transform these relatively benign, self-limiting diseases of childhood into their more serious counterparts in adolescents and young adults. Thus, rubella vaccine can actually increase the risk of birth defects.)[27]

One of the best places to pick up obvious and sometimes colorful examples of loaded words and pictures is your local health department. The folders are replete with most of the propaganda devices we have been discussing: post hoc reasoning, misleading statistics (Chapter 3), glittering generalities, appeals to authority, lumpism, two-valued thinking, card stacking, and loaded words and pictures. Another excellent source is your local newspaper, particularly articles celebrating the lifesaving virtues of some new vaccine or drug. In the literature from both these sources, words such as *dread, devastating, deadly, strike, danger, risk*, and *wipe out*, can usually be found, particularly at the beginning of the text. These are words calculated to get attention and arouse the reader, in this case, arouse fear and a subsequent dash to the doctor for "protection."

What about a word like *quack*? It is a label usually applied by the medical establishment to either an alternative healthcare system (quackery) or a healthcare practitioner who uses "unapproved" therapies; its purpose is to convince the reader to go only to standard brand (medical) doctors who use standard brand therapies. The word *quack* is associated with incompetence and deception and suggests a person who pretends to have knowledge or skill he or she doesn't possess. The label is derogatory and loaded—really old-fashioned name-calling.

Loaded labels like other loaded words can mislead—but sometimes even more so because labels are, in a sense, libels. When we label a person or a group, we tend to imply allness. We throw a person or a group into a category and "close the case." When we read or hear *incompetent* applied to someone or some group, we need to ask, With respect to what? Aren't we all incompetent with respect to something? Even relatively nonloaded labels, like *honest* or *intelligent*, when applied to someone, need to be questioned. Aren't we all honest or intelligent in some ways and in some circumstances and not in others?

Perhaps you have noticed that most of the propaganda techniques discussed are really different versions of the allness statement. The nature of language and the nature of human thinking tend toward generalizations. We couldn't communicate without them. We simply need to be aware that generalizing can be a trap. Overgeneralizing is, according to Stuart Chase, "probably the most seductive, and potentially the most dangerous, of all fallacies."[28]

Man's tendency to think that value can be measured in terms of popularity or consensus is, I think, part of this need to generalize. Let's look at one more propaganda technique that exploits man's need to identify himself with a group.

BANDWAGON

A recent editorial in our local newspaper that argued for the passage of a particular law began by pointing out that 16 states now have this law, and the use of seat belts mandated by this law is increasing. This is known as the bandwagon appeal, the appeal to join the crowd or be left out and "miss the boat." The spokesperson for the health department who said that 0.5 percent of the children eligible for vaccinations receive exemptions and 65,000 children were vaccinated in Virginia last year (Chapter 10) was suggesting that everybody's doing it, so it must be right: bandwagon.

The idea that something is right or good if enough people are doing it is one of the most seductive of mental traps. We don't have to go back very far in history to find that much of what most people thought and did was not necessarily good or true. Perhaps the seductiveness of "others, therefore me" lies in our human need to belong, to be accepted. This is our strength and our weakness: Our strength in that our group consciousness can help us be more aware of the needs of others; our weakness when we become mindless conformists.

And this is the problem with bandwagons. Because they are action- rather than critical-inquiry oriented, bandwagons can easily promote unconsciousness. They tend to accept the official version of the problem they are organized to redress, and the solutions they "demand" are nearly always quantitative—more of the standard brand solutions. Nowhere is this better illustrated than in the vaccination and AIDS bandwagons. With vaccinations it's more "education" and more legislation to get more people into the vaccine net. With AIDS it's more money for more research into more drugs and vaccines. Thus, bandwagons can easily become part of the problem.

THE WORLD AS PROCESS

"We can never step into the same river twice," Hereclitus said. "The only constant is change."[29] As the river changes from moment to moment, so does the world. Obvious, yes, but easy to forget. We tend to assume, for instance, that the person we saw yesterday is the same person today, or that a particular magazine we read five years ago has the same editorial policy today. We forget that people and objects have a uniqueness in time as well as in space.

When we enter the microscopic and submicroscopic worlds of molecular and atomic energies, the world as process becomes more apparent. On this level, change is continuous and instantaneous; we can see ourselves and the universe as a process in space-time. On the level of ordinary reality, however, our senses record only gross differences that are apparent only with relatively long lapses of time. Subtle changes that occur from moment to moment usually escape us.

To illustrate the distortions of time and our senses, my friend, who taught General Semantics, had her classes do some simple experiments. One of them, which was quite a source of merriment for the class, was to have each person at the end of a row whisper into the ear of his or her neighbor some simple message. The message was repeated in this way to each person in the row (about 8 times). The person at the other end told the class what the message was. What that person said was such a distortion of what the first person had said that everybody laughed. When the experiment was repeated using a single message for the whole class—about 30 repetitions—the distortion was so great the original message was almost unrecognizable.

Most of what we know of the world is based on reports, and each report has been filtered through the motives, biases, and conditioning of different reporters. Even two people witnessing the same event will describe and interpret it differently, as the Japanese film *Roshomon* illustrated so well. My friend would illustrate this point for her class by holding up a drawing of a scene in a department store. After a few minutes, she put the picture down and asked some questions about it. As you might guess, there were almost as many different answers as there were students in the class.

Do these experiments tell us something about the nature of language—and the nature of knowledge? For a starter, we might ask, Is the noun or object centeredness of our language partly responsible for our tendency to regard processes as things? We speak of diseases as though they were entities rather than processes. Microorganisms are labeled as though they were microentities rather than stages of an evolutionary cycle. A doctor frequently conducts tests to determine how the patient's disease "entity" can be labeled. Diagnosing and labeling disease entities is an important part of medical practice. A number of people have observed that this preoccupation tends to promote the treatment of labels, not disease processes, and certainly not people. Nowhere is this better illustrated than in mass immunization programs.

THE WORLD AS PROJECTION

"We see what we know," Johann Wolfgang von Goethe said. "It is our theories that determine what we see," Albert Einstein reminds us.[30] We do not live in a world of "hard facts" but a world of perceptions and interpretations. Believing is seeing. The microbial world, for instance, looks like this to some researchers:

These "microscopic biochemical components . . . constantly are at war between themselves and their external and internal environment.

"Like the humans of which they are integral parts, they form and break alliances with each other. Some, following the pattern of international intrigue, act as double agents, scientists report.

"In this never-ending battle, evolutionary changes constantly take place which enable the microscopic participants either to play more effective roles, or to become the slaves of more dominant factions, or even to be absorbed and become a part of them, research shows."[31]

Other researchers have seen molecular and bacterial interactions suggestive of cooperative, even self-sacrificing behavior.[32]

We project onto the world our beliefs and assumptions about it. For instance, if we start with the assumption (or premise) that vaccinations "protect" health, we can find "evidence" to support this idea, particularly if we have a vested interest in it. General Semantics might put it this way: We abstract from a multitude of details those that fit into our frame of reference—and, I would add, our ego needs.

Facts and values are mutually dependent. There is evidence, for instance, that the "objective" observations of scientists—as well as the theories they create, prove, or disprove—reflect the subjectivity of the scientist as well as the value system of the society in which the science operates.

There is also evidence that human beings, in a scientific investigation, tend to behave in a manner consistent with the observer's theory. They respond to the expectations of the observer.[33] We know plants and animals respond to color and sound vibrations as well as human thought and intention. Likewise, experimental animals. We need to recognize ourselves in the world we see and interpret.

THE WORLD AS SYMBOLS

Man is an ''amphibian'' he lives in two worlds—the world of physical reality and the world of symbols. The latter is supposed to communicate information about the former; however, as we have pointed out, it doesn't always do this. A primary reason it doesn't—and one we haven't discussed yet—is that we fail to check our verbal maps by going to the territory (Korzybski's terms). Languaging tends to get divorced from experiencing. Obviously, we can't experience directly all our assumptions about the nature of the world. I assume England is there, and I'm not going to go there to see if it is. I'm going to rely on reports and reports of reports, and so on.

We should be aware, however, that when we read a report we tend to assume its truthfulness. And that is the problem. Propaganda masquerades as news and information. For instance, I have a copy of a section of a university newsletter warning people about the hazards of a particular food (raw milk) and recommending a particular course of action (pasteurization).[34] The article refers to ''studies'' to support its position but gives no specifics other than to mention the group (Centers for Disease Control) who conducted the studies, a group long associated with the position taken by the article. Advocates of a different persuasion (the nutritional superiority of raw milk) are given short shrift with expressions such as ''no evidence'' and ''no way.'' The ''news'' item is one-sided and deals in generalities—the essential coin of propaganda.

When we read a report of an experiment or a study, we should at least ask who funded it and where and when it took place. Technical and professional publications usually include a reference as to where more particulars such as size, duration, and controls can be found.

When we see a set of statistics, we might want to know how some of the figures were arrived at. Numbers can vary considerably from source to source. Conclusions and interpretations of the same studies and experiments can also vary from one researcher to another. For instance, we read glowing reports of the cost-effectiveness of vaccinations—that for every $1 spent on vaccines, $10 is saved on later medical costs. Neither the vaccine failure rates nor the awards of the federal Vaccine Injury Compensation Program (VICP) are factored into this cost-benefit analysis. As of March 1993, this compensation program has awarded $329.5 million for vaccine injury or death with a predicted shortfall of $171 million for fiscal year 1993. The government's estimated future liability for pre–1988 injuries exceeds $1.7 billion. Factoring in these figures would more closely approximate the real cost of vaccines, but even this would exclude the cost from private settlements and families dependent on public assistance for medical and living expenses.[35]

One of the most effective tools the propagandist uses to support his or her argument is to compare two or more groups of people and point out that only the group that has or does what he or she recommends shows the desired result. If we look closely, however, we will find that only one or two factors among many significant factors have been considered. The variables have not been controlled.

An article on heart disease, for instance, points out the flaws in some of the studies upon which a prestigious scientific group (National Institutes of Health [NIH]) bases its position.[36] The studies involve comparing several population groups. However, only two factors (amounts of saturated fats and cholesterol in the diet) among many significant factors were studied and a casual relationship attributed to these two factors. This particular scientific group has held the same position for many years, and, I suspect, they approach their "research" deductively—that is, they attempt to find more "evidence" to support a conclusion already formulated and hardened into official policy.

This is one of the problems with scientific research. Science pretends to be inductive, to search for answers by examining facts and deriving principles from them. Too often, however, money and vested interests indicate the most profitable answers and fund scientists to search for evidence to support them. Thus, politics can masquerade as science.

THE WORLD AS CONSTRUCT

What we call the "real world" is largely a human construct. Beyond our sensory programs are the programs of our culture whose "truths" color and even determine our perceptions and hence our reality. In our present culture, the electronic and print media play primary roles in creating our reality. For instance, I'm old enough to remember when childhood diseases—measles, mumps, rubella, chickenpox—were merely episodes that my friends and I almost welcomed. There was the drama of the health department coming out and putting up the quarantine sign, giving us a chance to stay home from school, be fussed over, and have something to talk about. In some windows, we would occasionally see the whooping cough sign, and we knew that those within who had whooping cough would be absent from school longer than they would with the other diseases. The only disease that was kind of scary was scarlet fever and the occasional rumor of some classmate who had almost died from it. This was in the 1930s. Now, of course, these same diseases—with the exception of scarlet fever, which has apparently disappeared sans vaccinations—are threatening, causes for alarm. This is largely the creation of the media and, to a lesser extent, vaccinations themselves (see Chapter 2).

Not that my corner of the universe is definitive, but it is suggestive. The essentially benign, self-limiting nature of these childhood diseases has been articulated by a number of doctors, some of whom I have referred to earlier. For instance, of the 3,394 cases of measles in Ohio between 1987 and 1991, there were no deaths and no serious complications. The 29 hospitalizations were for observation only and lasted from one to three days.[37]

I'm also old enough to remember when immunizations were called *vaccinations* or *inoculations*. When did they become immunizations? As pointed out in Chapter 3, the term *immunization* suggests that vaccines produce genuine immunity.

Did you know that the term *herd immunity* originally meant freedom of a group from disease that was brought about by sanitary measures such as providing pure water, milk, and drainage?[38] When did it come to mean freedom of a group from disease as a result of vaccination?

Changing our perception of reality by changing terminology or changing the meaning of old terminology is a well-known ploy of public relations (propaganda?). Both medicine and the military use it regularly: for example, *death*—"a mortality experience" or "negative patient outcome"; *bombing*—"coercive diplomacy"; *explosion*—"energetic disassembly." This linguistic sanitizing has been called "doublespeak." When we refer to the bankrupting costs and inequities of our healthcare system, are we really referring to health care? Is health care bankrupting and inequitable? No. It's diseasecare, medically managed diseasecare that is bankrupting us. Is health care doublespeak for what we really have—a diseasecare system?

And do we really have health departments? Do they use their resources primarily to promote health measures, such as clean air, pure water, an unpolluted, whole foods diet, good hygiene—physical *and* mental, a balanced lifestyle, and basic sanitation? Or do they use their resources primarily to promote diseasescare and its usual panacea—vaccinations? The *H* word can hide the essential fear motif: *Give Your Child A Shot... At Good Health* reads the title of a pamphlet from the Bureau of Immunization at the Virginia Department of Health (1992). On the first page we read: "Is your child's health at risk?" "Yes—unless he or she is protected with shots! Shots (immunizations) prevent illnesses that cause: pain, fever, rashes, coughs, sore throats, hearing loss, blindness, crippling, brain damage, death." Has the Health Department mutated into the Diseasescare Department?

For those concerned with vaccine damage, vaccinations can be called "A Healthy Risk" (see note 14, Chapter 11). And for the environmentally minded, I've heard vaccinations promoted as "protecting our greatest [or most precious] resource." There's an appeal for everybody, as language—and clever illustrations—design our reality.

Another way of reinventing reality is, as we said earlier, via the one-sided presentation, the deletion of any evidence or ideas from the public forum (media) that would seriously challenge the set of assumptions that support the official position. This used to be called *censorship*. Now it's called *policy*. Paul Meier, biostatistician from the University of Chicago, addressed this problem in a panel discussion of the polio vaccine in 1960. He pointed out the discrepancy between the doubts expressed by members of the panel and the glowing reports of the Salk vaccine that were appearing in newspapers across the country. He said that the reason for this discrepancy was in the attitude of public health and publicity men: "It's hard to convince the public that something is good. Consequently, the best way to push forward a new program is to decide on what you think the best decision is and not question it thereafter, and further, not to raise questions before the public or expose the public to open discussion of the issues."[39]

So instead of open discussion of "sensitive" issues such as vaccination, the media gives us single-sided messages. What passes as discussion, if it does occur, is a group of people coming from the same mindset whose comments are variations on the same theme. This repetition of single-sided messages moves us toward unconsciousness because it closes the mind to other possibilities, making it incapable of thoughtful inquiry and discussion. Thus, gullibility, zealotry, and finally tyranny take root, and our humanity is diminished.

This is why recognizing propaganda is so crucial to our survival as humane and fully rational beings. (See Table 5.)

BACK TO PRINCIPLE

If knowledge, as this entire discussion has suggested, is tenuous—and picking our way through a maze of propaganda and misinformation is tricky—are there some relatively simple and straightforward ways we can recognize that which has genuine worth? Here are three:

1. We can unmask propaganda by asking questions that uncover basic assumptions behind a statement. Many of these have already been pointed out, but because vaccination propaganda is so rampant in our society, a brief recapitulation seems appropriate here. To illustrate the cost-effectiveness of vaccination, one medical doctor has stated that the shot which includes vaccination against whooping cough costs $20, while treating the disease costs $500 per day for weeks in an intensive-care ward.[40] Four assumptions jump right out at us, don't they?

First, vaccinations are always successful—no injuries, no failures. Second, whooping cough is always a serious and life-threatening disease. Third, there is no remedy except the intensive-care ward of a hospital. Fourth, there is nothing we can do to prevent the disease or mitigate its seriousness except get vaccinated. Allness statements and either/or thinking that create the false dilemma are the coin of propaganda. Doctors who make statements like this are probably sincere. They've simply been indoctrinated to think this way.

2. We can look for the "tape"—the automatic response, the official line, the formulaic thinking that is activated by a challenge. Remember, the tape is designed to sell a product or course of action that secures the propagandist's

TABLE 5. EDUCATION OR INDOCTRINATION?

INDOCTRINATION (PROPAGANDA)	EDUCATION
1. One-sided: Different or opposing views are either ignored, misrepresented, under-represented, or denigrated.	1. Many sided: Issues examined from many points of view; opposition fairly represented.
2. Uses generalizations, "allness" statements: Lacks specific references and data.	2. Uses qualifiers: Statements supported with specific references and data.
3. Card Stacking: Data carefully selected —even distorted—to present only the best or worst possible case. Language used to conceal.	3. Balanced: Presents samples from a wide range of available data on the subject. Language used to reveal.
4. Misleading use of statistics.	4. Statistical references qualified with respect to size, duration, criteria, controls, source, and subsidizer.
5. Lumpism: Ignores distinctions and subtle differences. Lumps superficially similar elements together. Reasons by analogy.	5. Discrimination: Points out differences and subtle distinctions. Uses analogies carefully, pointing out differences and non-applicability.
6. False dilemma (either/or): There are only two solutions to the problem or two ways of viewing the issue—the "right way" (the writer's or speaker's way) and the "wrong way" (any other way).	6. Alternatives: There are many ways of solving a problem or viewing an issue.
7. Appeals to authority: Statements by selected authority figures used to clinch an argument. "Only the 'expert' knows."	7. Appeals to reason: Statements by authority figures used to stimulate thought and discussion. "Experts" seldom agree.

TABLE 5. (Continued)

INDOCTRINATION (PROPAGANDA)	EDUCATION
8. Appeals to consensus (bandwagon): "Everybody's doing it," so it must be right.	8. Appeals to fact: Facts selected from a broad data base. Logical, ethical, aesthetic and psycho-spiritual aspects considered.
9. Appeals to emotions and automatic responses: Uses words and pictures with strong emotional connotations.	9. Appeals to people's capacity for thoughtful, reasoned responses: Uses emotionally neutral words and illustrations.
10. Labeling: Uses labels and derogatory language to describe proponents of opposing viewpoint.	10. Avoids labels and derogatory language: Addresses the argument, not the people supporting a particular viewpoint.
11. Promotes attitudes of attack/defense. Aim is to sell a position or product.	11. Promotes attitudes of openness and inquiry. Aim is to discover.
12. Ignores assumptions and built-in biases.	12. Explores assumptions and built-in biases.
13. Language usage promotes lack of awareness--unconsciousness.	13. Language usage promotes greater awareness—consciousness.
14. Can lead to tunnel vision and bigotry.	14. Can lead to breadth of vision and understanding.

position, status, or advantage. This product or course of action nearly always creates dependency. The vaccination tape goes something like this:

A. *The disease is more dangerous—deadly or risky—than the vaccine.* This statement is usually followed by numbers—usually large, round ones called . . .

B. "*Statistics.*" These are designed to show maximal possible damage from the disease and minimal possible damage from the vaccine. One in a million, for instance, is the figure currently bandied about for serious reactions from the MMR vaccine.[41] Other fantastic figures: "Brain infection, which may result in seizures or mental retardation—with measles, 1 per 1,000 cases; with vaccine, 1 per 1,000,000 (million) vaccinations. Death—with measles, 1 per 500 to 10,000 cases; with vaccine, not one reported case."[42] This same doctor points to "ear infection or pneumonia—with measles, 10 percent; with vaccine, 0 percent." Notice the extremes—0, not 1. The editorial goes on to point out how devastating measles was before the vaccine appeared: "Thousands were hospitalized or became mentally retarded as a result, and 100–200 children died each year from the disease." As a result of the measles vaccine, the article points out, the incidence of measles has been reduced to 2 percent of previous levels (500,000 to 800,000 cases in the United States before the vaccine).[43]

These figures, of course, don't square with the figures in this book or even the ones quoted in note 37. Remembering that adverse reactions to vaccines are very underreported—only 10 percent of physicians report them, and the FDA and CDC do not thoroughly investigate the nearly 1,000 reports collected monthly[44]—any set of figures will be very approximate. But to keep it simple, let's look at the 1 in 1 million "statistic" and compare it with the figures in note 37.

In 1991, the population of persons under 17 in the state of Ohio was 2,819,000,[45] and claims from injuries from the MMR vaccine were 15 and 1 death, making a total of 16 injuries, that is, 1 in 176,187 injured by the vaccine. The number of children under 5 (when most of the injuries are recognized and reported) was 796,000, that is, 1 in 49,750. On a national level the population of persons up to 14 was 55,129,000, and the claims of damage from the MMR vaccine totaled 378, including 27 deaths, that is, 1 in 145,844. The number of persons under 5 was 19,222,000, which comes to 1 in 50,852. Hardly 1 in 1 million!

How does officialdom respond to these challenges? By . . .

C. *Denial and discredit.* When the NVIC, for example, reported 17,221 illnesses and injuries and 360 deaths from vaccines in the last 20 months, the CDC countered by pointing to "statistics" showing much higher rates of death from the diseases. "The CDC is thoroughly familiar with the National Vaccination Information Center and contends that this group is mistakenly blaming vaccines for deaths in children who are dying from pneumonia, sudden infant death syndrome and other diseases when, in most instances, there is no relationship to the administration of a vaccine," one doctor writes.[46]

Recently I talked with a public health officer in Richmond about the discrepancy between the much lower figures for vaccine damage issued by the health department and the much higher figures from other sources such as the NVIC. He replied in much the same vein: Other sources were including illnesses that had nothing to do with vaccination. When I cited clear instances of neurological damage occurring after vaccination, he replied, "That would have happened anyway."[47]

This position is bolstered by . . .

D. *More statistics* designed to show the effectiveness of vaccines: When vaccination rates decline, epidemics and subsequent damage and death from the disease increase, and vice versa. One "old saw" that I thought was laid to rest in 1982 by the *DPT: Vaccine Roulette* program is still trotted out to make this point. This is the British whooping cough "epidemic" in the 1970s that was supposedly the result of a drop in vaccine acceptance from about 80 to 30 percent. The figures quoted by our government sources are not only much higher than the official government figures of the United Kingdom, but British epidemiologist Gordon Stewart said that "the death rate in the height of that so-called epidemic . . . was the lowest ever and hospital admissions in Scotland continued to fall."[48]

In short, the tape reads: (A) formula statement supported by (B) "creative" statistics, (C) ignoring or denying conflicting data, (D) discrediting opposing viewpoints and/or organizations, (E) slight variation of (A), and (F) more "creative" statistics.

So if we can't depend on the media to give us accurate, impartial reportage, what can we depend on? A friend of mine, who was in the newspaper business for 15 years and now does freelance investigative reporting, gave me a tip. She said, "If you read the newspapers, use them as guides for further research, not as sources of information. When you come across something that interests you, make a note to research it." You'll need to access sources that are usually nonmainstream, preferably primary, and sometimes less than respectable. She also said that to read newspapers is to get caught up in illusion and ignorance. I would add that it is also to get caught up in a corporate-designed world, which is the same thing.

3. And finally, and probably most important, we can become more holistic in our approach by activating other faculties of the inquiring self. Besides the purely rational faculty, which thrives on fact and reason, we can call into play our intuitive and aesthetic faculties. We can then uncover operative principles by asking questions that reveal the larger implications behind a claim or system of thought. To do this we need to look at other systems, other claims, particularly those that contrast with the one we are considering. Then we can ask, Is the operative principle behind this system essentially positive, or is it negative? That is, is it based on preventing an undesirable condition, or is it based on creating a desirable condition? Does it build on fear and avoidance or on creating harmony and connection? If the former, the paradigm and the solutions it suggests will be fragmented, out of context, and alienating. If the latter, the paradigm and the solutions will point in the direction of holism/contextuality and connectedness.

We might say, positive is beautiful. Surely the vision of a desired condition has more aesthetic potential than the vision of an undesired condition. So the other side of the coin of "back to principle" might be "back to beauty." As we pointed out in Chapter 9, the aesthetic criterion is a very valid one. We are drawn to the beautiful in other areas of life—why not scientific paradigms that are beautiful? Physicist, author, and distinguished historian of science, Thomas S. Kuhn has written that there is "another sort of consideration that can lead scientists to reject an old paradigm in favor of a new. These are the arguments, rarely made entirely explicit, that appeal to the individual's sense of the appropriate or the aesthetic. . . . The importance of aesthetic considerations can sometimes be decisive."[49]

So when we are choosing between two or more conflicting claims or systems of thought, why not choose the one that pleases us aesthetically? As Dr. Kuhn points out, scientists may do this. If this seems capricious because ideas of beauty are subject to personal bias, what isn't subject to this bias? Surely the paradigm that points in the direction of greater freedom, holism, and harmony is more beautiful than one that points in the direction of dependency, fragmentation, and alienation. On a practical level, this means that the natural would take precedence over the artificial, the whole would take precedence over the part, and self-help would take precedence over institutionalized help.

But then, this is my bias. Yours may be something else—hence the need for choice.

NOTES

1. Quoted by Gina Cerminara in "Two Courses in General Semantics—Beginners and Advanced," Virginia Beach, May 1–August 28, 1975.

2. Alfred Korzybski, *Science and Sanity* (International Non-Aristotelian Library Publishing Co., distributed by the Institute of General Semantics, Lakeville, CT, 1984).

3. Sir William Osler, "Introduction" to *The Life of Pasteur*, Rene Vallery-Radot, quoted by J. I. Rodale, "Bechamp or Pasteur?" *Prevention*, August 1956, p. 71.

4. Marcia Dunn, "Nation Marks 30th Year Free from Specter of Polio," *Virginian-Pilot*/EXTRA, April 17, 1985, p. 2.

5. Maureen Salaman, *Nutrition: The Cancer Answer* (Menlo Park, CA: Statford, 1984), p. 10; Robert S. Mendelsohn, *Confessions of a Medical Heretic* (Chicago, IL: Contemporary Books, 1979), p. 36.

6. "Doctors and Dollars," *Health Quarterly*, WHRO-TV, January 5, 1993.

7. Patricia Namen reporting on *Morning Edition*, WHRV-FM, January 11, 1993.

8. Morton Walker, "Chinese Seafood Eases Arthritis," *Natural Health*, March–April 1993.

9. *Morning Edition*, WHRV-FM, February 23, 1994.

10. *Virginian-Pilot*, January 18, 1988, p. A7.

11. Cancer Research Foundation of America, Alexandria, VA, September 1993; also Peter Barry Chowka, "Cancer 1988," *East West Journal*, December 1987. Chowka gives the figure of over a half a million. Since cancer has increased, the figure is probably well over a half a million.

12. Christopher J. Hegarty, "Eating the 'Wright' Way," *Health Consciousness*, October 1991.

13. Harvey Diamond and Marilyn Diamond, *Living Health* (New York: Warner Books, 1987), p. 409.

14. Max Ricketts, "Neurotoxicity: A Threat to Survival," *Health Freedom News*, October 1990, p. 30.

15. *Virginian-Pilot.*

16. Chowka, "Cancer 1988," p. 47.

17. Deepak Chopra, "Quantum Healing" (talk given at Visions of the Future Conference, Seattle, May 18, 1991).

18. *Friends of Peace Pilgrim, Newsletter*, no. 1, Autumn 1987. Extrapolated from the figure $17 billion a year to provide adequate food, water, education, health, and housing for everyone in the world. The $17 billion figure is an estimate.

19. Modern physics tells us that "this world does not exist in itself . . . [but] only as that met with by an ego." See Herman Weyl, *Mind and Nature* (Philadelphia: University of Pennsylvania Press, 1934), p. 1. Not only is the event dependent on a mind (or ego) to give it reality, but mind shapes the event itself. The Heisenberg uncertainty principle states that the observer always interacts with the observed, and the modes of perceiving alter the forms perceived.

20. Thomas Preston, M.D., *Donahue Show*, Virginia Beach, VA, January 7, 1982.

21. Gertrude Stein, "Sacred Emily" (poem).

22. Roger J. Williams, *You Are Extraordinary* (New York: Pyramid Books, 1974).

23. Ibid., p. 17.

24. Paavo Airola, *Everywoman's Book* (Phoenix, AZ: Health Plus, 1979), p. 289.

25. House Committee on Interstate and Foreign Commerce, *Hearings on H.R. 10541*, 87th Cong., 2nd sess., May 16, 1962, p. 86.

26. Gordon Stewart, *British Medical Journal*, January 31, 1976; reprinted by Glen Dettman and Archie Kalokerinos, " 'Mumps' the Word But You Have Yet Another Vaccine Deficiency," *Australasian Nurses Journal*, June 1981, p. 17.

27. Richard Moskowitz, *The Case Against Immunizations* (Washington D.C.: National Center for Homeopathy), p. 19.

28. Quoted in *You are Extraordinary*, p. 193.

29. Cerminara, "Two Courses in General Semantics."

30. Quoted by Patricia Anne Randolph Flynn, *The Healing Continuum* (Bowie, MD: Robert J. Brady, 1980) quotes are from the introduction.

31. Julian DeVries, medical editor, *Arizona Republic*, March 29, 1976; reprinted by William A. McGarey, "Medical Research Bulletin," *Pathways to Health*, August–September 1979.

32. Marilyn Ferguson, *The Aquarian Conspiracy* (Los Angeles, CA: J. P. Tarcher, 1980), p. 165.

33. George S. Howard, "The Role of Values in the Science of Psychology," *American Psychologist*, March 1985.

34. "Tufts University Diet and Nutrition Letter, "News from the World of Medicine,' " *Reader's Digest*, April 1985.

35. Kristine Severyn, "Parents 'Shut Out' of Congressional Vaccine Hearings"; reported by Barbara Mullarkey, "Government Support of Vaccinations Continues to Prick Parents," *Wednesday Journal*, June 9, 1993.

36. Ruth Adams, "Is Cholesterol the Villian?" *Better Nutrition*, May 1985, pp. 26–28.

37. See Kristine Severyn, "Vaccinations Fail, Hurt in Many Reported Cases," *Columbus Dispatch*, February 20, 1993. Unfortunately, recipients of the MMR vaccine did not fare so well. The VICP recently reported 378 claims—351 injuries and 27 deaths—

related to the MMR vaccine or one of its components (measles, mumps, or rubella). In Ohio there were 15 injuries and 1 death. See idem, "Vaccines May Do More Harm Than Good," *Dayton Daily News*, May 19, 1992.

38. *Dorland's Medical Dictionary*, 1944, s.v. "immunity," subheading is "herd immunity."

39. *Hearings on H.R. 10541*, pp. 90, 100.

40. Jon King, "Government-Paid Vaccines: Bargain for All," *Virginian-Pilot/Ledger-Star*, May 19, 1993. The doctor referred to is Howard Pearson, spokesperson for the American Academy of Pediatrics.

41. Diane Tennant, "A Healthy Risk," *Virginian Pilot/Ledger-Star*, August 14, 1993.

42. Nancy M. Welch, director, Chesapeake Health Department, "Risks: Measles Vs. Vaccination," *Virginian-Pilot/Ledger Star*, November 4, 1993.

43. Ibid.

44. Mullarkey, "Government Support of Vaccinations."

45. Population figures are from the *Statistical Abstracts of the United States*, 1992.

46. Harry D. Cox, "Immunizations Save Lives, Health-Care Costs," *Virginian-Pilot/Ledger-Star*, June 6, 1993.

47. Per phone call about November 4, 1993.

48. *DPT: Vaccine Roulette*, broadcast April 19, 1982. Richmond Health Department ("Immunizations") used this "epidemic" as an example, as have other doctors I've read.

49. Thomas S. Kuhn, *The Structure of Scientific Revolutions* (Chicago, IL: University of Chicago Press, 1970), pp. 155–156.

SUGGESTED ADDITIONAL READINGS

Cerminara, Gina. *Insights for the Age of Aquarius*. Englewood Cliffs, NJ: 1973.

Cerminara, Gina. "Two Courses in General Semantics—Beginners and Advanced." Virginia Beach, May 1–May 29, 1975, and June 19–August 28, 1975.

Fearnside, W. Ward, and William B. Holther. *Fallacy—The Counterfeit of Argument*. Englewood Cliffs, NJ: 1959.

"How to Say What You Mean." *Nation's Business*, May 1957.

Korzybski, Alfred. *Science and Sanity*. Lancaster, PA: Business Press, 1948.

Lynton, Alice. *Skills Basic to Improvement in Reading in the Secondary School*. Los Angeles City School District's Division of Secondary Education, September 1963.

13   The Coming Revolution in Healthcare

Man was created for the sake of choice.

—Hebrew saying

FROM EITHER/OR TO MULTIPLE OPTION[1]

"All progress has to do with increasing choices and options. If you talk about one society being more progressive than another, you talk about a society in which citizens have a greater freedom and greater range of choices and possibilities," Nathaniel Brandon, author and psychologist, told his audience. He pointed out how biological and evolutionary development is founded on the increase of options and choices.

If you talk about progress in the biological or evolutionary sense from an amoeba up to man, you're looking at organisms with increasing variability of response. They are able to do more and more things in response to the environment. The range of possibility keeps growing. If you think of people who do bodywork, any kind of opening of the body, working with blocks, whether it be Rolfing or any of the other types of work, it is always to make it possible for the body to do more things. . . . Think of psychotherapy, where a person we say is stuck or rigid. What do we call progress? It always has to do with increasing the ranges of choices and options.[2]

Options and choices will be central to the health care system of tomorrow. Choice is essential, not only to the health of a democratic society but to the health of the person as a whole. Knowing that we have choice empowers us, makes us feel responsible for our condition, and augments our impulse to participate in both our own healing and the healing of our society. There is "overwhelming evidence that the mind is a key controlling factor (if not *the* key controlling factor) in virtually all disease," Edgar Mitchell, former astronaut and founder of the Institute of Noetic Sciences, tell us.[3] To deny choice is to deny the role of the mind in the healing process. In fact, recent research "assures that any medicine that ignores the power of the conscious mind will ultimately be declared unethical."[4]

We are moving from a society with few choices to one of many—from either/or to multiple options, according to John Naisbitt.[5] What does this mean with respect to health care? We will see more growth in the alternative health care fields such as physiotherapy, homeopathy, naturopathy, herbology, chiropractic, acupuncture, and midwifery. This is already happening. A recent newspaper article discussed the impending doctor glut and the steady decline in the demand for physicians while nonmedical healthcare specialists are experiencing a boom cycle. Compared with 1960, for instance, by the year 2,000 the number of chiropractors and nurse-midwives is expected to triple.[6]

The results of a national poll in which over 50 percent of the respondents said they would seek treatments rejected by the medical community if they were stricken by serious disease were reported in another recent article. In the same poll, 50 percent of the respondents approved of allowing clinics to operate in the United States that treat cancer and other diseases in ways opposed by mainstream medicine.[7] This is remarkable considering the vigorous propaganda of the medical establishment damning "unproven" remedies and the near blackout of positive reportage on these remedies—remedies that generally offer no profit for drug companies.

Are we witnessing the beginnings of the dissolution of the great American medicine show? Certainly, increasing numbers of Americans are becoming disenchanted with the institution of diseasescare, symptom management, and complicating side effects, not to mention the skyrocketing price tag. More Americans are even beginning to suspect much of the literature emanating from authoritarian institutions, such as the medical establishment, as being possibly propaganda. We as a people are outgrowing authoritarian institutions and their style of relating, a style assumed by people whose assumptions about human nature and the natural world are negative and narrow. If the future belongs to democracy—and I think it does—it belongs to those people and those institutions whose assumptions about the nature of themselves and their world are essentially benign and life affirming. What could be more life affirming than the assumption that men are essentially good and capable of deciding what is best for themselves? This, of course, is the assumption behind the democratic ideal and the founding documents of this country. When enough people can open themselves to develop democratically, that is, become freer, less obstructed, and less attached to authority—titles and precedents—we will have a democratic society.

It is already happening. Healthcare practices are well into reflecting megatrends six and eight—movements from institutional help to self-help and from hierarchies to networking.

FROM INSTITUTIONAL HELP TO SELF-HELP

Television actress Linda Evans told a packed audience in the Senate Hearing Room how she had overcome severe allergies with the help of a nutritional counselor after she had been unsuccessfully treated with dangerous drugs like cortisone.[8] Thousands of people, including myself, could tell similar stories, stories of healing a chronic ailment by changing eating habits and otherwise adopting a healthier lifestyle. In my own case, which I mentioned in Chapter 4, I took courses from doctors who used natural methods of healing; I read books and was counseled by others who were knowledgeable in these methods. Like Linda Evans, I, too, first went the conventional medical route. My childhood days were punctuated by regular visits to the allergy specialist for shots. The result: The hayfever of my childhood became the asthma of my later adolescence and early adulthood.

Be Your Own Doctor is the title of a book by nutritionist and naturopath Ann Wigmore.[9] "Everyone over forty should be his own doctor," Dr. Jensen used to say.[10] Presumably, it takes that long to learn how to live healthfully. The idea of being our own doctor—except for accidents—has been echoed by many other healthcare practitioners. Learn how to live and forget doctors, they say. Megatrend number six (from institutional help to self-help) suggests that this may indeed be the wave of the future.

FROM HIERARCHIES TO NETWORKING

"The new healthcare model will be people helping people," Roger Jahnke, multidisciplinary healthcare practitioner, told his class. "We need to be health-care practitioners for each other."[11] Since this was a class in body therapies—neuromuscular release facilitated by working with partners and using such modalities as reflexology, bodywork, and acupressure—this statement was particularly apropos. We are the only culture—and this is true of industrial cultures generally—that depends on experts for healthcare, he said. In earlier cultures, people took care of each other.

What, then, is the role of the "expert"? Increasingly, I think, we are going to turn to the expert or medical specialist only for crisis situations, such as mechanical and chemical accidents, and to ourselves and to each other for health maintenance and working with chronic ailments. The healthcare professional will become more of a teacher and counselor and only secondarily a dispenser of pills and potions. The holism that was lost during the Middle Ages will return, and the practitioner not only will work with the patient as a mental, spiritual, and physical being but will himself be a spiritually conscious person. Assembly line health care—treating labels and symptoms—will be confined to crisis situations.

I look forward to the day when the philosopher-physician, like Plato's philosopher-king, will be the ideal, if not the norm. This is a person so spiritually attuned that knowledge, virtue, and love are fused. Knowledge of this caliber is experientially derived insight into the values and principles embedded in the very structure of the universe.

At the least, we will expect a healthcare practitioner to be an example of health and to have a "healing presence." As we move from the model of physician as technician and symptom manager to the model of physician as teacher and healer, those healthcare professionals who are skilled in working with their hands, such as body therapists, chiropractors, and acupuncturists, will be in greater demand. Because many of these skills—for example, massage, polarity, shiatsu, acupressure, and bodywork—do not require large investments of time and money to learn, we will see more people becoming skilled practitioners of these healing arts. As we learn to help ourselves and each other by sharing knowledge and skills, healing will become democratized.

FROM SHORT TERM TO LONG TERM

Expedient or "quick-fix" solutions that create long-term damage are losing ground to less expedient, long-term solutions. When we talk about long-term solutions, we are talking about those that involve whole systems rather than parts of systems. The quick-fix solution seeks to isolate and alter a part. The long-term solution works with wholes—whole systems and whole persons. In an interview, Dr. Michael Smith, who uses herbs and acupuncture to treat drug addicts, said, "Pharmacological science always seeks to alter just one thing—a bacteria or a nerve, for example. The drug is supposed to have this single effect; although in practice, it always has twenty other effects—side effects. The whole process is totally separate from the way life works."[12] From the short term to the long term—from the part to the whole—is the trend away from treating effects toward removing causes.

"Art is simple, but art is long," a music teacher friend of mine used to say. Substitute the word *healing* for the word *art*, and we have the essence of natural healing and the new paradigm shift in healthcare. As disillusion with symptom-treating, technological medicine increases, we will see more people opting for the simpler but more long-range solutions of natural and holistic healing.

No discussion of long-term solutions would be complete without mentioning agriculture because many of the principles that apply to creating health in humans—and animals—apply to creating health in plants. Healthy plants, like healthy humans, do not attract pests nor do they get diseases. Many experiments have demonstrated that plants grown on organically mineralized and balanced soil do not attract pests, nor do they get diseases as do plants grown on deficient and chemically fertilized soil.

One example among hundreds that could be cited is described by horticulturist Sand Mueller: "I had read claims by organic gardeners saying their healthy plants had no insect problems. I believed these assertions were preposterous, as did every horticulturist I knew." He then describes how the bug problem in his garden completely disappeared after using compost. His first composted garden coincided with a year of cutworms. The cutworms were everywhere—except in his garden.

His second composted garden coincided with the year of the locusts. Swarms of grasshoppers severely damaged the alfalfa in the surrounding fields before coming to his garden. "For five days they buzzed around my lettuce, tomatoes, beans, peppers, and cabbages. Then they all left," he tells us. Although every part of the garden was swarming with grasshoppers, the only damage they did was to eat five small cabbages. In a quarter of an acre of tender garden plants, not a single leaf, other than the five cabbages, was damaged, and he had used no poisons of any kind.[13]

A number of studies have shown that insects can detect subtle mineral imbalances in plants and devour only those plants that are out of balance. "Satellite photographs of Africa have shown how gigantic flights of locusts will cover thousands of miles ignoring healthy vegetation, then descending and destroying fields where the soil is worn out."[14] Again we see that "pests," like bacteria, are nature's undertakers, returning the unfit to the elements for recycling.

Over a hundred years ago, the great German pathologist Rudolf Virchow said germs "seek their natural habitat," that is, diseased tissue. As mosquitoes seek the stagnant water but do not cause the water to become stagnant, germs seek diseased tissue, but do not cause the tissue to become diseased.[15] With Kirlian photography and other energy-measuring devices, we now know that the cells of every form of life—plant, animal, human, and microorganismic—emit radio signals as well as photons (light).[16] A strong, healthy plant radiates wavelengths of a different frequency from that of an imbalanced, unhealthy one. Strong, virile plants—plants nurtured in soils mineralized and rich in humus—"broadcast" wavelengths harmless to humans and animals but that act like a protective screen against pests.[17] Another way of interpreting this might be that balanced and unbalanced plant cells emit different signals, which are detected by insects. Could we infer that something similar happens on a human level?

Poisoning crops with pesticides is a bit like driving our car and shooting the oil gauge when the red light goes on. We're treating an effect, an indicator. As our understanding of ecology and the interdependence of all life increases, these shortsighted solutions will wane. We will seek life-enhancing solutions that work with whole systems, not isolated parts. We will respect all forms of life, knowing that each in some way contributes to the welfare of the whole.

FROM MASS TO ENERGY

Instead of physical examinations and checkups, will we go to the doctor for "energy field studies"? We know that sickness shows up in the energy field before it shows up in the physical body, and early detection shortens and simplifies therapy. "Gradually, human anatomy will be recognized as energy anatomy, and physiology as energy physiology, when medicine catches up with physics," Harvey Grady, director of the John E. Fetzer Energy Medicine Research Institute, points out.[18]

As we move from an object-oriented consciousness to an energy-oriented consciousness, we will think of the body more in terms of energy fields than of a composite of physical and biochemical parts. Actually, noninvasive electrodiagnostic and therapeutic techniques are being used now. Europe has been using electrodiagnosis for 20 years, and we in the United States are using low-frequency electro- and electromagnetic therapy for pain relief, regaining function of paralyzed or weakened nerves or muscles, and accelerating the healing of cataracts and other ailments. Electromagnetic currents have also been used to regenerate limbs; grow severed nerve cells; and accelerate repair of skin ulcers, wounds, and bone fractures in rats and salamanders. "Many ancient civilizations used energies in sophisticated forms of healing, such as Chinese acupuncture 5,000 years ago," Dr. William McGarey reminds us. "Now is the time to reclaim that heritage."[19] Part of reclaiming that heritage will be learning to utilize therapeutically the energies of sound (including music), light (including color), and heat as well as the more subtle energies of thought, feeling, and visualization.

Energy balance and imbalance on a cellular level seem to be the primary signifiers of health and disease states. Electrodiagnosis uses very sensitive instruments to detect energy imbalances as they manifest in various organs of the body. Energy therapies seek to redress these imbalances. Are we returning to earlier researchers such as Bechamp, Rife, Koch, and Enderlein who told us that disease begins in unbalanced cell metabolism, which, of course, reflects some kind of unbalancing influence in the life of the host organism? And isn't the transition from an object-centered consciousness to an energy-centered consciousness an aspect of the transformation from fragmentation to holism and from isolation to connectedness? For it is on the level of energy—information-bearing energy, electricity, consciousness—that we are whole and connected and that our mind-body is one.

FROM SUBSTITUTION TO REGENERATION

"Plato said, more than two thousand years ago, that what is honoured in a country, will be cultivated there," warned the Executive Board of the World

Health Organization. "We may have to take a second look at what we honour."[20]

The evening news features an item on the progress of the latest heart transplant recipient; the local newspaper tells a "heartrending" story of a child who needs a liver transplant; a popular magazine tells the story of the "heroic" boy who saves the life of his brother by giving him his healthy kidney. The story of the man who regenerates his heart by diet, herbs, cleansing, exercise, and other modalities is not news; neither is the story of the child who regenerates a failing body by a change in lifestyle. Enlightened self-discipline is not the stuff of high drama. It is also not the stuff of large investments in expensive technology. In short, it is not the stuff of big money and our cultural penchant for magic and melodrama.

As our diseasecare system grows more expensive and inefficient and as our awareness of the pressing human needs of the larger global community grows, we are going to ask ourselves some searching questions such as: Does the enormous expense of high-tech, high-drama diseasecare, which at best can benefit a very few, justify itself? How can we transform expensive diseasecare into cost-efficient healthcare? How can we reorient our thinking to move from doctor dependency to self-reliance, and from drug and surgical intervention to self-regulation and organ regeneration?

RECYCLING DINOSAURS

"B Complex, Inositol—Nature's Tranquilizers."

"Herbal Formula Helps Regenerate Pancreas"

"Aluminum, Fluoride Implicated in Alzheimer's"

Headlines of the future? When the trends toward self-care and networking, holistic and ecological thinking, and long-term solutions that are simple and harmless reach a critical mass, we will see headlines such as these. When the trend toward multiple options reaches a critical mass, we will read articles in the popular press about the research and discoveries of natural schools of healing such as herbology, homeopathy, and chiropractic. And when the current peace movement becomes perceptive enough to see that peace begins in consciousness and the language that reflects that consciousness, then the healing of our planet, our language, and ourselves will begin. Bellecose rhetoric such as "battle of the budget" and "keeping the democratic knives from cutting too deeply," typical of the rhetoric of politics, will be replaced by metaphors suggesting connection and cooperation.

"The future exists in language," Werner Erhard told his audience. "Where being shows up is in language."[21] Linguistic violence reflects mental violence which becomes physical violence. A harmonious consciousness reflects itself in peace-oriented language. Here we must begin if we would have healing for ourselves and our planet.

How can we recycle the military metaphors of the medical model to suggest an ecological and essentially harmonious relationship with microorganisms and the health and disease processes to which they are related? What metaphors can we use that will suggest harmony, interdependence, and stewardship rather than conflict, alienation, and victimization? What metaphors will help us to think of our bodies as extensions of our consciousness and the world around and within them as a continuum of life-support systems?

We might begin by referring to our illnesses as a reaping of imbalances or unwise choices instead of something that "strikes" us or that "bug going around." Instead of saying, "I caught a cold," say, "I created a cold." This helps us to be aware that we are responsible, empowered beings. Louis Pasteur used to refer to the "invaded patient." I suggest we use the term *client* rather than *patient* because it connotes working with rather than working upon—a partnership rather than a paternal or administering relationship. And, of course, we are not invaded; we create conditions that produce consequences.

The military metaphors describing the immune system and its functions need to be recycled to suggest an ecological system within a larger ecological system, instead of a battlefield within a larger battlefield. Instead of terms such as *building defenses* and *conquering disease*, we could use terms such as *enhancing health*, *creating harmony*, and *cleansing and balancing*. These terms are more bland and don't pack the adrenal charge as do the old metaphors. Perhaps someone with a more poetic gift than mine will come along and give us metaphors that are more incisive and dramatic.

What about the term *immune*? It comes from the Latin *immunis*, which means safe, untaxed, free from, and has come to mean free from disease. Not a bad term, but is there one that could suggest some of the more affirmative aspects of immune function such as (1) its establishment and maintenance of molecular identity (Varela), and (2) its role as a "barometer" of the integrity and vitality of the body? (See Chapter 7.)

I remember a TV program, *The Body in Question*, in which we saw a leukocyte (white blood cell) surround and devour a foreign object. The narrator, Dr. Jonathan Miller, told us that white blood cells are nature's garbage collectors. So instead of white blood cells being "warriors" and first lines of defense," they were cleanup crews. They clear out morbid or toxic matter. Could we find a name that suggests cleanliness or honors the capacity of cells to transform their environment and in turn be transformed by it? We learned earlier that germs are not only pleomorphic; every germ has both its healthy and unhealthy form (Rife and Enderlein). (See Chapters 5 and 7.) Is there a term that would suggest these more assertive and creative functions of the immune system?

Once we begin using more affirmative metaphors, the idea of injecting poisons into one's body for the purpose of "building defenses" to "fight disease" becomes ludicrous. I predict the time will come, perhaps in our lifetime, when the administration of toxins—drugs and vaccines—either for the prevention or treatment of disease will be looked on much as we now look on the practice of bloodletting. Doctors will attempt to justify the practice of vaccination long after it has been discredited, much as they attempted to justify bloodletting for many years after it was discredited. However, the justification for the practice of vaccination will be particularly tenacious, because another element has entered the picture: Unlike the old practitioners of bloodletting, the vaccinators have gone to the state and enlisted its police powers to enforce obedience to their dogma.

What about the term *preventive medicine*? Both words need recycling. When we think in terms of prevention, we focus energy on preventing an undesirable condition instead of creating a desirable condition. What we give energy to expands. Do we want to expand more undesirable conditions and more ways to prevent them? What about the term *medicine*? To most of us, it suggests using something unpleasant to get rid of something bad. How can we change this negative into a positive? If our goal is the creation and enhancement of health, why not call our healthcare program simply that: a healthcare program? (See Table 6.)

But more important, the term *medicine* has been overdone in our culture. It has been used to refer to a system of healthcare that has too long monopolized the healthcare market. *Medical research, medical science, medical advice, medical authority,* and *medical supervision* are terms we use automatically as though the medical model were some kind of absolute—the way things are. Using other terms such as *healthcare research* or *healthcare supervision* might help to open us to the possibilities of other models, other approaches.

Once we begin to recycle language, our fascination with pathology and its classification will yield to a more holistic perception of the relationship between health and disease. "Disease is nothing but life under altered conditions," pathologist Rudolf Virchow reminds us. And it is conditions that should be the object of therapy, not diseases, he added.[22] The myriad possibilities of the whole, the healthy, the optimal, and the conditions that produce them will be the occupation of the healthcare system of tomorrow.

What about recycling some of the more destructive elements of the medical-pharmaceutical and agrichemical industries? How can these industries be retooled to produce biologically and ecologically supportive commodities such as compost, organically grown food, natural and organic food supplements, ecologically supportive energy sources, and training for health-oriented healthcare practitioners? We could extend this redirection, of course, to include other businesses such as the food-processing business, the media, and the military.

When the adversarial consciousness and the language habits that feed it are recycled, the destructive elements within the social institutions of a culture also will be recycled. Form follows consciousness.

TABLE 6. OLD VERSUS NEW HEALTHCARE MODELS

OLD OUTER-DIRECTED DISEASECARE	NEW INNER-DIRECTED HEALTHCARE
1. Palliative: Emphasis on removing symptoms. Aims for quick results.	1. Educative: Emphasis on removing causes through knowledge and its integration into living habits. Aims for long-term results.
2. Authoritarian: Emphasis on management and control. Professional "manages" disease; patient "follows doctor's orders."	2. Egalitarian: Emphasis on patient participation and recovery. Professional gives guidelines; patient directs his own therapy.
3. Assembly line methods geared for profit.	3. Client-centered methods geared for autonomy.
4. Relies on technological intervention and substitution, e.g., organ transplants, insulin injections, synthetic and frequently toxic drugs, and vaccinations. Focuses on replacing organs or their functions.	4. Relies on harmless, noninevasive therapies and substances, e.g., food—including herbs and supplements; water—used both internally and externally; visualization—meditation; body movement and alignment. Focuses on regenerating organs and restoring their functions.
5. Cost and dependency escalating.	5. Cost and dependency de-escalating.
6. Disease and disability seen in terms of victimization and melodrama.	6. Disease and disability seen as self-created and preventable, the natural consequences of violating principles.
7. Mechanistic: Body seen as mass, an object containing discrete parts.	7. Organic: Body seen as energy, living patterns and interacting fields.
8. Fragmented: Body and mind treated separately. Parts of body regarded separately and treated singly.	8. Holistic: Body-mind treated as a unity. Parts of body treated in relation to other parts and aspects of the body-mind.
9. Atavistic: Disease seen as entity separate from patient.	9. Contemporary: Disease seen as process, inseparable from patient.

TABLE 6. (CONTINUED)

OLD OUTER-DIRECTED DISEASECARE	NEW INNER-DIRECTED HEALTHCARE
10. Adversarial: Disease seen as enemy.	10. Unifying: Disease seen as corrective.
11. Externalizes causality: Focus is outside the patient: viruses, bacteria, poisons, and stresses in the environment.	11. Internalizes causality: Focus is on the patient: his choices, attitudes, habits, and reactions to environmental influences.
12. Disease oriented: Focuses on labeling and controlling or destroying disease entities. Research focuses on prevention and elimination of disease. Absence of disease seen as the result of technological intervention.	12. Health oriented: Focuses on supporting the natural healing energies of the body-mind. Research focuses on what creates optimum health. Absence of disease seen as by-product of health.
13. Uses military rhetoric: "Building defenses," "fighting," "battle against," "strike," "attack," "weapons," etc.	13. Language suggests harmony and cooperation such as referring to disease as a healer, and detoxification as a cleanser.
14. Monolithic and coercive.	14. Pluralistic and voluntary (multi-optioned).
15. Negative: Builds on fear and distrust of the natural world. A system of "diseasescare."	15. Positive: Builds on rapport and cooperation with the natural world. A system of healthcare.

FULL CIRCLE

> The universe, like a bellows,
> Is always emptying, always full . . .
>
> Life and death, though stemming from each other, seem to conflict as
> stages of change.
>
> —Laotzu,
> *Tao Teh Ching* (Witter Bynner, translator)

The idea of the universe as a bellows and life and death as complementary cycles of a larger whole recurs perennially throughout religious, philosophical, and mythical literature. From the days and nights of Brahman to the yin and yang of Taoism, man intuited that the universe was a living entity with cycles of inhalation and exhalation, expansion and contraction, growth and decay, creation and dissolution. Now physics is discovering that pulsation, a dynamic expansion and contraction, is indeed the core of all experience.[23] On the human level, we are rediscovering that good health depends on balancing these forces—the anabolic and the catabolic—within the body.[24] Dr. Emanuel Revici has, for instance, developed a system of medicine utilizing these concepts and has had remarkable success using it in treating seriously ill patients.[25]

Have we forgotten something, something man has known intuitively for thousands of years? In our fixation on dissection and analysis, we see fragments—opposition where there is complementarity, dissolution where there is cleansing, death where there is renewal. Shiva, for instance, the third member of the Hindu trinity, represents the aspect of destruction or dissolution and is recognized by the Hindus as part of the life process. (The other two aspects of God are Brahma and Vishnu, the creator and preserver.) Because our inclinations and our instruments predispose us to see only one half of the cycle, we fear the other half; that half we see darkly. And so we fight it.

"From the most primitive life forms, viruses and bacteria, to the most evolved body cells in the cerebrum, our bodies include a constantly evolving continuum of life forms," writes Leonard Jacobs in his explication of the macrobiotic point of view. "The primitive forms are not our enemies, but constitute the evolutionary origin of our body cells and the eventual future of our bodies returning to the soil in the grave."[26]

Substituting *microzymas* (small ferments) for *viruses* and *bacteria* in the above quotation, we get a simplified idea of what is meant by the phrase "ecology of the body." We could think of disease symptoms as the body's attempt to rebalance an internal ecology that has become imbalanced through unwise choices and living habits. "Perhaps one day our medical schools will start paying due attention to the person, realizing that the human being is the only reality, and that disease is born out of the malfunctioning life that dwells within that individual," Dr. William McGarey tells us.[27] As we have seen, that malfunctioning life resonates on many levels.

What will future historians call our age, an age when people used the same shortsighted application of technology to pollute their bodies as they did to pollute their planet, an age when the body and its infirmities were exploited for profit, an age when the fascination with and fear of pathology reached epic proportions (witness the current AIDS hysteria), an age when the earth and its resources were treated as if they were insensible and infinitely expendable commodities, an age when the universe and most of its life forms were seen as hostile and people fought diseases as they fought each other?

Currently we are enmeshed in an ecological crisis. In fact, some have called our age the environmental age. This means that the frontiers of awareness are pushing toward the recognition that everything is connected to everything else. On a personal level, this translates into holistic health and healing.

We are also in the information age, sometimes called info-glut, meaning we have a surfeit of information, misinformation, and dysinformation. This surfeit creates its own crises—that of discriminating among the valid, the valuable, the trivial, and the specious. Could we also call our age the age of discrimination? This again has its personal, physiological counterpart: the immune system. We learned earlier that on a molecular level the immune system is both a cognitive and a cleansing system. As such, it is a system that discriminates. Could our current epidemic of immune disorders symbolize our inability to discriminate?

Developing our powers of discrimination is one of the ways we become adults. If we as a nation are going to pass from adolescence into adulthood, we must learn how to ask questions that uncover principles and implications behind tribal mores and mandates. Then we can enter what some have called the Age of Enlightenment or the New Age. These terms refer to a new awareness of our connection to a larger whole and a new ethic that recognizes that the well-being of the personal, the interpersonal, the transpersonal, and the planetary are inseparable. When our ecological awakening includes the mental and microscopic universes, we will graduate from the model of a mechanical, mindless, threatening universe to a model of a living and loving one. Then the mentality of attack, defend, and coerce will be outgrown, and we will enter the adulthood of humanity.

NOTES

1. John Naisbitt, *Megatrends* (NY: Warner Books, 1984). See Contents and text for this and other megatrends discussed in this chapter.

2. Nathaniel Branden, talk recorded in Del Mar, CA, 1981, by Mandala Outer Circle (tape untitled).

3. Edgar D. Mitchell, form letter sent during the mid–1980s to prospective members of the Institute of Noetic Sciences, undated. Edgar D. Mitchell is the former astronaut who founded the Institute.

4. Catalog of Omega Institute, Summer 1986, p. 37. This page described the background of the leaders of a course given at Omega Institute, July 26–27, 1986.

5. Naisbitt, *Megatrends*.

6. Don Colburn, "Doctor Supply Outpaces Nation's Growth," *Washington Post News Service*; reprinted by *Ledger-Star*/EXTRA, December 12, 1985.

7. Lawrence Kilman, "Permit Unproven Cancer Clinics to Operate, 50% Say in Survey," *Ledger-Star*, February 6, 1986.

8. Clinton Ray Miller, "The Washington Report," *Health Freedom News*, January 1986, p. 27.

9. Ann Wigmore, *Be Your Own Doctor* (St. Paul, MN: Dan Palla Printing, n.d.).

10. Remembered from lectures about 45 years ago.

11. Roger Jahnke, Workshop and Lecture on Body Therapies, Association for Research and Enlightenment, Virginia Beach, VA, May 10, 1983.

12. Peter Barry Chowka, "The Organized Drugging of America," *Health Freedom News*, October 1983, p. 9.

13. Sand Mueller, "A Horticulturist Speaks Out on Health," *Health Science*, April–May 1980, pp. 27–31.

14. Ibid., p. 28.

15. C. Norman Shealy, *90 Days to Self-Health* (New York: Bantam, 1980), p. 19.

16. "Living Cells Emit Light, German Scientist Reports," *Brain/Mind Bulletin*, August 19, 1985, p. 1.

17. *Organic Consumer Report* (Topanga, CA), January 26, 1982.

18. A.R.E. Clinic, *Pathways to Health* (Phoenix, AZ), September 1984, p. 1.

19. Ibid.

20. *Organic Consumer Report* (Topanga, CA), December 14, 1976.

21. Werner Erhard, *Taking a Stand for the Future* audiocassette, 1983.

22. Rudolf Virchow, quoted by Karl Menninger, *The Vital Balance* (New York: Viking Press, 1963), p. 41. (Book written with Martin Mayman and Paul Pruyser.)

23. "Movement Psychology: Freeing 'Postural Beliefs,' " *Brain/Mind Bulletin*, April 18, 1983, p. 1. (Idea is from psychologist Stuart Heller.)

24. In this context, *anabolic* refers to processes that are constructive and proliferative, and *catabolic* to processes that involve the liberation of energy and the utilization of stored resources.

25. "Emanuel Revici: Evolution of Genius," *Impact* (special supp.), spring 1985.

26. Leonard Jacobs, "Menage," *East West Journal*, September 1977, p. 14.

27. William McGarey, "Medical Research Bulletin," *Pathways to Health* (Phoenix, AZ), June 1985, p. ii.

SUGGESTED ADDITIONAL READINGS

Borg, Gavin. "Sounds Foretell Disease." *Moneysworth*, winter 1986.

Douglass, William Campbell. "Employee Health and the Tomato Effect." *Health Freedom News*, February 1986.

"Germanium—Element #32." *Organic Consumer Report* (Topanga, CA), June 14, 1983.

Matchan, Don. "Hierarchy Halts Treatment of Cataract with Low-Pulse Energy." *National Health Federation Bulletin*, October 1980, pp. 22–24.

"Radionics—By Any Other Name." *Organic Consumer Report* (Topanga, CA), July 29, 1980.

"What's in a Name?" *Organic Consumer Report* (Topanga, CA), July 23, 1985.

14   Reclaiming Our Heritage:
What You Can Do Now

Ours was the first society openly to define itself in terms of both
spirituality and human liberty.

—Jimmy Carter,
Inaugural Address

Liberty don't work as good in practice as it does in speeches.

—Will Rogers,
American humorist

WHAT YOU CAN DO UNTIL THE PARADIGM SHIFTS

Legal Power

If you do not want your child vaccinated, first find out where you stand legally
with respect to (1) state law and (2) federal law. Virtually all states have a
compulsory immunization law requiring children to be vaccinated against certain
childhood diseases: diphtheria, pertussis, tetanus, measles, mumps, rubella, and
polio. By now, your state probably requires hepatitis B and Hib vaccinations.
Because the law changes frequently, you will need to get a copy of the latest
version of the vaccination code of your state. The easiest way to get one is to
call (1) your state representative or (2) your state or county health department
and request a copy of the vaccination laws of your state. If time "is of the
essence," go directly to the law library or the reference section of your local

library and ask for the revised statutes under Public Health Law or Communicable Disease sections. The vaccination requirements will appear first and then the exemptions.

You will find there are two and sometimes three exemptions: medical, religious, and personal belief. To qualify for the medical exemption, a doctor must certify in writing that vaccines would be detrimental to your child's health. To qualify for the religious exemption, a parent or guardian must sign a notarized affidavit stating that vaccinations conflict with the parent's or guardian's religious beliefs. If your state is one with the personal belief exemption, simply write on a piece of paper that vaccinations are contrary to your beliefs. As of April 1994, the following states have the personal belief exemption: Arizona, California, Colorado, Idaho, Indiana, Louisiana, Maine, Michigan, Minnesota, Nebraska, New Mexico, North Dakota, Ohio, Oklahoma, Rhode Island, Utah, Vermont, Washington and Wisconsin. As mentioned earlier, the law changes frequently, so by the time you read this book, your state may or may not be on this list. Ohio, for instance, technically has a personal belief exemption, but so far the courts have not recognized it (see "What You Can Do to Help the Paradigm Shift"). Also, the personal belief exemption clause in Indiana, I was told recently, was threatened by the health department. It seems that most health officials want to exert as much control as possible while assuming as little responsibility as possible. It's important to be firm with them by knowing the law, but don't be antagonistic.

When we read of most European countries having freedom of choice with respect to vaccinations, this does not necessarily mean that compulsory vaccination laws are not on the books. It simply means that there is an "escape" clause, namely, the personal belief exemption. Actually, in Germany there are no mandatory vaccinations, and in Western Europe, only the tetanus and oral polio vaccinations are "required."[1]

All states except Minnesota, Mississippi, and West Virginia have a religious belief exemption clause. Some states apparently require that the parent belong to a church whose religious beliefs specifically oppose vaccination. This is clearly unconstitutional because the state is then defining what is and is not a religion.[2]

"The right to claim exemption from immunization based on religious beliefs is available to all persons who hold religious beliefs against immunization regardless of what any state statute may say regarding the necessity for membership in any particular religious group or church," James Filenbaum, a New York attorney who has won many key cases, said. He continues:

The First Amendment to the U.S. Constitution prohibits states from discriminating between people based on their religious beliefs. If there is any state law which allows for exemption based on religious beliefs, it is available to all those people who hold religious beliefs against immunization even if their beliefs are personal and unique to them alone.

These rights have been firmly established by numerous decisions of the U.S. Federal Courts.

We have been able to convince the court that a whole body of law which prohibits religious discrimination applies to those who have personal religious beliefs against immunization.[3]

Since 1983, there have been a series of decisions by federal district and appellate courts that have clearly established the rights of parents to have their children exempted from vaccination based upon their *personal* religious beliefs.

What constitutes a personal religious belief? It must be paramount in your life, and you must live by those beliefs. It does *not* have to include a belief in a diety. It may or may not be consistent or coherent or understandable to others.[4]

It is also possible "for parents to file as conscientious objectors with the state health department, although this choice is not advertised," Carol Horowitz tells us. She says that several people she knows who are conscientious objectors state that it is their "God-given right to refuse to immunize my child." Any lesser statement is legally unacceptable. You cannot say, for instance, that you read so many articles in newspapers and medical journals or saw some documentary on television.[5]

In his book *Dangers of Compulsory Immunizations, How to Avoid Them Legally*, attorney Tom Finn describes some legal tactics that may be used but do require the services of a lawyer.

Some attorneys have successfully prevented litigation by demanding from the school board, the hospital, and the physician administering the vaccine a guarantee that the vaccine will not cause disease, death or injurious side effects. The guarantee usually states that the vaccine will prevent the particular disease for which it is given to prevent. It is worded in such a way so as to make the persons signing it not only liable as a representative of the school district or hospital but also individually for damages should any damage in fact occur. To my knowledge no one has ever signed such a document and in each case in which it was used the child has been allowed to return to class without the vaccination.[6]

Certainly, compulsory immunization laws raise constitutional issues such as violation of the First, Ninth, and Fourteenth Amendments as well as violation of civil tort law.

How to Legally Avoid Unwanted Immunizations of All Kinds, a booklet published by the Humanitarian Publishing Company in Pennsylvania (see Appendix G), is another good source of information on avoiding vaccinations.

If your doctor or the school authorities insist on vaccinating your child against your will, contact the National Vaccine Information Center (NVIC), 512 West Maple Avenue, #206, Vienna, VA 22180, 703-DPT3, also the National Health Federation, P. O. Box 688, Monrovia, CA 91016, (818) 357–2181. These organizations may be able to help you. For more information and guidance regarding vaccination of school-age children, including exemption letters based on state laws, contact the American Natural Hygiene Society, P. O. Box 30630, Tampa, FL 33630, (813) 855–6607.

International Travel

When you receive your passport, it might be wise to request a copy of Foreign Rules and Regulations, Part 71, Title 42, on immunization. The World Health Organization (WHO) in Geneva grants American visitors the right to refuse vaccinations when traveling internationally. Remember the basic rule: No one will vaccinate you against your will, because by so doing that person assumes full responsibility for the consequences, both legal and medical.[7]

When traveling abroad, you may secure exemptions from vaccines by using Clause 83 of the International Sanitary Code, issued by the World Health Organization and adopted by all its members. It states, in effect, that only when coming from an infected area are vaccinations necessary *or* the traveler could be quarantined for up to 14 days from the time he left the infected area *if* the health department deems it necessary. If you come from an area where there has been an epidemic, you will probably be put under surveillance (close watch). This simply means that together with the local health officer you must keep a close watch for any suspicious signs or symptoms. You will probably be required to report periodically to your local health officer for a period of up to 14 days from the time of departure from the infected area. If you notice any outbreak or symptom, you must immediately turn yourself in and submit to quarantine or isolation.

In actual practice, not only is this possibility very remote, but if it should occur, the vaccinated person may be required to submit to the same surveillance as the unvaccinated! Remember, every year, thousands of unimmunized tourists travel in and out of the United States with little or no inconvenience or embarrassment.[8]

But laws change. In this country, power and money can circumvent them, even create them. Even though the Constitution clearly protects religious freedom (First Amendment rights), several states have deleted the religious exemption clause from their compulsory vaccination code. Even though the Supreme Court has ruled that no one can invade your body without your consent,[9] we still have compulsory vaccination laws and penalties—sometimes severe—for noncompliance. Even though attorney Thomas G. Finn has stated, "Legally no state has the right to force citizens of the United States to have a substance injected into their children's bodies without their permission,"[10] states have taken children away from parents who objected to vaccinations, charging them with medical, or even child, neglect and had them vaccinated. Clearly, something more is needed.

WHAT YOU CAN DO TO HELP THE PARADIGM SHIFT

> Never doubt that a small group of thoughtful, committed citizens can change the world; indeed it's the only thing that ever has.
>
> —Margaret Mead

People Power

It is axiomatic that a few people organized around a powerful idea have changed the world. The American Revolution and the founding of our country was the result of just such an idea—freedom. More recently, the deescalation and final cessation of the Vietnam War were the result of people organized around a powerful idea—peace. But peace is not possible without freedom. Nor is justice or brotherhood. Liberty, equality, fraternity—the rallying cry of the French Revolution—suggest their interdependence. Because these ideas are more than intellectual propositions and have universal or spiritual underpinnings, they can be called ideals. And this is what we are about.

Get Clear with Yourself. The issue is compulsory vaccination. How do you really feel about it? Check the statement that most closely describes your position:

1. Compulsory vaccination laws are necessary to "protect" the community.

2. Some vaccinations are good, others questionable.

3. All vaccinations are inherently harmful and should be banned.

4. Counseling and presentation of "truthful" information should always precede vaccination.

5. Vaccinations, like any other invasive medical procedure, must always be subject to choice.

If you checked any statement but number 5, you don't really have an issue. If you checked number 4, thinking number 5, is implied and therefore ensured, you may find that in practice this does not necessarily follow. For instance, to protect themselves from litigation, public health clinics and many pediatricians present the parent with a "consent" form to sign. The form states that the parent has read and understood the information in the form pertaining to the benefits and risks of the vaccine and that he or she authorizes and requests that the vaccine be given. If the parent doesn't sign, he or she is breaking the law unless the state has a philosophical or personal exemption clause. Also, what constitutes "truthful" information can be very debatable and difficult to enforce.

If you checked number 1, you're comfortable with the way things are and don't need to read or investigate further. It might help, however, to read books such as this one simply to expand your horizons and arena of rapport to include those of a different persuasion. Being able to see the world—or an issue—from different perspectives is part of the maturation process.

If you checked number 2, you're still caught in the net of the vaccine doctrine. You may or may not agree with number 5.

If you checked number 3, no matter how thoroughly you have investigated the subject or how strongly you feel about it, you're not on solid ground. On the immediate, practical level, the chances of banning vaccinations or even suspending them for a period of time are extremely slim. The medical-pharmaceutical industry would throw its weight against this because it would delegitimize its power over the American people (think of the lawsuits that would occur if this industry admitted that vaccinations were inherently damaging!). Besides, the conditioning, the indoctrination, of the American public has been so thorough (as has that of medical professionals) that most people feel the need for "protection" and believe that vaccinations are the "magic bullet" that will provide it. We must respect that need and their right to choose. Not to respect that right is to be on the same level as the opposition which doesn't respect your right. (The right to choose can be legitimately abrogated only if a decision would result in an action that is unequivocally and demonstrably harmful or violates another person's right to choose.)

Choice, which is the heart of freedom, is wrapped in responsibility. Perhaps this is why most people avoid it. Any number of doctors have testified that most of their patients want to be told what to do. The authoritarian model is comfortable for most people. But that "most" is shrinking. The major cause of the shrinkage, I think, is that more people are becoming aware of other "realities," among them other models of healthcare. And they are demanding the right to choose other models, particularly models that do not include disease prevention via drugs and vaccines and, in fact, eschew them. They are ready to accept full responsibility for the consequences of their decisions, just as the person who chooses to vaccinate must accept full responsibility for the consequences of his or her decision. Not to have the option of choosing is not to have the option of taking responsibility, which, in a very real sense, deprives a person of the opportunity to fully mature.

So our issue is really freedom, the opportunity to choose among a number of positive alternatives. Freedom is of the spirit. To understand and experience it requires alignment with the spiritual dimension. This is no doubt why it has been so difficult to secure and yet has been such an insistent theme throughout human history. The ability to choose, sometimes called free will, is an aspect of the soul and is implied in the great spiritual traditions of the world as well as clearly stated in the Cayce readings. It is also implied in the founding documents of our country.

Organize. Multiply your ability to make a difference by uniting with others who share your concerns. As we said earlier, a small group of thoughtful, committed citizens can change the world.

Begin by contacting people. Contact people you know who share your concerns with the compulsory vaccination issue. These people will frequently have valuable suggestions as to time and place for your meetings. You may want to have the first meeting at your own home. Certainly, a private residence is more inviting than the impersonality of a room in a public building. You don't need many people to begin with—as few as three or four is enough.

First, agree on a purpose, a name, and officers or job titles and descriptions. Once you have clarity of purpose, your group will organize itself. (This is the principle of living systems.) Since most people are busy, as you no doubt are, keep your objectives simple. Have a single agenda, but not so narrow that it becomes too confrontational and looses sight of larger principles. If your purpose is to change or influence legislation, you'll need to broaden your base by getting more people involved and informed. You'll want to reach as many people as possible with the least amount of time and energy expenditure, so put a notice in the paper in the community events section announcing the time, place, speaker, and program of your first public meeting. If room permits, include the purpose of your organization. It may help to post notices on bulletin boards in health food stores or other suitable places. If your local paper has recently published articles on healthcare reform or vaccinations, write letters to the editor, including the name of your group and your title. At this point, it is very important to have official stationery stating the name of your organization and the name, address, and phone number of the president. It is also important that any correspondence such as a letter to the editor be professional, that is, fact-filled and literate. Also, sum up by relating facts to a larger principle.

Generally speaking, avoid using the terms *immunization* and *immunized* because they are misleading, for reasons discussed in Chapter 3. Use instead the terms *vaccination* and *vaccinated*. And never say a person is *unimmunized*; he or she is *unvaccinated*.

You may want to align yourself with a national organization such as the National Health Federation (NHF) and open a local chapter of that organization. The NHF can give you advice and support. Their phone number is (818) 357-2181.

If crucial legislation is pending such as the deletion of the personal exemption clause or, worse, the deletion of the religious exemption clause (yes, it has happened here!), you need to act immediately to expand your base and contact your representatives. It makes a stronger impression if several of you go to meet with your legislators. It makes a still stronger impression if you can contact parents with a vaccine-damaged child and have them come with you with their child.

If you or some member of your group is being taken to court because of refusal to get his or her child vaccinated, be sure to get the media involved. The American public is generally sensitive about government abuses of power and violations of civil rights. Even though compulsory vaccinations have as yet not been viewed as a violation of civil rights, there are a surprising number of people, including doctors, who believe in vaccinations but not compulsion. The compulsory aspect alone sullies the vaccine doctrine, as well as organized medicine.

Have one of your officers, preferably the president or director, phone your local newspaper and TV stations, making a statement to this effect: On Tuesday, October 14, at the County Courthouse, Jane Jones, vice president of [name of state] Parents for Healthcare Choice, will appear in court for refusing to have her 4-month-old baby vaccinated with DPT. A particularly disturbing aspect of this case is that the child was born with epilepsy, a neurological disorder specifically contraindicated for this vaccine in both the packet insert and the *Physician's Desk Reference.*

(This incident, though fictitious, is similar to an actual case. In February 1994, a woman phoned from a personal exemption state telling me that the director of the health department as well as her neurologist were hassling her to get her 4-month-old epileptic daughter vaccinated. She said the health department and other medical groups were working to get the personal belief exemption clause deleted.)

First public meeting. Before the meeting, arrange a table with pertinent books (see Appendix G) and articles for purchase as well as free leaflets informing people where they can get more information. It might be wise to begin this initial meeting by having a short talk—about 30 minutes—explaining the purpose of the organization and why the right to choose or refuse any or all vaccinations is so important. The rest of the meeting might best be used for answering questions and signing people up and getting them to write or meet with their representatives. You may feel it more expedient at this time simply to have a petition for people to sign. Remember, it is easier to maintain an existing law than it is to get a new law passed, particularly if the old law has been in place for many years.

If your group decides to have regular monthly or even weekly meetings, you may want to have a series of lectures, each focusing on different aspects of the vaccination issue, such as (1) the inherent harmfulness of vaccinations, (2) the ineffectiveness of vaccinations, (3) the germ theory and monomorphism versus evidence for pleomorphism and the existence of an elementary life particle, (4) the meaning of illness or disease from the point of view of different schools of healing and what this implies for the use of vaccines, (5) natural ways of treating children's diseases and other illnesses, (6) compulsory vaccinations versus holistic healthcare, (6) vaccinations, vegetarianism, and animal rights, (7) using general semantics to recognize medical propaganda, and (8) compulsory vaccinations and the spiritual ideals embodied in the founding documents of our country.

However, don't lose sight of your central objective, which is to secure freedom to practice your own kind of healthcare. Part of every meeting needs to at least mention some kind of political action. You may want to have bumper stickers with such phrases as "Education—not Medication" or "Education—not Indoctrination." You might even want to have a second bumper sticker with the phrase "Education—Not Vaccination." This latter is probably too confrontational. After all, vaccination is almost a religion, certainly a sacred cow. Most people's belief in it runs deep, and any direct challenge to the doctrine is offensive.

Other organizations. Although every situation is different, we can learn from organizations that have been successful in changing legislation to protect people from the "vaccine machine."

Ohio Parents for Vaccine Safety (251 West Ridgeway Drive, Dayton, OH 45459), founded and directed by Kristine Severyn, a registered pharmacist with a degree in biopharmaceutics, was successful in getting the Ohio House of Representatives to reinstate the personal exemption clause by a vote of 93 to 3, even adding the words "moral and philosophical" to the exemptions. However, the bill was held up in the Ohio Senate because of opposition by the "health" (diseasescare?) department, where as of this writing it is still pending. Even though exemption #3 of the Ohio Code reads that a parent or guardian may object "to the immunization for good cause, including religious convictions," Kristine Severyn told me that only medical and religious exemptions have been recognized by the Ohio courts.

The group's purpose is to ensure that (1) truthful information be given to the parents (i.e., risks versus "benefits" of the vaccine), and that (2) vaccines be given only with the informed consent of the parent. Because both vaccine safety and effectiveness are in question, and public health officials are not held accountable for the results of their policies, the informed consent of the parent is essential.

Kristine Severyn has appeared before a number of legislative committees and writes professional, fact-filled editorials. She also puts out a professional newsletter filled with vaccine information from all over the world.

The *National Health Federation*, founded in 1955 to promote freedom of choice in health matters, was responsible for getting the personal belief exemption clause inserted into the vaccination code of California. The NHF promotes its agenda via a magazine (see Appendix G), national and regional conferences, regional chapters, maintaining a speaker's bureau, and legislative action including member contact with legislators.

The *National Vaccine Information Center* (NVIC) was founded in 1982 to prevent vaccine injuries and deaths by educating the public to make informed, independent vaccination decisions free of government interference. The NVIC was largely responsible for getting the Vaccine Adverse Event Reporting System (VAERS) passed (Public Law 99–660), which created the Vaccine Injury Compensation Program. This bill also set up improved vaccine safety mechanisms to help monitor and prevent vaccine-associated injuries and deaths. I was initially very opposed to this legislation because it sticks the taxpayer with the compensation bill, which I thought the vaccine manufacturers should pay. But then I realized that if the government mandates, the government should pay. This group publishes literature (see Appendix G), and its president, Barbara Loe Fisher, speaks before many different groups.

Mention should be made of the important work of the *National Anti-Vaccination League of Great Britain*, which was able to keep vaccinations free from compulsion—but not pressure—in Great Britain. (Today, their National Health Service actually pays a "bonus" to doctors with documented vaccination rates above specified percentages).[11] The league—though apparently no longer extant—was founded during the latter half of the nineteenth century. Its success was probably due to (1) distribution of literature that was informative, literate, and sometimes witty, (2) speakers who appeared before a wide range of groups, and (3) the consciousness of much of the British public. This awareness is due in part to the British experience with smallpox epidemics during the nineteenth century, which demonstrated that vaccinations not only didn't prevent but actually increased the incidence of smallpox as well as caused many disabilities and deaths, and in part to the recognition of the value of natural health and healing or "Nature Cure."

Two Common Objections. Your group needs to have speakers. Because your organization is not national, one or two good speakers are probably enough. You may have occasion to speak to persons or groups who are thoroughly entrenched in the vaccine doctrine. You'll probably find as I have that two objections repeatedly come up, so be prepared to answer them as directly and simply as possible.

A. If vaccinations were not compulsory then many people wouldn't vaccinate, and old plagues and diseases would return.

B. If vaccinations aren't effective, why did polio disappear?

Question A: This, of course, is the herd immunity idea again—vaccination in the line of duty to protect the community. Don't bank on opening people up to the reasonableness of voluntary vaccinations by pointing out the inherent contradiction of this kind of thinking with the premises of vaccination. Once people are thoroughly indoctrinated, they can become psychologically deaf to hearing other points of view. One woman said to me after I pointed out the contradiction, "If your child wasn't vaccinated and my child caught German measles after playing with him, I'd take you to court!"

The same kind of circular reasoning that the vaccinators use today to justify forced vaccinations was used a hundred years ago to justify vaccine failure. If you were vaccinated for smallpox and got smallpox anyway, you would have gotten it worse if you weren't vaccinated. If you almost died of smallpox, you would surely have died if you weren't vaccinated. "And if you have the impudence, after you have been vaccinated, to go and die outright, then, 'You could not have been vaccinated properly.' "[12]

Second point: Diseases for which vaccinations are given were 90 to 95 percent eliminated before vaccinations were introduced, and other diseases such as cholera and tuberculosis disappeared without vaccinations (see Chapter 3). Charts illustrating this decline as well as the epidemics of smallpox and diphtheria, which occurred *after* mass vaccinations, can be helpful. You might want to reinforce this point by adding that, contrary to popular belief, smallpox has not disappeared. It is still appearing among vaccinated people. Usually, these cases occur among relatively isolated groups, many and sometimes most of whose members have been vaccinated.[13]

Third point: Patterns of health and disease reflect the living habits of a person or a community (see Chapter 4). You may want to dramatize this idea by telling your audience how we love to romanticize the Middle Ages with their beautiful costumes and later with the elaborate dress and high-piled hair of the upper-class ladies. What we don't see—and smell—is the ever-present filth, not only from human and animal fecal matter all around but the lack of bathing. The high-piled hair of the upper-class ladies was not taken down for shampooing for a very long time—not "until they became so offensive to themselves and everyone else that no one could get within several yards of them."[14] And clothing? It was not only unwashed but usually infested with vermin.[15]

It has been said that during the Middle Ages Europe went a thousand years without a bath. "Saint Francis of Assisi considered an unwashed body a stinking badge of piety. Queen Isobella of Castile boasted that she had had only two baths in her life—at birth and before her marriage."[16] In colonial America, leaders discouraged bathing. Laws in Pennsylvania and Virginia either banned or limited bathing, and for a time in Philadelphia, anyone who bathed more than once a month faced jail. Why the prejudice against bathing? It was thought to promote nudity, which could only lead to promiscuity.[17]

One of the major but usually hidden heroes of the nineteenth-century health revolution was personal hygiene wherein the simple act of handwashing sharply reduced maternal and infant mortality. Sometimes people need to be reminded with a few dramatic examples that the conditions which spawned the epidemics of history—even recent history—no longer prevail and that diseases reflect conditions, not lack of vaccines.

Now we have mass vaccinations which themselves can cause epidemics (Chapters 2, 3, and 8).

Question B: Naturally occurring paralytic polio was always a rare disease (see Chapters 3, 4, and 6 and statements by Drs. Ratner, Moskowitz, and Ritchie). The high prevalence and subsequent demise of polio as a result of the Salk vaccine (and later the Sabin) was the creation of statistical artifact (Chapter 3) and media hype. Changing patterns of living may also be involved (Chapter 4).

Media hype: The extent and intensity of the hype engineered by the National Foundation for Infantile Paralysis in the 1940s and early 1950s is without parallel in my experience. Even the AIDS hoopla doesn't compare with it. The March of Dimes campaign (the fund-raising arm of the foundation) was kicked off by the annual Birthday Balls on January 30, and all over the nation mothers began marching for money to support the research that would produce the miracle vaccine that would save the children. Letters, phone calls, March of Dimes banks on store counters and other public places, and posters and billboards featuring a beautiful child wearing braces and/or crutches seemed to be everywhere—all reminding us to give, give, give. And give we did—$500 million in 15 years,[18] a remarkable sum for that time. Even the warnings from the health department urging parents to keep their children away from swimming pools and other such public places during the polio season were part of the blitz. Polioscare was everywhere.

When the "miracle" vaccine, whose research was subsidized by the National Foundation for Infantile Paralysis, made its long-awaited appearance in 1954, its developer, Jonas Salk, became an instant celebrity. But when the vaccine failed to live up to its promise and in hundreds of cases produced instead of prevented polio, this fact was gradually censored out of the media. For instance, on May 6, 1955, the *News Chronicle* reported that "the numbers developing polio were far greater than had no inoculation been given" and that in Idaho "polio struck only vaccinated children in areas where there had been no cases of polio since the preceding autumn."[19] (Interestingly, the same article reported that the interval between inoculation and the first sign of paralysis ranged from 5 to 20 days and that in 9 out of 10 cases the paralysis occurred in the arm in which the vaccine had been injected.) By June 23, 1955, the American Public Health Service announced that there had been "168 confirmed cases of poliomyelitis among the vaccinated, with six deaths."[20] But by November 15, 1955, the "U.S. Public Health Service released a report declaring that a single inoculation of the Salk vaccine used in 1955 was sufficient to give 50 to 80 percent protection against paralytic poliomyelitis," and two days later it issued another report stressing the safety of the vaccine.[21] Glowing reports of the safety and effectiveness continued even in the face of a 179 percent increase in cases of the triply-vaccinated (up to September 20) in the years 1957 and 1958.[22] In fact, by 1958, the U.S. Public Health Service claimed the vaccine 87 percent effective, and the AMA recommended that "every physician see to it that every person he examines be vaccinated fully."[23]

Could this contradiction between policy and reality have something to do with the condemnation of the Cutter laboratories in June 1955 which caused its stock to drop from $15.50 to $8.75 per share and the fact that it had over $1 million worth of Salk vaccine on hand?[24] (The Cutter laboratory manufactured the vaccine that paralyzed hundreds of babies and their contacts during the first two weeks of the mass introduction of the Salk vaccine in the United States in 1955.)[25] Could it have something to do with the other five laboratories whose $8 million supply of Salk vaccine[26] might have to be discarded? Could it have something to do with the National Foundation for Infantile Paralysis and its credibility? In December 1958, this foundation announced that inasmuch as poliomyelitis had been conquered, it was changing its name to the National Foundation and turning to "a broadened attack—arthritis and 'birth defects.' "[27] Worth noting is the statement made in March 1959 by Basil O'Conner, president of the National Foundation, that because of the Salk vaccine "no child . . . in the world need ever again suffer the paralysis of one disease—polio."[28] But in the first quarter of that same year, there were 83 percent more cases of paralytic polio than in the first quarter of 1958; three weeks later, it had grown to more than 100 percent.[29] One month later, Dr. Herman Bundesen, president of the Chicago Board of Health, extolled the effectiveness of the Salk vaccine, saying, "Widespread use of the vaccine is undoubtedly the reason why not a single case of polio has been reported here since January 1."[30]

In the face of the marked increase in paralytic polio in the United States—many of whom were triple vaccinees and many who died—Dr. A. D. Langmuir of the U.S. Department of Health, Education and Welfare still wrote of the "marked downward trend of poliomyelitis in the past four years" and that "completion of the immunization program should lead to the essential elimination of paralytic poliomyelitis from the United States."[31]

Now that the Sabin has replaced the Salk vaccine, is a similar kind of lying and censorship going on? Most of the negative reportage I have heard is another variation of the old scare tactic: Because both vaccines can create carriers in the recipients, meaning the virus can be excreted, unvaccinated persons may contract polio and become paralyzed. So everyone needs to be vaccinated to protect themselves from the vaccinated! Several years ago, I saw a television program illustrating this idea. One case was an elderly man with an already compromised immune system who "caught" polio from changing the diapers of his recently vaccinated grandson (Sabin oral vaccine). So now instead of the vaccinated being threatened by the unvaccinated, the unvaccinated are threatened by the vaccinated!

But is polio really contagious? Prior to the March of Dimes hoopla, the paralytic form of polio was considered by many doctors to be a rare, idiosyncratic disease, the virus being produced within the body when certain biochemical conditions prevailed, namely, poisoning and nutritional deficiencies (see Chapter 4). Carl S. Frischkorn, who investigated many cases, said that polio is "neither contagious nor infectious, as case after case can be cited where the victim had been sleeping with other children and had played with other children, being the only one struck."[32] Many other doctors have said the same thing. In fact, the noncontagious nature of polio was one of the central arguments Don Matchen, who represented the National Health Federation, used in California to secure the personal belief exemption clause in the compulsory polio immunization bill (A.B. 1490) when he appeared before the Assembly Public Health Committee on March 29, 1961.[33] Australian researcher Viera Scheibner also cites doctors who point to the essentially endogenous (originating from within) origin of polio.[34] Has the polio vaccine transformed an endogenous disease into something more exogenous (originating from without)? Returning to principle (Part II of this book), we might ask, Is there such a thing as a contagious disease, or is it a "contagious" compromised immune system?

And finally, did polio disappear? No, according to Dr. Scheibner, it has simply been renamed: "Aseptic (or viral) meningitis, often followed by residual paralysis, and affecting hundreds of vaccinated children every year in the so-called developed countries, is just one of the fancy names for paralytic poliomyelitis."[35] And now we have a fancy name for meningitis vaccine: Hib.

And the show goes on. Only the actors change. Will fact and reason abate, or at least, diminish the production? For well over 150 years, people, including many distinguished doctors and researchers, have been trying to do just that, but the show continues becoming more entrenched, intrusive, and tentacled.

Why? For one, it's very easy to counter one set of facts with another set of "facts" and build theoretical structures based upon those "facts," particularly when other facts and reality models are not readily accessible. And this, I think, is the nub of the problem. As long as we attempt to solve a problem on its own level, that is, the level of consciousness (or thinking) that created the problem in the first place, we will merely create "head-ons"—attacks and counterattacks, facts and denial of facts, evidence and counterevidence. No, we have to move to higher ground.

Here in the United States—"the land of the free"—the best the dissenters have been able to do is to create a small space for exemptions from the compulsory vaccination laws, but the floodwaters of coercion continually threaten to overwhelm that space. Can't we do better than this? Fact and reason, while essential, cannot work alone. Something else is needed, and, I believe, that something else will open the gates to freedom.

THE PARADIGM SHIFTS

The power of the visible is the invisible.

—Marianne Moore,
American poet

Consciousness Power

"Don't speak to him personally. Don't listen to him speak from a crowd." Because he said "always ally yourself with the part of your enemy that knows what is right" and he knew how to do it. He knew that what is right is inherently possible, and he'll make you think that, too. These were the instructions given to new British officials in old India as they were told to "stay away from Gandhi" because "he'll get you."[36]

What was the secret of Gandhi's power? What transformed this shy, tongue-tied "average" little man into a leader of 100,000 people in South Africa and later the entire nation of India in one of the most remarkable experiments in history—a war without violence? What changed Mohandas Karamchand Gandhi into a Mahatma, "great soul," a man whom even those who opposed him called a saint?[37]

In 1908, in South Africa, Gandhi coined the word *satyagraha*, which he defined this way: "Truth (satya) implies love, and Firmness (agraha) engenders and therefore serves as a synonym for force. I thus began to call the Indian movement 'satyagraha': that is to say, the force which is born of truth and love or nonviolence."[38] The power of Truth or Satyagraha, literally "Truth Force," was the theme of the mature Gandhi's life and the source of his power. In fact, the subtitle of Gandhi's autobiography is *The Story of My Experiments with Truth. Truth* with a capital *T* refers to ideas that transcend the limitations of time and space, ideas that come from a universal or spiritual dimension. When we access this dimension, we access what Deepak Chopra calls the Cosmic Self, the field of all possibilities. To know this dimension is to experience the inherently right and the power that makes it inherently possible.

These Truths—the inherently right—are, I believe, the source of the genius and the power of the ideals behind the founding documents of our country. When the leaders of the American Revolution and the signers of the Declaration of Independence wrote "all men are created equal" and are "endowed by their Creator with certain unalienable Rights" which derive from the "Laws of Nature and Nature's God"—truths held "to be self-evident"—what did they mean? They meant that all men come from the same Source and contain within themselves the divine nature of that Source and are therefore entitled to equality and justice, which I might translate as Respect actualized.

How can I be so sure? Because 51 of the 56 signers of the Declaration of Independence were members of the Freemasons and/or Rosicrucians,[39] ancient Mystery Schools that acknowledged the power and importance of the invisible realms through their sacred rituals. The reality of these nonvisible realms of being has always been an integral part of human understanding. Only in the past 200 years with the rise of scientific materialism has our picture of reality been confined to the visible, tangible world.[40] But this is changing. Witness the rise of parapsychology, transpersonal psychology, deep ecology, and quantum-relativistic physics, which are returning us to a more holistic, less sense-bound awareness of ourselves and our universe. And it is this new awareness that floodlights the limitations of the conventional medical model and its primary cornerstone—compulsory vaccinations. Based on diseasescare and diseasefight, the vaccination paradigm epitomizes nineteenth-century mechanical, reductionist ideas of ourselves and our universe. Its coercive aspect also epitomizes the degeneration of a supposed healing profession into fear-mongering and policing, one of the many examples of the enantiodromias of history, whereby the supposed intent and ideals of a profession turn into their opposite.

How can we apply Gandhi's "experiments with Truth," which pioneered a worldwide consciousness that delegitimized nation-state imperialism, to pioneering a consciousness that delegitimizes medical-pharmaceutical imperialism? As Gandhi legitimized the recognition of the inherent worth and dignity of every human being and his or her right to self-determination—which are the cornerstones of democracy—we must legitimize the right of every human being to self-determination with respect to healthcare. But there are differences between his situation and ours, and these can be daunting: (1) The wrongs that Gandhi sought to right were visible and obvious, and (2) he had the consciousness of the great majority of Hindus behind him. We have neither. The evils of forced medical treatments, that is, vaccinations, are not obvious, nor does it appear that the majority of Americans are behind the idea of self-determination with respect to them. Never mind that democracy does not mean the dictatorship of the majority (or vested interests) but the protection of the rights of the minority. Never mind that ideas like multiculturalism, pluralism, diversity, and alternatives are "in"; these ideas are "out" with respect to nonvaccinations and nonmedical options. (Have you ever heard of a parent charged with naturopathic neglect or chiropractic neglect?) Never mind that the Constitution forbids state-supported religion; the religion of Modern Medicine is exclusively and generously supported by the state and federal government. Never mind that the mind-body is a continuum and mind must believe in a treatment before it can be effective; the vaccine machine doesn't know this. Here is the robotic giant's Achilles' heel and our first and probably greatest ally.

Holistic medicine is "in" and growing. The talk is about the infusion of spirit and consciousness into the healing process—indeed, the necessity of it. Conscious participation of the patient is a given. One of the principles behind the founding of the American Holistic Medical Association is that man is a spiritual being and that treatment must be directed toward the total person—body, mind, and spirit. Another tenet says, in effect, that the patient has an inalienable right to share in the decision-making processes pertaining to a medical treatment.[41] The contradiction between these ideas and the compulsory vaccination laws is obvious.

We now have the key that will eventually open the lock: consciousness.

What if we regarded "the other" as a holy being, as the term *holism* implies (Chapter 8)? It would revolutionize not only health care but all our other institutions as well. We would finally begin to respect each other, even nonhuman others. We would be capable of "listening." Our minds would open to other possibilities, other approaches, other ways of experiencing and being in the world. Conventional medicine (drug and surgery oriented) would be seen as one of many approaches and vaccinations one of many possible solutions (assuming it is a solution). This brings us to our second ally—General Semantics (see Chapter 12).

General Semantics is usually thought of as a purely intellectual discipline, but it can also expand the consciousness. By making us aware that our reality is created largely by the processes of abstracting and projecting, we become less "stuck," more open, and flexible. As just pointed out, we will see Modern Medicine as simply one of many possible ways of constructing reality.

Did you know that at one time this idea was a given? "Before 1910, many systems of healthcare co-existed in America. These included nutrition, homeopathy, herbal medicine, osteopathy [the classical, nondrug, manipulative osteopathy], allopathy, chiropractic, and hydrotherapy. Each had its own schools. At the turn of the century, America was among the healthiest nations."[42] What happened? In 1910, Congress accepted the Flexner Report on Medical Education. Sponsored by the American Medical Association, this report declared allopathic or drug medicine to be superior. "Congress enacted laws to regulate medical education that in effect eradicated all but the drug medical schools. Taxpayer dollars began to flow to the allopathic schools, making it even more difficult for the competition to survive."[43] Today, we have the most expensive healthcare system in the world and yet we lead the world in degenerative disease (Chapter 12). Now we come to our third ally—ecology.

The relatively recent development among "white man" of an *ecological consciousness* has opened him or her to the subtleties of the long range, the less visible, and the multidirectional. We now know that living systems are self-regulating and that the introduction of a foreign element into that system can have far-reaching consequences, vaccination being a prime example of this (Chapter 2).

Have you ever wondered what really happens when teams of "health" workers go into Third World countries and vaccinate large numbers of mostly under- and malnourished populations? Have you ever wanted to get behind the glowing reports of diseases being "wiped out" by their "tireless efforts"? We got a hint in Chapter 3 with the *Science* report of a poliolike disease affecting large numbers of vaccinated children in China and Latin America, and in Chapter 8 with the report of AIDS affecting large numbers of vaccinated people in Africa and Haiti. Even the World Health Organization has withdrawn from use a measles vaccine strain because it resulted in increased deaths from other causes in Third World children.[44] But no one seems to give credit to the civil and sanitary engineers who usually accompany the teams of health workers and who create infrastructures to bring potable water and sanitation to the community. Sometimes there are organic agriculturists who show people how to grow "nutrition-dense" crops. These are the real heroes who bring about the reduction of diseases. So interventions into a living system can be salutary as well as damaging. It's important to know the difference. Now our fourth ally—animal rights.

The animal rights movement, which is really an extension of the emerging holistic and ecological consciousness, is another powerful but as yet untapped (in this country) source of support for liberation from forced vaccinations. The number of animals sacrificed every year for medical research in the United States has been estimated at anywhere from 22 million to 60–100 million.[45] Of this number, a conservative estimate finds that about 10 percent are used in the research and production of vaccines. I remember seeing a National Geographic Special on primates used in medical research for an AIDS vaccine. We were shown a compound of white, irregularly shaped buildings where the monkeys were caged. Inside we saw tiers of small cages and rows of expressionless eyes staring out at us. I recall one commentator saying the monkeys were psychologically brain dead. This "concentration camp" is but one of many examples of animal cruelty in the name of medical "progress."

Discussions on this subject invariably, in my experience, degenerate into an either/or, us-or-them parody of inquiry. This is, of course, because most people are stuck in the tunnel of the medical model, which sees health as a commodity and disease as an adversary. A discussion of plant-based and other natural remedies for ills that animal research and products have been touted to relieve or prevent goes beyond the scope of this book, but once we get out of the medical tunnel, a new world of thinking and being will open up to us.

This brings us to our fifth and leavening ally—humor.

Wearing his khadhi loincloth and shawl to Buckingham Palace, Gandhi was asked by a reporter afterwards, "Mr. Gandhi, don't you think you were a trifle underdressed for the occasion?" "His Majesty," Gandhi answered, "had enough clothes on for both of us."[46]

A *sense of humor* is essential to give us perspective; otherwise, we can slide into depression, myopia, and even stridency. When the "enemy" works against universal principles, it will eventually hang itself. Did you know that biologists are now working on genetically altering fruits and vegetables to serve as edible vaccines? Mitch Hein, a scientist at Scripps Research Institute, for instance, is currently working on an alfalfa seedling "he has genetically engineered to contain just enough of the deadly cholera toxin he thinks will confer immunity on anyone who eats enough of it."[47] The same article describes another scientist, Charles Arntzen at Texas A & M University, who is trying to develop a banana that can prevent hepatitis B, and a biology professor, Roy Curtis at Washington University in St. Louis, who is engineering vaccines that use broccoli, turnips, and Brussel sprouts. Will we soon have recipes featuring polio turnips, measles broccoli, and hepatitis bananas? Will "pass the cholera sprouts or pertussis potatoes" be part of our dinner parlance?

There is a sort of theater-of-the-absurd humor about this, but there is also a glimmer of hope. If vaccine foods actually come to pass, it will be next to impossible for the medical-pharmaceutical industry to force vaccinations. They could enforce purchase of a vaccine veggie, but are they going to dispatch troops to our dinner tables to see to it that we eat our veggies?

Begin where you are. First, where are you in your life? Do you use prescription drugs? Do you patronize drug- and vaccine-promoting doctors? Do you or your children use some vaccines and not others? Do you give to charities that support vaccinations, synthetic and toxic drugs, and/or research on them? Do you use insecticides and chemical fertilizers? If you answer yes to any of these questions, you might want to take a second look at your choices. Why? Because every time you use one of these products or support organizations that do, you are contributing to the medical and petrochemical industries and the hold that they have over our lives and our planet.

A husband and wife chiropractic team in our area, Drs. Patricia and Michael McLean, have stated the case very pointedly:

We must demand that our birthright—total unimpaired health—be supported both within ourselves and by our society. Let's begin by refusing to be held hostage to the petrochemical and medical industries. Let's free ourselves from drug dependency by refusing to medicate ourselves and our babies. Free our earth from toxins and poisons that are the by-products of these industries. Call your legislators and ask for more research for health, not for disease. Realize that you can be healthy and find the courage to take back your life.[48]

We must get the government out of the drug- and vaccine-promoting business by pointing out that besides the misinformation and fear-mongering that has accompanied the promotion of vaccinations, this doctrine represents only one school among many schools of healing and should not be supported unless other models of health and healing are also supported.

Besides writing to legislators to encourage them to support or veto a particular piece of legislation, we must write to congratulate them when they vote for freedom of choice and reducing government subsidies for promotion of drugs and vaccines. We must also write to "nonprofit" organizations that ask for our contributions but support vaccinations and explain why we can't support them. You can make a difference. One highly respected organization, for instance, sent us a sample copy of their newsletter, which featured an editorial extolling the benefits of infant vaccination. I wrote back saying that I had associated their organization with the more enlightened ecological and planetary awareness but couldn't support them because their claim of "thorough research and analysis" of issues was contradicted by their uncritical acceptance of the party line of the medical-pharmaceutical industry. After pointing out the central controversies surrounding vaccinations, I recommended some books for them to read. While I have never received another free copy of their newsletter, I have noticed that subsequent literature they have sent has said nothing about vaccinations or even the WHO.

Our goal, like Gandhi's, must be the elimination of tyranny. As Gandhi's goal was the elimination of the tyranny of the British raj, our goal must be the elimination of the tyranny of the compulsory vaccination laws. If just a small group of "vaccine-touting doctors" actively pressuring "every state legislature in the country" could get the compulsory vaccination laws passed,[49] surely a much larger group could get them rescinded.

We need to contact and work with other practitioners of natural therapies and the schools and organizations representing them, for example, naturopathy, homeopathy, chiropractic, herbology, and acupuncture. Even though many of these practitioners may still believe in vaccinations, their concerns are much the same as ours, namely, securing an open, multioptioned system of health care, so they would be open to rescinding the compulsory vaccination laws. When our support reaches a "critical mass," we can directly challenge the compulsory vaccination laws. This shouldn't be as difficult as it might at first appear. According to a 1990 survey, one out of every three Americans uses alternative methods of healthcare,[50] and that number is increasing. Student enrollment at the three existing naturopathic medical schools is soaring to an all-time high.[51] (When a naturopathic doctor opened an office in our area, she was booked up for four months!) There was even an article from the Associated Press recently titled "Link Is Possible Between Shots and Brain Damage."[52] So there is a gradual change of consciousness with respect to vaccinations and a demand for nontoxic, noninvasive ways of caring for the body-mind.

The time is ripe to pioneer the new healthcare consciousness. This is the consciousness that recognizes the interdependence and purposefulness of all life forms. It, therefore, recognizes that diseases and the microorganisms associated with them have necessary functions (Chapters 5, 6, 7, 9). This consciousness also recognizes that "enemy making" (seeing something or someone as an enemy) is separative and distancing, taking us away from the very thing we need to get close to in order to understand it. And, of course, this consciousness recognizes the creative power of the mind (Chapter 8) and the uselessness of coercion to force the "correct" response. Even more important, this consciousness recognizes the disrespect, nay, the irreverence, of forcing one's will upon another. "The greatest sins in the world today," Edgar Cayce said, "are selfishness and the domination of one individual will by another will." Earlier in the same talk he said, "as our information says [information from his psychic readings], anyone who would force another to submit to his will is a tyrant!"[53]

Nonviolent noncooperation with evil was the hallmark of the Gandhi-inspired satyagraha movement in India. This means delegitimizing exploitive industries and governments by withdrawing our support for them. We do this by not purchasing their products or consenting to their "services" and creating instead products and services that are life supporting and life respecting.

Nonviolent noncooperation with evil also means having the courage to "just say no" to an unjust law. Forced vaccinations are just such a law.

The satyagrahi doesn't take refuge in numbers but begins with one person's refusal to obey an unjust law. The movement itself began in Africa in 1893 when Gandhi refused to give up his reserved seat to a white man and was thrown off the train. More than 60 years later in our country, the civil rights movement began when Rosa Parks refused to give up her seat to a white man and was arrested for it.

In keeping with the spirit of the new healthcare consciousness and the model Gandhi has given us, we will love our opponents and go out of our way to offer them every courtesy. Establishing trust through sympathy and patience are "the main 'weapons' with which the satyagrahi transforms his opponent and alters the nature of the conflict relationship. From mistrust and enmity, the relationship evolves to trust, respect and cooperation," and an enemy becomes an ally.[54] Today this is called conflict resolution where everybody wins.

But what is a righteous cause? According to Gandhi, it is a cause with the power of Truth behind it, and this Truth can only be known by the systematic reduction of self-interest. "Reduce yourself to zero," he used to say.[55] The reduction of self-will is the discipline necessary to know Truth. Without this discipline, the search for Truth becomes "impure, unethical" and can lead to "self-righteousness, arrogance, and tyranny."[56] I'm reminded of Professor Embler (Chapter 3) who said that self-interest can so distort our judgments that we can prefer the "monstrous to the beautiful and good."

That small group of "vaccine-touting" doctors who managed to get the compulsory vaccination laws passed probably had no idea that this violation of the most fundamental of human rights—the right to have control over what is put into our bodies—would open the door to other related and, if possible, even more monstrous violations. I refer to the systematic warping of the human mind by insistent, persistent media blitzes promoting a single idea, one that brooks no discussion, no critical inquiry, no serious questioning—one that demands that we all line up and march to the same drummer.

"Today, a massive nationwide public misinformation campaign led by the federal government is underway to convince the American public that vaccines are totally safe and effective, do not cause death or injury, and must be used by everyone in order to protect the public health," Barbara Loe Fisher tells us. "Led by the federal government with the enthusiastic cooperation of the drug companies and physician organizations, there is a concerted effort to hide the truth about vaccine risks and convince state legislators to pass oppressive mandatory vaccination laws to force all children to be vaccinated with each new vaccine the drug companies produce."[57]

Did you know that parents are being charged with child neglect for failing to vaccinate their children with all federally recommended vaccines? Did you know that in Wisconsin the Milwaukee Public Schools, the City Health Department, and the district attorney joined forces and announced that parents who refuse to vaccinate their children will be fined $25 per day until the children are vaccinated? Did you know that in this same state immunization courts are being set up to handle prosecution of parents for noncompliance on the grounds that those who remain unvaccinated threaten public health?[58]

Is this America where the most fundamental human right, the right to refuse to be injected with foreign substances that have the potential for long-term damage and even death, shouldn't have to be debated or fought for? Or is this a bad dream of the Salem witchcraft trials where intolerance and stupidity sat in the seats of power?

But, as Barbara Loe Fisher points out, those who profit from the violation of this most basic human right have become very wealthy and politically powerful.[59] And, I would add, the tentacles of this self-interest extend into every organization within the Medical Industrial Complex, for example, the American Medical Association (AMA), the American Academy of Pediatrics (AAP), the federal Centers for Disease Control (CDC), the Food and Drug Administration (FDA), and the World Health Organization (WHO). Self-interest has indeed, in Professor Embler's words, "changed the face of reality altogether" so that each of us is inherently dangerous to each other, a source of disease and infection. We must be decontaminated by being injected with toxic material to make us less toxic to each other. If some of us die or are seriously injured, we are merely good soldiers who must be sacrificed in the line of duty for the public good. We have indeed embraced the monstrous over the beautiful and good.

I hope you're as outraged as I am at this betrayal of the public trust by our government leaders. I hope you're as outraged as I am at our complacency which has allowed this to happen. These perverted herd immunity theories were introduced back in 1962 in the congressional hearings referred to in Chapter 3, as was evidence of a possible connection between the SV–40 virus, found in both the Salk and Sabin vaccines, and cancer.[60] (See Chapters 3 and 8.)

But ultimately we have no one but ourselves to blame. Our ready gullibility and need to blame something or someone—for example, a virus, a "carrier" of contagion—for our misfortunes has made us easy pawns. Yes, we have lacked vigilance in protecting the liberties our founding fathers fought so hard for. But we have also lacked a discriminating and enquiring mind.

For instance, I heard on the radio (September 2, 1994, WHRV-FM): "Federal health officials are blaming 247 cases of measles in 10 states on one of 25,000 skiers who spent spring break at a Colorado resort." The broadcast went on to say that the Centers for Disease Control in Atlanta said the unidentified skier (source of contagion) was probably free of symptoms and that most of the victims were unvaccinated high school or college students. The skier passed the disease to 5 others, including a girl "whose family follows Christian Science, a religion that shuns medical care, including inoculations." She started an outbreak that infected 51 people in her hometown and 156 people at her boarding school. "The outbreak eventually spread to 7 other states as vacationing skiers returning home infected family and friends who were not vaccinated."

Now, the unvaccinated are not only at risk themselves, but are a danger to others, and even unidentified, symptom-free persons can be blamed for spreading disease. Thus, a relatively mild disease (for healthy persons) is cast into the den of ignominy and vaccine failure becomes invisible.

I'm reminded of something Hermann Goering, one of the Nazi leaders, said at the Nuremberg Trials: "Voice or no voice, the people can always be brought to the bidding of the leaders. That is easy. All you have to do is tell them they are being attacked and denounce the pacifists for lack of patriotism and exposing the country to danger. It works the same in any country."[61] Now let's reword the next to last sentence to read: All you have to do is tell them they are being attacked by disease and blame the unvaccinated for exposing the country to danger.

And we thought it couldn't happen here! Or is it our witchcraft heritage resurfacing?

Did you know that the much-tougher National Vaccine Initiative in our country is "part of a worldwide vaccine initiative being underwritten by the largest banks in the world, including the World Bank?"[62] Did you know that there is a global infrastructure being set up wherein the United States will serve as a leader and the mass, mandatory vaccination program here will serve as the prototype for the rest of the countries? And who is leading this effort? Besides the U.S. federal health agencies, this initiative is being led by physicians in the WHO, UNICEF (recently changed to UNCF—United Nations Children's Fund), and UNDP (United Nations Development Program) and is being underwritten by the Rockefeller Foundation, the World Bank, and the world's major pharmaceutical companies.[63]

And what about adults? Did you think they were exempt from this physiological assault? According to Fisher, "There are indications that there is a plan to eventually force adults in the U.S. to be vaccinated with government-recommended vaccines and use economic sanctions to enforce vaccination, including making it impossible to attend college, get health insurance, file your income taxes or get a job if you cannot show proof you have been a good citizen and have received all the recommended vaccines."[64] This has already been adumbrated in the recommended adult immunization schedule and the poster advertising "Shots Are Not Just for Kids" mentioned in the preface of this book.

And how is such a mass manipulation and control system going to be implemented? It has already been implemented to a 95 percent–plus degree in the childhood vaccination programs;[65] but the national vaccination computer tracking system that is being set up to enforce childhood vaccinations will help close the few breathing spaces people have left. "This national vaccination tracking system could eventually be linked up with an international vaccination tracking system,"[66] which is one reason we need an international organization to protect people from this massive assault on human rights. But, first, we must succeed at home.

If our task seems overwhelming, even intimidating, we must remember that the power of truth and love, which Gandhi called soul or truth force, is on our side, and evil, which is related to manipulation and control of others, eventually overreaches itself and becomes an ally. When adults begin to realize that they, too, will be caught in the vaccination net, they will begin to question. It is already happening as more and more people are becoming informed. Recent reports of serious symptoms—for example, pains, nausea, hair loss, tumors, memory loss—suffered by thousands of Gulf War veterans given an experimental oral vaccine to prevent anthrax and nerve gas poisoning[67] are accelerating public awareness of the dangers of vaccines. What about a possible AIDS vaccine and mandatory AIDS vaccinations? This, I think, will be the turning point, but I hope it will happen long before this as more people not only become informed but open themselves to other approaches. But most important, there is a new spiritual awakening in our country, a new consciousness of the essential divinity of the human person and the importance of mind and spirit being supportive of a treatment in order for it to be effective.

But to the vaccine machine, human beings are ciphers, objects to be manipulated and controlled. Did you know that this reduction of human beings to something less than fully human is akin to the assumptions undergirding the politics of the ancient world and, in particular, the Middle Ages? To those in power, the average man was naturally foolish and needed to be watched, controlled, regimented, and scared half out of his wits or he would get into mischief and damage himself or other people in some way.[68] Did you know that our Constitution assumes exactly the opposite? It assumes the average man is to be trusted, not only with the formation of his own opinions but with a disposition to self-reliance, responsibility, resourcefulness, self-determination, and sensible

compromise where there can't be complete agreement. Did you know that our
system of government, which is based on the existence of a vital spiritual presence in its citizens, is, as far as I know, without precedence in recorded history?[69]
The onslaught of the vaccine machine is one of the pivotal tests of whether this
noble experiment will succeed or fail.

I hope the discussions, here and elsewhere in this book, of the spiritual and
political as well as medical dimensions of the vaccination issue have aroused in
you some sense of outrage and that you and I together can conserve our anger,
as Gandhi did, and transmute it into soul or truth force. Gandhi said it best:
"As heat conserved is transmuted into energy . . . anger controlled can be transmuted into a power which can move the world."[70]

NOTES

1. Harris L. Coulter, *Vaccination, Social Violence and Criminality* (Berkeley, CA:
North Atlantic Books, 1990), p. 262. Information about vaccination laws in Germany are
from Brandt Schenkel, *International Vaccination Newsletter*, December 1993, p. 16.

2. Bonnie K. Miller and Clinton Ray Miller, "Personal Religious Beliefs Are Constitutional Protection Against Compulsory Immunizations," *Health Freedom News*, July–
August 1989, pp. 35–41.

3. Ibid., pp. 31–32.

4. Ibid., p 35.

5. Carol Horowitz, "Immunizations and Informed Consent," *Mothering*, winter
1983, p. 38.

6. Thomas Finn, *Dangers of Compulsory Immunizations, How to Avoid Them Legally*
(New Port Richey, FL: Family Fitness Press, 1983), p. 39.

7. *How to Legally Avoid Unwanted Immunizations of All Kinds* (Quakertown, PA:
Humanitarian), p. 5.

8. Clinton R. Miller, "Your Right to Refuse Immunization in International Travel,"
National Health Federation Bulletin, July–August 1968, pp. 13–16.

9. C. David Finley, *Decisions on Death and Dying,* Chautauqua Lectures, WHRV-
FM, March 22. 1993.

10. Thomas G. Finn, "How to Avoid Compulsory Immunizations," *Vegetarian
Times/Well-Being*, no. 48, 1981, p. 77.

11. Richard Moskowitz, "Vaccination: A Sacrament of Modern Medicine" (speech
given at the Annual Conference of the Society of Homeopaths, Manchester, England,
September 1991); cited by Neil Z. Miller in *Vaccines: Are They Really Safe and Effective?* (Santa Fe, NM: New Atlantean Press, 1992), p. 70.

12. W. R. Hadwen, "The Vaccination Delusion" (a public lecture given on May 1,
1902, and later published by the National Anti-Vaccination League, Strand, W.C., England, 1912), p. 18.

13. Viera Scheibner, *Vaccination: The Medical Assault on the Immune System* (Maryborough, Victoria, Australia: Australian Print Group, 1993), chap. 9.

14. Hadwen, "The Vaccination Delusion," p. 16.

15. Jay Stuller, "Cleanliness Has Only Recently Become a Virtue," *Smithsonian*,
February 1991, p. 133.

16. Ibid., p. 127.

17. Ibid. These attitudes and proscriptions against bathing had their genesis in the excesses of the public baths in Rome. Beginning as a hygienic and social ritual wherein the body was steamed, rubbed, annointed with fine oils, and plunged into cool and refreshing water, the baths eventually became hotbeds of promiscuity and vice, some being adjuncts to brothels. The early church fathers equated bodily cleanliness with the materialism, paganism, and what has been called "the monstrous sensualities of Rome" (p. 130).

18. Basil O'Connor, president of the National Foundation for Infantile Paralysis, cited by Ernest B. Zeisler, "The Great Salk Vaccine Fiasco," *Minority of One,* June 1960: reprinted by *Herald of Health,* December 1960. Dr. Zeisler, a private practitioner, scholar, and clinical associate professor of medicine at the Chicago Medical School who contributed many articles to medical journals, said that "no newspaper, periodical or medical journal" would "touch this article."

19. M. Beddow Bayly, quoted by Leon Chaitow, *Vaccination and Immunization: Dangers, Delusions and Alternatives* (Essex, England: C. W. Daniel Company Limited, 1987), p. 40. Also reported by Eleanora McBean, *The Poisoned Needle* (Mokelumne Hill, CA: Health Research, 1956), p. 102. McBean reprints an entire paragraph from the *News Chronicle* from which I quoted.

20. Dr. Bayly goes on to say that the report also included 149 cases and 6 deaths among contact persons.

21. Zeisler, "The Great Salk Vaccine Fiasco."

22. Ibid.

23. Ibid.

24. *Time,* June 20, 1955; cited by McBean, *The Poisoned Needle,* p. 102.

25. Viera Scheibner, "Is There Such a Thing as Vaccine-preventable diseases?" *International Vaccination Newsletter* (Belgium), December 1993.

26. McBean, *The Poisoned Needle.*

27. *Journal of the American Medical Association,* December 25, 1958; cited by Zeisler, "The Great Salk Vaccine Fiasco."

28. Ibid.

29. Ibid.

30. *Chicago Tribune,* May 24, 1959; cited in ibid.

31. A. D. Langmuir, "Progress in Conquest of Paralytic Poliomyelitis," *Journal of the American Medical Association* 171 (1959): 271; cited by Zeisler, "The Great Salk Vaccine Fiasco."

32. Louis LaVine, "Infantile Paralysis Can Be Prevented," *Scientific Chiropractor,* June–July 1942.

33. "California Compulsory Polio Immunization Bill," *National Health Federation Bulletin,* May 1961. Some of the doctors cited by Don Matchen were Ralph R. Scoby, *Archives of Pediatrics*; J. E. R. McDonagh, *The Universe Through Medicine*; Joseph Melnick, *Tidskrift for Halsa* (Danish medical publication); and journalist John A. Toomey, *Science.* Other doctors cited who believed polio was essentially a nutritional disease included W. J. McCormack, Toronto; J. F. Edwards, Manitoba; C. W. Jungeblut, Columbia University; William Albrecht, University of Missouri; and Virgil A. Davis and M. H. August, New York City.

34. Scheibner, *Vaccination,* pp. 147–148. Also Chapter 7 of Scheibner's book on the polio vaccines indirectly suggests the endogenous origin of polio.

35. Scheibner, "Is There Such a Thing," p. 4

36. Anne Herbert, "Gandhi on Non-Violence," *Essential Whole Earth Catalog*, 1986.

37. Eknath Easwaran, *Gandhi, the Man* (Petaluma, CA: Nilgiri Press, 1983).

38. Ibid, p. 150.

39. Robert William Krajenke, *The Psychic Side of the American Dream* (Virginia Beach: A.R.E. Press, 1976), p. 12.

40. Shirley Nicholson, *Ancient Wisdom—Modern Insight* (Wheaton, IL: Theosophical Publishing House, 1985), p. 121.

41. "A.R.E. Members Head American Holistic Medical Association," *A.R.E. News*, August 1978, pp. 1–3.

42. Lawrence D. Wilson, "Healing the Health Care System," *Health Freedom News*, August 1993, p. 17.

43. Ibid.

44. Kristine M. Severyn, "Ohio Parents for Vaccine Safety," Autumn 1993, p. 2.

45. CBS News, September 27, 1988 (the 22 million figure), and People for the Ethical Treatment of Animals (PETA), *Animal Liberation*, 1993 (the 60–100 million figure).

46. Easwaran, *Gandhi, the Man*, p. 76.

47. "Genetically Altered Food May Serve as Vaccines," *Los Angeles Times* (San Diego); reprinted in the *Virginian-Pilot/Ledger-Star*, November 25, 1993.

48. Melissa Gregory, editor, "Bill Signed for Chiropractors in Military But No Action Taken," *Navy News*, December 23 and 30, 1992.

49. Robert S. Mendelsohn, *The Risks of Immunizations and How to Avoid Them* (Evanston, IL: The People's Doctor Newsletter, 1988), p. 90. This "small group of vaccine-touting doctors" succeeded because "a much larger group of doctors who were uninformed about and often indifferent to vaccines insured passage of these laws by their own inaction," Dr. Mendelsohn tells us. He goes on to say that "only a handful of doctors spoke out against mandatory immunizations."

50. *New England Journal of Medicine*, Spring 1992; cited by Bill Moyers in an interview with Studs Terkel on *Studs Terkel's Almanac*, WHRV-FM, August 12, 1993.

51. Stephanie D. Story, "Alternative Medicine/Naturopathic Medicine," *Dimensions*, March 1994, p. 9.

52. Associated Press, Washington, "Link Is Possible Between Shots and Brain Damage." *Virginian Pilot/Ledger-Star*, March 1994. (A friend gave me the article, but the date and name of the paper were torn off. He gave me the month and said it was the local paper.)

53. Edgar Cayce, "Mental Telepathy" (talk given in Virginia Beach, February 15, 1931); reprinted in *The Searchlight*, January 1962.

54. Easwaran, *Gandhi, the Man*, p. 163.

55. Ibid., p. 151.

56. Ibid.

57. Barbara Loe Fisher, "Vaccination and Public Health," *International Chiropractic Pediatric Association* (Atlanta, GA), March 1994.

58. Ibid.

59. Ibid.

60. House Committee on Interstate and Foreign Commerce, *Hearings on H.R. 10541*, 87th Cong., 2nd sess., May 15 and 16, 1962, pp. 84, 116, 120.

61. Quoted by Peace Pilrim, *Her Life and Work in Her Own Words* (Santa Fe, NM: Ocean Tree Book, 1982), pp. 114–115.

62. Interview with Barbara Loe Fisher, *International Vaccination Newsletter* (Genk, Belgium), December 1993.

63. Ibid.

64. Interview with Barbara Loe Fisher, *International Vaccination Newsletter* (Genk, Belgium), March 1994, p. 7.

65. Centers for Disease Control; cited by *Washington Post*; reprinted in *Health Freedom News*, August 1993, p. 7. Figure doesn't include the two newest vaccines.

66. Interview with Barbara Loe Fisher, March 1994, p. 7.

67. WHRV-FM, May 6 and 7, 1994; WNIS-AM, May 6, 1994.

68. Emmet Fox, *The American Spirit*; cited by Robert William Krajenke, *The Psychic Side of the American Dream* (Virginia Beach, VA: A.R.E. Press, 1976), p. 13.

69. Krajenke, *The Psychic Side*, p. 14. Some of these concepts are taken from Thomas Jefferson and Emmett Fox, which are cited by the author.

70. Easwaran, *Gandhi, the Man*, p. 74.

Appendixes

A. Keys to a Healthy Immune System (A Holistic Approach)

I. Physical

A. Keep the body alkaline by:

1. Eating plenty of fresh fruits and vegetables. For most people the proportion should be 80 percent alkaline-forming food to 20 percent acid-forming food. In general, fresh fruits and vegetables are alkaline forming, and starches and proteins are acid forming. The more physically active a person is, the more acid-forming foods his body can handle.

2. Eating only whole, natural foods. As much as possible, eat food that is fresh, in season, organically and locally grown. Eat most food raw or slightly steamed with an emphasis on green leafy vegetables.[1]

3. Chewing food well; saliva alkalinizes food.

4. Eating whole grains that have been germinated. Germination makes them more alkaline, easier to digest, and increases protein and enzyme content.

5. Keeping eliminative organs working well and periodically going on short cleansing regimes.[2]

6. Getting adequate rest, exercise, pure water, and fresh air.

B. Avoid:

1. Refined sugar.

2. Refined, chemicalized, stale, and overcooked food.

3. Poisons such as drugs, vaccines, insecticides, Xrays, and radioactivity.

4. And, of course, coffee, tobacco, and alcohol.

C. Take supplements as needed. The following nutrients specifically support the immune system:

1. Vitamins C, A, E, and the B complex.

2. Minerals zinc, calcium, magnesium, iodine, iron, and selenium.

3. Herbs such as garlic, alfalfa, echinacea, yarrow, gingerroot, cayenne, and taheebo.[3]

4. Lemons, acidophilus culture (for colon).

For more information on dosage and preparation of herbs, see the following references:

Airola, Paavo. *Everywoman's Book.* Phoenix, AZ: Health Plus, 1979.

Christopher, John. *Childhood Diseases.* Springville, VT: Christopher Publications, 1978.

Kloss, Jethro. *Back to Eden.* Coalmont, TN: Longview Publishing House, 1950.

Sultanoff, Barry. "How to Strengthen Your Immune System." *East West Journal,* 1986.

II. Mental

A. Practice:

1. Moderation: Do nothing in excess.

2. Positive thinking: Give energy to the desired condition.

3. Open-mindedness: Believe you can have the desired condition.

4. Visualization: See the desired condition.

5. Balanced living: Balance physical, mental, social, and spiritual activities.

B. Avoid:

1. Reacting negatively or stressfully to a situation.

III. Spiritual

A. Practice:

1. Seeing yourself as part of an "unbroken wholeness" in which every part supports every other part.

2. Seeing the universe as harmonious and life affirming.

3. Seeing your body as an energy field, an extension of your consciousness that responds to your thoughts and feelings.

4. "Centering" and getting in touch with your transpersonal self and its life-affirming energies.

NOTES

1. Some writers and therapists, such as those of the macrobiotic and Natural Hygiene school of thought, maintain that childhood diseases can be avoided by eliminating dairy products (in the context of a health-promoting lifestyle, of course). I suspect that it isn't the elimination of dairy products per se that produces results but the elimination of adulterated dairy products—pasteurized, homogenized, chemicalized—that are consumed.

2. A cleansing regime consists of certain dietary restrictions along with bowel cleansing, exercise, rest, pure water, and fresh air. The dietary restrictions consist primarily of eliminating concentrated proteins and starches and living on fresh fruits and vegetables and/or their juices. The duration is usually from 1 to 11 days.

3. Special mention should be made of the remarkable herb pau d'arco, or taheebo, from the bark of a South American tree. Unlike most medicinal herbs, taheebo is eminently palatable. A delicious tea that can be given to children is made by simmering the bark and adding a little peppermint tea and/or honey.

B. Some Natural Remedies for Children's Ailments

The following information was obtained from a local nurse-midwife who has worked for two pediatricians who used nutritional therapy. By following these "rules," she told me, her own children have never been ill for more than one day.

Rule No. 1: If child is sick, take him off dairy and flour products. Of course, nothing made with white sugar is ever permissible.

Rule No. 2: Give child large doses of vitamin C with pantothenic acid and calcium.

Rule No. 3: Keep the bowels open with either an enema or an herbal bowel cleanser such as Herb-Lax.

Rule No. 4: If possible, fast the child and give him or her herb teas such as camomile, catnip, fennel, and peppermint.

For a sick child in general: Diet of green beans, celery, zucchini (Bieler broth). Broth is made by steaming the above vegetables and liquefying them.

For diarrhea: Brown rice and steamed carrots. For small child, liquefy.

For colds: Fasting and vitiman C—1,000 milligrams of vitamin C for every year up to age 10. The addition of pantothenic acid makes this therapy even more effective. If the child is very young and whines for food, give him or her some fresh fruit.

For general mucous conditions such as earache, bronchitis, and sinus: Give child fresh fruits and vegetables, chicken,[1] and peanut butter. (Can fill celery sticks with peanut butter.) No dairy products and no flour products.

To these general remedies herbalists might add lemon, garlic, capsicum, alfalfa, and high doses of vitamins A and C for both prevention and treatment of infectious diseases. Besides the books mentioned in Appendix A, there are a number of excellent books outlining naturopathic and herbal remedies for specific ailments. Here are some we have found particularly helpful:

Bieler, Henry G. *Food Is Your Best Medicine*. New York: Random House, 1969.[2]

Tenney, Louise. *Today's Herbal Health*. Provo, UT: Woodland Books, 1983.

Tierra, Michael. *The Way of Herbs*. Santa Cruz, CA: Unity Press, 1980.

Nothing said here, of course, is meant to substitute for consultation with a healthcare professional who is knowledgeable in natural methods of healing.

NOTES

1. Because commercial chicken is so polluted and the chickens are treated so inhumanely, I would substitute vegetable proteins such as lentils, tempe, tofu, seeds, and nuts for chicken.

2. More recent books include Janet Zand, *Smart Medicine for a Healthier Child* (Garden City Park, NY: Avery Publishing Group, 1992), available from New Leaf or your bookstore, and Stan Malstrom, *Natural Treatment for Childhood Diseases*, available from Economy Herbs, Box 587, Melbourne, AZ 72556.

C. What You Can Do for a Vaccine-Injured Child

First, don't accept the idea that the injury is permanent or irreparable. There is help even for the severely neurologically damaged. To grasp these therapies, one must move in consciousness to think in terms of subtle or soul energies rather than purely physical manifestations and biochemical equations. I've read about, as well as known personally, many cases where the energies of mind and spirit have regenerated destroyed tissue. To access these energies to heal and regenerate the physical body, the following organizations and resources can be helpful:

1. *ARE (Association for Research and Enlightenment; 67th Street and Atlantic Avenue, P. O. Box 595, Virginia Beach, VA 23451; [800] 428–3588 or [800] 333–4499).* This organization was founded to research, study, and apply the spiritual principles found in the Edgar Cayce "readings" (psychic dissertations given by the late Edgar Cayce when he was in a self-induced altered state of consciousness). The ARE also makes available and works with material from other sources that work through the same principles. A central tenet of the Cayce readings is that spirit is the life force, mind is the builder (creates from the energies of spirit), and the physical is the result. The causal level, therefore, is spirit working through mind. This level must be accessed before real healing can take place. Some of the modalities used are prayer and meditation, presleep suggestion, castor oil packs, wet cell appliance, spinal adjustments, massage, colonics, diet, deep breathing, getting close to nature, and working with dreams, cycles, and spiritual ideals. Two medical clinics that work with the Cayce principles are: (1) ARE Clinic in Phoenix, AZ; (602) 955–1551, and (2) Scottsdale Holistic Medical Group; (602) 990–1528.

2. *Signature Sound Works (Colorado office: P. O. Box 12184, Denver, CO 80212–0184. [303] 458–6072. Ohio office: P. O. Box 706, Athens, OH 45701; [614] 698–7117).*

This organization was founded to research and apply the healing principles discovered by Sharry Edwards, who not only could hear beyond the range of "normal" hearing but could vocally produce pure tones,—sine waves that she discovered produced remarkable healing in cases of injury, disease, poisoning, and mental retardation. The work of Sharry Edwards has been the subject of five books, a 10-part TV series, and two documentaries. Besides researching in her own facility, Dimensional Resources, she teaches parapsychology at Blue Ridge Community College in Virginia and is working on her doctorate.

3. *Barbara Brennan School of Healing (P. O. Box 2005, East Hampton, NY 11937; [516] 329–0951).* As a former NASA (National Aeronautics and Space Administration) scientist and author of the best-selling *Hands of Light*, Barbara Ann Brennan is "gifted" with clairvoyant sight that enables her to have "internal vision" and see the human energy field or aura. She observed that various colors and patterns in the aura corresponded to different physiologic and psychologic states and learned to work with these energy fields to heal people. One of her therapies, bioenergotherapy, is particularly effective for nervous system disorders.

4. *The Synergy Company (83 Bailey Lane, Box 2901, CVSR, Moab, UT 84532; [801] 259–5366).* This company was founded by Mitchell May, who in 1972 was so severely injured in an automobile accident that it took rescuers 45 minutes to free him from the wreckage and left him with many critical injuries. His legs sustained over 40 fractures, as well as severe nerve and muscle damage. Doctors insisted he would never walk again and, in fact, wanted to amputate his legs. He refused and, with the help of a psychic healer from the parapsychology department of UCLA, began his own healing program, eventually regenerating nerve, bone, and muscle and making medical history. Today, Mitchell racewalks, backpacks, and hikes in the canyons near his home. He teaches healing and has developed a food supplement, Pure Synergy, made from completely natural substances, whose purpose is to foster chi, the life energy.

5. *Physicians Association of Anthroposophic Medicine (P. O. Box 269, Kimberton, PA 19442).* Works with the spiritual aspects of the patient and the meaning of the disease process. Supports healing with homeopathic remedies.

Other energy-based therapies:

6. *Homeopathy.* Homeopaths can give nosodes, highly dilute vaccine or disease products, and other homeopathic remedies for vaccine injuries. Some homeopaths, I have been told, specialize in vaccine injuries. For a homeopath nearest you, you may want to contact the National Center for Homeopathy, 1500 Massachusetts Avenue N.W., Suite 41, Washington D.C. 20005.

7. *Other energy-based therapies.* These include acupressure, acupuncture, polarity therapy, radionics, Reiki treatments, massage therapy, music therapy, and chiropractic and osteopathic adjustments.

8. *Other natural therapies.* I have heard of remarkable improvements in neurologically damaged children by the use of hydro- and nutritional therapies—for example, colonics; cleansing diets; whole foods, preferably organically grown; and food and herbal supplements. Also movement therapies such as repatterning and yoga—stretching and deep breathing. Getting close to nature such as gardening and walking in the woods and on the seashore can also be helpful.

D.   Instead of Sugar

Because refined sugar consumption weakens the immune system and has been implicated in a number of serious diseases such as cancer and mental illness,[1] we should replace this nonfood with real food. A ''sweet tooth'' is generally indicative of a vitamin B deficiency; the craving for sweets usually disappears when adequate amounts of a natural source of vitamin B complex, such as nutritional yeast, are taken. Nature provides an abundance of fruits to satisfy our need for sweets, so when we need a sweetener or something ''sweet,'' why not try the following:

FRUITS AND FRUIT CONCENTRATES

Fruit concentrates using fruits such as pear, pineapple, grape, and peach juices are now being used by a number of producers of natural foods to sweeten drinks, cookies, cereals, candy bars, and even chocolate sauce. In our family, we usually use apple juice as a sweetener for lemonade and for the iced herbal teas we drink in the summer. We use about two thirds tea and one third apple juice. Mint, lemon grass, and wintergreen are particularly refreshing with apple juice.

For popsicles, dissolve 1 tablespoon of gelatin in a scant ¼ cup cold water. When softened, add about ¼ cup boiling water and stir until dissolved. Add this mixture to about 1½ pints of unsweetened fruit juice such as pineapple, orange, or grape. Mix in a blender, pour into popsicle molds, and put in freezer.

Fruit juice–sweetened syrups are available and make delicious toppings for cereals, pancakes, and ice cream. Date sugar made of dehydrated, pulverized dates makes a good sweetener for baking, as do raisins and currents. These more concentrated sweeteners should generally be used in colder weather when we need more concentrated foods.

GRAIN SWEETENERS

Although expensive, barley malt, rice syrup, and amazake are composed largely of maltose, which is released into the blood more slowly than the sugars of other natural sweeteners, which are largely sucrose and fructose. This slower release time helps to stabilize the blood sugar.

MAPLE SYRUP AND BLACKSTRAP MOLASSES

Maple syrup is regarded by many as the premier, gourmet sweetener among natural sweeteners. Although less processed and more expensive than blackstrap molasses, it, like blackstrap, does require boiling to produce. Unlike the grain sweeteners, these both have a strong flavor that can limit their use.[2]

HONEY

Of all natural sweeteners, other than fruit, honey—natural, raw, unheated, unfiltered, unprocessed—is the only one that could be called a medicinal food. Pollen-rich honey, Dr. Airola tells us, (1) increases calcium retention; (2) increases hemoglobin count, thus preventing or curing nutritional anemia; (3) is beneficial in kidney and liver disorders, colds, poor circulation, and complexion disorders; (4) has a beneficial effect on healing processes in such conditions as arthritis, constipation, poor circulation, weak heart, and insomnia; and (5) retards aging. In one study of longevity, Russian biologist Dr. Nicolai Tsitsin found that a large number of centenarians were bee keepers, and all of the centenarians, without exception, said their principal food was honey![3]

So we see that $sugar_1$ is not the same as $sugar_2$ which is not the same as $sugar_3$, and so on. Table 7 comparing the differences in the way our bodies handle refined white table sugar and unrefined, raw, unfiltered honey illustrates this point. We could even construct a table comparing different natural honeys. Generally, the darker the honey, the richer it is in minerals.

To substitute honey for sugar in cooking, use ¾ cup honey for every cup of sugar and reduce other liquid ingredients by ⅕. Ice cream is probably the easiest dessert to make with honey. Use the same recipe as for making popsicles except use top milk (unhomogenized, of course) instead of fruit juice and from ⅓ to ½ cup of honey and 2 teaspoons of vanilla. For chocolate ice cream, I use carob powder, and for fruit and nut flavors, I use natural fruits and nut flavors. To make the ice cream richer, I add several tablespoons of skim milk powder (noninstant). My daughter, Ingri, makes a delicious ice cream using lecithin granules instead of gelatin. Her recipe is this:

In a blender, mix in order the following: 2 eggs, 1 cup cream, 3 heaping tablespoons lecithin granules, 2 teaspoons pure vanilla, ½ cup honey, 1 cup cream. To make a full quart, add a bit more milk-cream and pour into freezing trays. When frozen, cut mixture into strips and homogenize in the Champion Juicer. Serve with ground almonds. To make the ice cream less mucus forming and to give it a delicious maple flavor, add 3 tablespoonful of slippery elm powder and eliminate the eggs (I use 1 egg).

Because obtaining quality milk and cream—unpasteurized and unhomogenized—is for most people in the United States very difficult, if not impossible, many health-minded consumers are substituting nut and seed milks. We make a delicious ice cream using

TABLE 7. COMPARATIVE NUTRITIONAL VALUES OF SUGAR AND HONEY

SUGAR*	HONEY**
acid reacting	alkaline reacting
supports bacterial growth	kills bacteria
oxidizes or burns intensely in the body, producing a shock effect on the nervous system and vital organs	gradual and even absorption by the body
intense stimulation followed by a slump	no letdown
addictive	contains built-in satiety factor, self-limiting
druglike effect	food
empty calories—leeches vitamins and minerals (particularly calcium and vitamin B_1) from the tissues to metabolize itself	contains vitamins, enzymes, minerals, utilized by the body as a food
primary cause of many diseases such as poliomyelitis, diabetes, arthritis, heart disease, ulcers	has been used to prevent and treat certain diseases such as polio, diabetes, arthritis
stimulating	relaxing and mildly sedative
contributes to constipation	mildly laxative
forms toxic metabolites such as pyruvic acid and abnormal sugars containing 5 carbon atoms which interfere with cell respiration in the brain, blood, and nervous system.	burns clean— no toxic metabolic residue

*Sugar refers to refined, white, table sugar (sucrose).
**Honey refers to raw, unfiltered, unpolluted (no chemical additives) honey.

Sources: William Dufty, *Sugar Blues* (New York: Warner Books, 1975).
Bodog F. Beck, *Honey and Your Health* (New York: Bantam Books, 1971).
John Yudkin, *Sweet and Dangerous* (New York: Bantam Books, 1973).
Benjamin P. Sandler, *Diet Prevents Polio* (Milwaukee, Wisconsin: The Lee Foundation for Nutritional Research, 1951).
D.C. Jarvis, "The Use of Honey in the Prevention of Polio," *American Bee Journal*, August 1951, pp. 336-337.

sesame seed milk. To a quart of sesame seed milk, add about 3 heaping tablespoons of lecithin granules, 2 teaspoons vanilla, and about ½ cup honey. Blend in liquefier. Pour in ice tray and place in freezer. When frozen, put cubes through the Champion Juicer. To store, put in plastic containers and place in freezer.

To make nut or seed milks, simply blend in liquefier about ¼ cup raw nuts or seeds— almonds, sesame, cashews—with 1 cup of water and add 1 or 2 tablespoons of honey or maple syrup. Blend until smooth—usually three or four minutes at high speed. To make milk richer, increase quantity of nuts or seeds. To make milk smoother, strain through a cheesecloth or fine strainer. Also soaking nuts or seeds overnight and/or grinding them in a grinder before liquefying helps to make the milk smoother and easier to liquefy. The skins of almonds can easily be pulled off after they have been soaked overnight, thereby producing a sweeter, whiter milk. (Hulled sesame seeds also produce a sweeter, whiter milk.) To blanche almonds before soaking them, simply boil water and immerse the almonds in it for 30 seconds. The skins will come off easily.

Sometimes we use apple juice as a sweetener, so we substitute ½ of the water with ½ apple juice. We also like a richer milk, so we use ½ cup seeds or nuts to 1½ cups liquid. Double this recipe for a quart of ice cream and liquefy about 8 or 10 minutes.

Flavors, of course, can be varied. For almond or lemon flavor, add 2 teaspoon almond or lemon extract. Different fruits and fruit juices such as banana or pineapple can be added. With a little imagination, you can make a variety of delicious, non-mucous-forming ice cream.

To make malts, put cubes of frozen ice cream mixture in a blender with enough milk to cover blades. Blend and eat. If the cubes are vanilla flavored, you can add carob or fruit to the milk to vary the flavor.

Here is our favorite cookie recipe, excellent for cold weather and so simple my 7-year-old grandson can practically make these cookies himself: In a fairly large bowl, mix the following ingredients: ⅔ cup oil (cold pressed—we use safflower, soy, or olive oil), ⅔ cup honey, 1 egg, 2 teaspoons lemon flavoring, ½ teaspoon cinnamon, ¼ cup whole wheat flour, ½ cup *fresh* wheat germ or a mixture of soy flour, bran and protein powder, 1 teaspoon salt, 3 cups oatmeal, 1 cup sunflower seeds, 1 cup raisins. If batter is too dry, add a bit of water. Drop by teaspoons onto greased cookie sheets and bake at 325° for 15 to 20 minutes.

Making candy with honey is simplicity itself. The basic recipe is this: Mix together equal parts of honey, nut butter, milk or protein powder (noninstant), nuts, and seeds. Roll in wax paper, put in freezer, and slice when frozen; or press into flat buttered trays, put in refrigerator, and cut into squares. Here is my daughter's favorite candy, which she calls "Super Fudge": Use equal parts of honey, peanut butter (smooth), and carob powder. Add chopped walnuts and/or sunflower seeds and enough shredded coconut (unsweetened) to make a thick consistency. Either roll in wax paper, put in freezer, and slice when frozen, or shape into balls, roll in coconut, and put in refrigerator.

MENTAL IMAGERY

Ever tried cutting carrots crosswise and calling them carrot cookies? Or slicing apples crosswise, coring them, and calling them apple doughnuts? Or cutting celery into three-inch pieces, filling the groove with peanut butter, and calling them celery boats? A little imagination can turn an ordinary vegetable into a gourmet adventure. It can even turn a disaster into a triumph. My daughter once made a supercake with all natural ingredients. It didn't rise. She forgot the baking powder. We called it rock cake and ate every "chip."

The suggestions here are just a few of the ways you can transform health-destroying sugar addiction into conscious choices that support health.

CAVEAT

Because refined sugar is bad, don't make the mistake of thinking chemical sweeteners are better. Did you know that the chemical sweetener aspartame—commercially known as NutraSweet and Equal—has been associated with depression, anxiety attacks, hearing loss, ringing in the ears, slurred speech, blurred vision, numbness in the extremities, breathing difficulties, seizures and dizziness, memory loss, coma, blindness, and death? These are just some of the most severe symptoms reported by the FDA as of April 3, 1989. This report is based on 4,915 aspartame complaints totaling 73 symptoms.[4]

Did you know that, like drugs and the chemicals from pesticides, cigarettes, and alcohol, artificial sweeteners have to be detoxified by the liver?[5] One study linked myasthenia gravis (fatigue, exhaustion of muscular system, and progressive paralysis of muscles) to artificial sweetners.[6]

Moral: Natural is best.

NOTES

1. A number of researchers and books have pointed out the deleterious effects of refined sugar consumption. A few of these are Emanuel Cheraskin and W.M. Ringsdorf, *Psychodietetics* (New York: Bantam Books, 1978); John Yudkin, *Sweet and Dangerous* (New York: Bantam Books, 1973); David Reuben, *Everything You Always Wanted to Know About Nutrition* (New York: Avon, 1979); William Dufty, *Sugar Blues* (New York: Warner Books, 1975).

2. An informative article describing the properties, uses, and methods of processing natural sweeteners is Richard Leviton's "A Shopper's Guide to Sweeteners," *East West Journal*, May 1986.

3. Paavo Airola, *Rejuvenation Secrets from Around the World*. (Phoenix, AZ: Health Plus, 1977), pp. 42–46.

4. *NutriVoice*, a Health-Watch Newsletter, edited by Barbara A. Mullarkey, spring 1989, p. 3.

5. Robert Rogers, interviewed by Gary Null, *Gary Null Show*, WNIS-AM, May 1, 1994.

6. *Gary Null Show*, WNIS-AM, September 5, 1993.

E.   Questions and Answers

The following are some of the questions I have been asked that have not been specifically discussed in the text. Since many of these questions are of general interest, I include them here.

I'm from Texas. People can become immune to snake bites by being bitten by snakes. Isn't immunization based on the same principle?

You can become desensitized to—sometimes called "building a tolerance for"—a toxin by gradually increasing your exposure to it. For instance, when a person first starts to smoke, it usually makes him or her sick, but gradually the body adjusts. Could you honestly say that person is healthier?

What we are talking about here—and throughout this book—is establishing "broad-spectrum" immunity rather than merely disease-specific immunity.

I don't want my children immunized, but our state has a compulsory immunization law. How do I get out of it?

This is the most commonly asked question. See Chapter 14.

My cousin had whooping cough, and it lasted almost four months. She almost died. Wouldn't the risk of shots be better than this?

This is a two-pronged question. First, you are assuming that vaccinations work, that they really do prevent the diseases for which they are given. Second, you are assuming that because someone else had a severe case of an illness, there is nothing you can do to prevent a similar occurrence except vaccinate. In answer to both of these, read this book. You may wish to pursue the matter further by reading some of the references I have used as well as some of the literature listed in Appendix G. Dr. Gordon Stewart said in the interview in *D.P.T.: Vaccine Roulette* that when children die of whooping cough, it is because they are severely disadvantaged in some way. Evidence suggests that a healthy child, properly cared for, will not die from whooping cough, nor will the disease be serious or protracted.

If you still feel uneasy about not having your child "protected," I would suggest you see a homeopathic doctor. He can give your child oral immunizing agents that are harmless. If you're still uneasy and want regular "shots," wait until your child is at least 2 years old.

Immunizations do have an effect. They work. How do you explain that commercial chickens that were dying by the thousands from some disease caused by the terrible conditions under which they were kept are no longer dying of it because of a vaccine that was developed?

Go back to principle. If you have an undesirable condition and you make it disappear without correcting the cause, watch out. It will surface later in another form—and one that is usually more serious or debilitating. In the healing arts, we call this the progression from acute to chronic to degenerative disease. Artificially raised animals are usually slaughtered before the chronic or degenerative form of the disease is visible. We eat the diseased flesh and become ourselves diseased. Some of the hormones used in feeding commercial animals, for instance, have been linked to cancer in humans.

I knew a young man years ago who worked for a while cutting up chickens in a meat-packing facility. He made the mistake of not wearing gloves, and he developed a painful and unsightly skin condition on his hands and forearms just from handling the meat! He told me horror stories of diseased animals in which the diseased parts were cut out and the rest cut and packaged for human consumption. Many think that practices like this contribute to our high rate of degenerative disease.

If doctors—chiropractors, naturopaths, homeopaths, herbalists, and others—using natural methods of healing are so effective, why don't we hear about any great contributions they have made? What research has been done to demonstrate that their methods work?

I once heard a chiropractor in a public lecture say that because chiropractic does not get funds from government and big corporations such as the pharmaceutical houses that he can't point to this or that controlled study and say this is what we found. In fact, he said, when a chiropractor goes out to practice, he is learning. "Every day I am learning and discovering the remarkable benefits of chiropractic. I treat for one condition, and other conditions seem to clear up in the process," he said. Other health care practitioners who use natural methods have made similar remarks. Obviously, their methods don't make money for pharmaceutical houses, surgeons, medical technicians, and manufacturers of expensive medical equipment. Hence, research in natural therapies is not financed by big-moneyed interests.

Also, who are the big advertisers? Industries engaged in the manufacture of hi-tech commodities that include drugs and vaccines. Advertising is the financial lifeline of the media, and stories that do not support the interests of their advertisers are not published.

But natural and holistic healing has a long and honorable history. The current interest in holistic healing, nutrition, body movement, and color and music therapies began with Pythagoras in 580 B.C. at least a century before Hippocrates. The latter carried on this tradition using herbs and diet and advocating a practice we today call chiropractic.

Another reason you don't hear about the breakthroughs in natural healing is that they are, for the most part, individual and anecdotal. Central to the philosophy of natural healing that is holistic, such as homeopathy, is that patients are people, not numbers, things, or mindless bodies. Illnesses are not entities that can be separated from the people who have them; hence, assembly line treatment as practiced by most of mainstream medicine has no place. Again, this latter style of health care is where the money is.

Until someone can figure out how to make substantial profits by selling such things as sunshine, fresh air, pure water, natural food and herbs, exercise, positive thinking, and self-sufficiency, you're going to have to be content with anecdotal evidence, and there is plenty of that.

Are you saying that vaccinations exist because drug companies and doctors make a profit from them?

There is no doubt that vaccines are big business. The research and administration of vaccines employ tens of thousands of people in drug companies, private research laboratories, universities, state health departments, public health clinics, the FDA, the CDC (Centers for Disease Control), hospitals, and doctors' offices. States obtain federal grants to hire additional personnel in their health departments to implement mass immunization programs.

The CDC estimates that the eight major vaccines distributed in the United States in 1981 generated more than $300 million for the drug industry.[1] For an industry that grosses sales in the tens of billions of dollars a year, this is not a significant amount of money. What is significant, though, is the mind-set that is promoted by this ritual. It is this mind-set that makes the money. It is a mind-set that sees disease as a frightening, foreign invader, an implaccable enemy whose mysteries can only be fathomed by men versed in a specific technology and whose defeat depends entirely on their ministrations.

Most medical doctors, being products of the system they serve, are probably sincere. They probably believe in what they are doing; however, I have read of studies and have heard of individual cases where doctors refuse to give their own children some of the vaccinations they give to other children. You have to remember medical doctors are under a lot of pressure from their local medical society. If they don't conform, they could be ousted or, at least, censured. How much their sincerity is distorted by pressure to conform is anybody's guess.

Do you know what Edgar Cayce said about immunizations?

One of the most valuable and interesting features of the Cayce health readings is their holistic nature. In an editorial of the *Journal of the American Medical Association*, John P. Callan said, "The roots of present-day holism probably go back 100 years to the birth of Edgar Cayce in Hopkinsville, Kentucky."[2] So when we read an Edgar Cayce reading, we must remember that we are reading a message that addresses the consciousness of the person requesting the reading. Cayce once used the term *castor oil consciousness*. Is it too much to use the term *vaccination consciousness*? And wouldn't his answers be somewhat different for someone with a strong vaccination consciousness than for someone with a different consciousness?

I have read quite a number of the Cayce readings on vaccinations, and the only consistency I can find is that he never recommended them as part of a health care program. His advice was always in answer to a question about some vaccination or vaccinations in general. Generally, he said that vaccines should not be mixed; give only one at a time. Sometimes he told parents to wait until a particular age to have it done, frequently saying that if the body were kept in an alkaline condition by the addition of carrots, celery, lettuce, and the like, each day, there would be no need for vaccinations. Sometimes he told people to stay away from them, particularly the smallpox vaccination. One parent who had given her child the diphtheria and whooping cough injections asked if they were "detrimental to the body," and if so, what could be done. Cayce advised her to "do the things that would be in keeping with making the normal conditions, overcoming the harm already done." He advised among others things better eliminations and circulation (3172-2).[3] I know one case of a child who had a vaccine injury, and he prescribed a purification regime and she recovered.

A quotation from a Cayce reading sheds a revealing light on this entire discussion:

Many times has the evolution of the earth reached the stage of development as it has today, and then [sunk] again, to rise again in the next development. Some along one line, some along others, for often we find the higher branches of so-called learning destroys itself in the seed it produces in man's development, *as we have in the medical forces* . . . as we have in some forms of spiritual forces, as we have in forms of destructive forces of the various natures.[4]

UPDATE

Because many people have asked me about shots for animals, this is what I tell them: I haven't studied animals, but I would guess that the same principles apply to them as to humans. An excellent book, *The Complete Herbal Handbook for the Dog and Cat*, by Juliette deBairacle Levy is full of valuable information for the natural care of dogs and cats. She quotes medical doctors, homeopaths, veterinarians, breeders, and dog owners who point to the ineffectiveness and harmfulness of vaccination for distemper. Levy describes herbal immunizations. One of them is an herbal compound made of minced garlic and eucalyptus oil rolled in whole wheat flour and honey and divided into pills. She uses one drop of eucalyptus oil to every tablespoon of the mixture. Other remedies include an herbal laxative and a half-day fast.

For forced vaccination, rub the site of the shot with the juice of a lemon using a whole lemon. Do this immediately after vaccination. (See Appendix G for publisher.)

NOTES

1. Harris L. Coulter and Barbara Loe Fisher, *DPT: A Shot in the Dark* (New York: Harcourt Brace Jovanovich, 1985), p. 406. A later figure is that the vaccine industry grosses $10 billion a year (Paul James,"Letter to the Editor," The *Virginian-Pilot/ Ledger-Star*, May 11, 1993).

2. John P. Callan, Editorial, "Holistic Health or Holistic Hoax?" *Journal of the American Medical Association*, March 16, 1979, p. 1156.

3. Edgar Cayce, reading #3172–2.

4. Edgar Cayce, reading #900–70 (italics mine).

F.   "I Have a Dream"

I have a dream that one day we will have temple-spas throughout the country where people will go to renew their spirits, nourish their minds, and regenerate their bodies. These temple-spas will be surrounded by gardens, fragrant with the scent of herbs and flowers, with pathways leading to nearby woods and meadows. Certain areas of the temple-spa will be set aside for specialized activities, each contributing to attunement to the Universal: (1) natural therapies such as music, color, massage, manipulation, and hydro- and heliotherapies; (2) body movement such as dancing, swimming, yoga, and tai chi; (3) programs such as music, drama, and lecture/discussion; (4) libraries for reading and research; (5) creative activities such as working with arts and crafts; (6) working with nature through gardening or study; (7) turning within through prayer and meditation. A common denominator of the temple-spa experience will be individualized therapeutic programs and a large, windowed cafeteria serving fresh, whole, unadulterated, organically grown food and pure, unpolluted water.

These temple-spas will be as much a part of our national life as hospitals and churches are today. An impossible dream? So were the airplane and the telephone—in fact, most of what we call modern civilization. Progress begins with "impossible" dreams. Except this time around, the impossible dream must be of a different nature, must move us in a different direction if we are to survive into the twenty-first century. The new direction will be toward health, wholeness, and harmony both within and without ourselves and our world. This is the peace we are seeking.

G. Resources

ORGANIZATIONS

The National Health Federation
212 West Foothill Boulevard
Monrovia, CA 91016
Mailing address:
P. O. Box 688
Monrovia, CA 91017
Phone: (818) 357–2181
    Works to protect our health freedoms in all areas. Has a vaccination kit for $25.00. Members receive 10 issues of *Health Freedom News*, which features articles on some of the latest investigative research in nutrition, medicine (including vaccines), and medical politics.

National Vaccine Information Center (NVIC)
512 West Maple Avenue #206
Vienna, VA 22180
Phone: (703) 938-DPT3
    If your child has been injured by vaccinations and you are seeking reparation, or if you want to prevent your child from getting vaccinated and are under pressure from your school and/or doctor to do so, the NVIC may be able to help you. Members of this organization receive a regular newsletter that includes legislative updates.

Vaccination Alternatives
Sharon Kimmelman, Director
P. O. Box 346
New York, NY 10023
Phone: (212) 870–5117

Has an introductory information packet on vaccines for $3.00 plus postage. Also stocks books and taped lectures on the subject.

Vaccine Research Institute
Josephine Szczesny
P. O. Box 4182
Northbrook, IL 60065

Provides lists of the latest published information, including books, and media presentations on vaccinations.

New Atlantean Press
New Atlantean Books
P. O. Box 9638
Santa Fe, NM 87504
Phone: (505) 983–1856

Publishes a comprehensive catalog of books on vaccinations as well as transcripts from interviews with and seminars by Neil Miller, author (see next section). Also features books on health and nutrition, natural child care, medical racketeering, home schooling, child rearing, and mind over matter. For $4.00 plus 7 percent shipping, you can get a copy of the exact vaccination laws of your state. *New Atlantean Press* is the newsletter that gives updates on the politics of vaccination.

National Center for Homeopathy
1500 Massachusetts Avenue N.W., Suite 42
Washington, D.C. 20005
Phone: (202) 223–6182

Information resource center for booklets, reprints of articles, and homeopathic medicine. Publishes a national directory of homeopathic practitioners.

BOOKS

A. For the general reader and open-minded professional: The three books in this category were selected for readability, easy access to information (each vaccine is discussed separately, comparing severity and frequency of the disease to the frequency of vaccine failure and adverse side effects) and thoroughness of documentation. All three books are available from New Atlantean Books (see above).

What About Immunizations? Exposing the Vaccine Philosophy
Cynthia Cournoyer
Nelson's Books (1991)
P. O. Box 2302
Santa Cruz, CA 95063
$8.95

Features psychological and philosophical aspects of vaccinations such as a personal question and answer inventory and discussion of different ways of interpreting disease symptoms and vaccine reactions. Also discusses ingredients of vaccines.

Vaccines: Are They Really Safe and Effective?
Neil Z. Miller
New Atlantean Press (1993)
Santa Fe, New Mexico 87504
$7.95

Packs a remarkable amount of information in less than 80 pages, something a parent can read in a couple of evenings. With 12 figures (diagrams, tables, and a waiver form), which make their point at a glance, this book, like the Cournoyer book, goes beyond the vaccine paradigm.

The Immunization Decision
Randall Neustaedter
North Atlantic Books (1990)
2800 Woolsey Street
Berkeley, CA 94705
$8.95

For the medically minded, this book will be valued for its "balanced" point of view and deference to the questioning, concerned parent. Although the author makes the case for developing a strong immune system by allowing the child to respond to infectious challenges naturally, he doesn't invalidate the vaccine model.

B. These three books focus on the short- and long-term effects of vaccinations in general. Contains some detailed, technical information.

Vaccination and Immunization: Dangers Delusions and Alternatives
Leon Chaitow
C. W. Daniel Company Limited (1987)
Saffron Walden, Essex, England

Includes history of vaccination, claims and counterclaims, and alternatives to vaccinations. Features much little known information. Available from New Atlantean Books.

Vaccinations and Immune Malfunction
Harold E. Buttram and John Chriss Hoffman
The Humanitarian Society (1982)

Points to connection between vaccinations and immune malfunction. Available from New Atlantean Books.

The Dangers of Immunization
Harold E. Buttram
The Humanitarian Society (1979)

Focuses on long-term effects of vaccinations, particularly with respect to evidence from molecular biology. Also points out differences between natural immunity and vaccinations as well as suggestions for maintaining a strong immune system.

Note: For $9.00 you can get the above two books plus another, *How to Legally Avoid Unwanted Immunizations of All Kinds*, by sending to Humanitarian Publishing Company, R.D. 3, Climer Road, Quakertown PA 18951. (Price may have gone up.)

C. These two books are outstanding for their scholarly research and startling conclusions. For the serious researcher and professional. Both are available from New Atlantean Books.

Vaccination, Social Violence and Criminality: The Medical Assault on the American Brain
Harris L. Coulter
North Atlantic Books (1990)
Berkeley, CA 94705

Points to connection between vaccinations and damage to the central and autonomic nervous systems resulting in disorders such as autism, mental retardation including learning disabilities, sociopathic personality, and criminality.

Vaccination: The Medical Assault on the Immune System
Viera Scheibner
Australian Print Group (1993)
Maryborough, Victoria, Australia
$30.00 (less from New Atlantean Press)

Presents evidence showing that vaccines do not immunize but sensitize, damaging both the immune and nervous systems. The result has been the enormous increase in the last 50 years of allergies, respiratory disorders including asthma, and brain damage including uncontrollable movements and fits. Contrasts the development of natural immunity with the effects of vaccines.

OTHER PUBLICATIONS

The Risks of Immunizations and How to Avoid Them
Robert S. Mendelsohn
The People's Doctor
Evanston, IL 60201
$18.00

Reprints of 13 newsletters dealing with vaccines published in 1976 through 1988. A newer version of this booklet plus other things Dr. Mendelsohn said about vaccines is available from New Atlantean Press under the title *Immunizations: The Terrible Risks Your Children Face That Your Doctor Won't Reveal*. Price: $12.00

"The Case Against Immunizations" (article reprint)
Richard Moskowitz
National Center for Homeopathy (1983)
1500 Massachusetts Avenue, NW, Washington. D.C. 20005
$2.25

Discusses immunosuppressive effects of vaccines as well as vaccine failure. Cases from the author's own practice are described.

"Vaccination—The Rest of the Story"
Article reprints from *Mothering Magazine*
P.O. Box 1690
Santa Fe, NM 87504
$14.95

Presents pros and cons of the vaccination issue. Includes Dr. Moskowitz's articles.

"A Shot in the Dark"
Richard Leviton
Yoga Journal, May/June 1992
2054 University Avenue
Berkeley, CA 94704
Reprints available $2.50 each; back issues available for $5.00 each.

Interview with Harris L. Coulter in which the division between the "Empirics" and the "Rationalists" is discussed. The former focuses on individuality, life force, and total organismic pattern and response. The latter focuses on specific, isolated pathology, symptom suppression, and microbial annihilation. This latter, of course, is the allopathic model that currently dominates the medical-political agenda of this country. Homeopathic alternatives to vaccinations are presented. Vaccine damage, politics, and the need to reclaim our immune systems are discussed.

What Every Parent Should Know About Childhood Immunization
Jamie Murphy
Earth Healing Products (1993)
Dennis, MA 02638
$13.95

A clear, easy-to-follow discussion of vaccines and immunity. Includes chapters on the immune system, animal experimentation, vaccine production, and ingredients. Available from the National Vaccine Information Center and New Atlantean Press.

A Shot in the Dark
Harris L. Coulter and Barbara Loe Fisher
Avery Publishing (1991)
Garden City Park, New York
$9.00

Shows how the pertussis (P) component of the DPT vaccine can be dangerous. Poignant cases of vaccine-damaged children presented along with history of pertussis and the vaccine. Available from National Vaccine Information Center and New Atlantean Press.

Dangers of Compulsory Immunizations, How to Avoid Them Legally
Tom Finn
Foreword by Robert S. Mendelsohn
Family Fitness Press (1983)
P.O. Box 1658
New Port Richey, FL 33552
$5.95

Harmfulness of vaccines, legal precedents, and strategies for avoiding vaccinations.

The Complete Herbal Handbook for the Dog and Cat
Juliette deBairacli Levy
Redwood Burn Limited (1985)
Trowbridge, Wiltshire
London, England

Has chapter on herbal "vaccines" and preventing contagious diseases naturally. Available from many public libraries.

PERIODICALS

The International Vaccination Newsletter
Kris Gaublomme, editor
Krekenstraat 4, 3600 Genk
Belgium
$35.00/year

The vaccination issue as reported by writers from around the world.

ATTORNEYS

James R. Filenbaum
2 Executive Boulevard

Suite 201
Suffern, New York 10901
Fax: (914) 357–7826
Phone: (914) 357–0020
    For vaccination information packet phone (800) 753-laws.

Tom Finn
6320 Rowan Road
New Port Richey, FL 34653
Phone: (813) 844–3466
    Has written booklet mentioned earlier.

Index

About the Author

WALENE JAMES is a freelance writer and lecturer. She has contributed articles to *Health Freedom News*, *At The Crossroads*, *Metro*, and *The International Vaccination Newsletter*. Her earlier book, *Handbook for Educating in the New Age*, was published in 1977.

ISBN 0-89789-359-X

HARDCOVER BAR CODE